Anxiety Disorders

Anxiety Disorders

An Introduction to Clinical Management and Research

Edited by

Eric J.L. Griez

Department of Psychiatry and Neuropsychology,
University of Maastricht, The Netherlands

Carlo Faravelli

Department of Neurology and Psychiatry,
Florence University Medical School, Italy

David Nutt

Psychopharmacology Unit, School of Medical Sciences,
University of Bristol, UK

and

Joseph Zohar

Department of Psychiatry and Anxiety Clinic,
Sheba Medical Center, Tel Hashomer,
University of Tel Aviv, Sackler Faculty of Medicine, Israel

JOHN WILEY & SONS, LTD

Chichester · New York · Weinham · Brisbane · Singapore · Toronto

Copyright © 2001 by John Wiley & Sons Ltd,
Baffins Lane, Chichester,
West Sussex PO19 1UD, England

National   01243 779777
International   (+44) 1243 779777
e-mail (for orders and customer service enquiries): cs-books@wiley.co.uk
Visit our home page on http://www.wiley.co.uk or http://www.wiley.com

Reprinted April 2002

Other Wiley Editorial Offices

John Wiley & Sons, Inc., 605 Third Avenue,
New York, NY 10158-0012, USA

WILEY-VCH Verlag GmbH, Pappelallee 3
D-69469 Weinheim, Germany

Jacaranda Wiley Ltd, 33 Park Road, Milton,
Queensland 4064, Australia

John Wiley & Sons (Asia) Pte Ltd, 2 Clementi Loop #02-01,
Jin Xing Distripark, Singapore 129809

John Wiley & Sons (Canada) Ltd, 22 Worcester Road,
Rexdale, Ontario M9W 1L1, Canada

Library of Congress Cataloging-in-Publication Data

Anxiety disorders: an introduction to clinical
  management and research / edited by E.J.L. Griez . . . [et al.].
    p. cm.
  Includes bibliographical references and index.
  ISBN 0-471-97873-6 (alk. paper)
  1. Anxiety. 2. Phobias. 3. Obsessive–comprehensive disorder. 4. Anxiety—Research.
  5. Phobias—Research. 6. Obsessive–compulsive disorder—Research. I. Griez, E.J.L.

  RC531.E94   2001
  616.85´22—dc21   00–069333

British Library Cataloguing in Publication Data

A catalogue record for this book is available from the British Library

ISBN 0–471–97873–6

Typeset in 10/12pt Baskerville from the author's disks by Vision Typesetting, Manchester
Printed and bound in Great Britain by Biddles Ltd, Guildford and King's Lynn
This book is printed on acid-free paper responsibly manufactured from sustainable forestry, in which at least two trees are planted for each one used for paper production.

Contents

Contributors

J.K. Abrams   *Psychopharmacology Unit, School of Medicine, University of Bristol, University Walk, Bristol BS8 1TD, UK*

Revital Amiaz   *Division of Psychiatry, Tel Hashomer and Sackler School of Medicine, Chaim Sheba Medical Center, Tel-Hashomer 52621, Israel*

Spilios V. Argyopoulos   *Psychopharmacology Unit, School of Medicine, University of Bristol, University Walk, Bristol BS8 1TD, UK*

F. Baeyens   *Department of Psychology, University of Leuven, Tiensestraat 102, 3000 Leuven, Belbium*

Laura Bellodi   *Department of Neuroscience, Fondazione Centro San Raffaele del Monte Tabor, Via L. Prinetti 27, Milan, Italy*

Michel Bourin   *Faculty of Medicine, University of Nantes, 1 rue Gaston Veil, 44035 Nantes Cedex, France*

Chantal I.M. Caes   *Centre for Gender and Diversity, Maastricht University, PO Box 616, 6200 MD Maastricht, The Netherlands*

Maria C. Cavallini   *Department of Neuroscience, Fondazione Centro San Raffaele del Monte Tabor, Via L. Prinetti 27, Milan, Italy*

Natalie Caycedo   *c/o Valencia 133, 08011 Barcelona, Spain*

Miriam Chopra   *Division of Psychiatry, Tel Hashomer and Sackler School of Medicine, Chaim Sheba Medical Center, Tel-Hashomer 52621, Israel*

J. Cottraux   *Hôpital Neurologique et Neuro-Chirurgical, Pierre Wertheimer, 59 Boulevard Pinel, Lyon-Montchat 69394, Lyon Cedez 03, France*

P. Dannon   *Division of Psychiatry, Tel Hashomer and Sackler School of Medicine, Chaim Sheba Medical Center, Tel-Hashomer 52621, Israel*

Benoît de Brettes   *Hôpital Fernand Widal, Service de Psychiatrie, 200 rue du Faubourg Saint Denis, 75010 Paris, France*

Philip A.E.G. Delespaul   *Department of Psychiatry and Neuropsychology, Maastricht University, PO Box 616, 6200 MD Maastricht, The Netherlands*

Wolter S. de Loos   *Psychotrauma Centre, University Medical Centre Utrecht and Central Military Hospital, PO Box 90000, 3509 AA Utrecht, The Netherlands*

Martin W. deVries   *Department of Psychiatry and Neuropsychology, Maastricht University, PO Box 616, 6200 MD Maastricht, The Netherlands*

Paul Eelens   *Department of Psychology, University of Leuven, Tiensestraat 102, 3000 Leyven, Belgium*

Carlo Faravelli   *Department of Neurology and Psychiatry, Florence University Medical School, Policlinico Careggi, 50134 Florence, Italy*

Ph. Fontaine   *Hôpital Neurologique et Neuro-Chirurgical, Pierre Wertheimer, 59 Boulevard Pinel, Lyon-Montchat 69394, Lyon Cedez 03, France*

Eric J.L. Griez   *Department of Psychiatry and Neuropsychology, Maastricht University, PO Box 616, 6200 MD Maastricht, The Netherlands*

D. Hermans   *Department of Psychology, University of Leuven, Tiensestraat 102, 3000 Leuven, Belgium*

Iulian Iancu   *Division of Psychiatry, Tel Hashomer and Sackler School of Medicine, Chaim Sheba Medical Center, Tel-Hashomer 52621, Israel*

Donald F. Klein   *New York State Psychiatry Institute, 1051 Riverside Drive, New York 10032, USA*

Jean Pierre Lépine   *Hôpital Fernand Widal, Service de Psychiatrie, 200 rue du Faubourg Saint Denis, 75010 Paris, France*

Harald Merckelbach   *Department of Experimental Psychology, Maastricht University, PO Box 616, 6200 MD Maastricht, The Netherlands*

E. Mollard   *Hôpital Neurologique et Neuro-Chirurgical, Pierre Wertheimer, 59 Boulevard Pinel, Lyon-Montchat 69394, Lyon Cedez 03, France*

Peter Muris   *Department of Experimental Psychiatry, Maastricht University, PO Box 616, 6200 MD Maastricht, The Netherlands*

David J. Nutt   *Psychopharmacology Unit, School of Medicine, University of Bristol, University Walk, Bristol BS8 1TD, UK*

Thea Overbeek   *Department of Psychiatry and Neuropsychology, Maastricht University, PO Box 616, 6200 MD Maastricht, The Netherlands*

A. Paionni   *Department of Neurology and Psychiatry, Florence University Medical School, Policlinico Careggi, 50134 Florence, Italy*

Giampaolo Perna   *Istituto Scientifico Ospedale San Raffaele, Vita-Salute University, Via Prinetti, 29, 20127 Milan, Italy*

A. Perone   *Department of Neurology and Psychiatry, Florence University Medical School, Policlinico Careggi, 50134 Florence, Italy*

V. Ricca   *Department of Neurology and Psychiatry, Florence University Medical School, Policlinico Careggi, 50134 Florence, Italy*

R. Salmoria   *Department of Neurology and Psychiatry, Florence University Medical School, Policlinico Categgi, 50134 Florence, Italy*

Yehuda Sasson   *Division of Psychiatry, Tel Hashomer and Sackler School of Medicine, Chaim Sheba Medical Center, Tel-Hashomer 52621, Israel*

E. Truglia   *Department of Neurology and Psychiatry, Florence University Medical School, Policlinico Careggi, 50134 Florence, Italy*

Kees Verburg   *Mediant, Locatie Helmerzijde, Broekheurnering 1050, PO Box 775, 4500 AT Enschede, The Netherlands*

Eric Vermetten   *Department of Psychiatry, Yale University School of Medicine, 47 College Street, Suite 212, New Haven CT 06510, USA*

B. Viviani   *Department of Neurology and Psychiatry, Florence University Medical School, Policlinico Careggi, 50134 Florence, Italy*

S.N. Yao   *Hôpital Neurologique et Neuro-Chirurgical, Pierre Wertheimer, 59 Boulevard Pinel, Lyon-Montchat 69394, Lyon Cedez 03, France*

Joseph Zohar   *Chaim Sheba Medical Center, Division of Psychiatry, Tel Hashomer and Sackler School of Medicine, Tel-Hashomer 52621, Israel*

T. Zucchi   *Department of Neurology and Psychiatry, Florence University Medical School, Policlinico Careggi, 50134 Florence, Italy*

Preface

There is ample evidence concerning the burden of anxiety disorders. We clinicians know the personal distress of those suffering with panic attacks, severe phobias or obsessive–compulsive disorder, not to mention people living with stigmas of traumatic experiences. In addition to psychic pain, pathological anxiety severely affects the patient's existence, causing a state of dependence which most often starts in early adulthood and has long-standing consequences, disrupting both family life and professional career. Anxiety disorders, in particular panic attacks, go along with various autonomic disturbances that trigger physical complaints and motivate medical procedures. Therefore, when not properly recognized, anxiety syndromes often induce useless and sometimes expensive complementary investigations, adding unnecessary strain for the patient and costs for the health care system. Finally, there is accumulating evidence that an anxiety disorder, when left untreated, may worsen the prognosis of a coexisting somatic condition. This has been clearly demonstrated in case of cardiac diseases. It certainly holds true in many other instances.

Overall, anxiety disorders represent an impressive burden of individual suffering, social impairment and economic costs. However, all too often the patient's symptoms are not properly interpreted. It has been estimated that in primary care, less than half of the subjects presenting with an anxiety disorder are recognized as having a clinically relevant condition. Only a subset of them will be diagnosed as suffering with an anxiety disorder. And again, only a small part of those with a correct diagnosis of anxiety will be fully informed and offered a state-of-the-art treatment.

Yet, the latest decades have witnessed an exponential growth of knowledge in the field of affective disorders, in particular anxiety. Since Klein's pioneering delineation of the concept of panic, and the subsequent adoption of a more empirically-based nosology of anxiety state, the impetus of research has produced a huge accumulation of data, based on scientific methodology rather than on a theoretical discourse. However, the new, fast-changing situation has produced some drawbacks. As in other fields of medicine, it has become increasingly difficult for the practicing clinician to keep abreast of ongoing developments. This knowledge helps us understand the present paradox: in spite of existing evidence indicating that they could be helped in a very effective way, a substantial proportion of patients with anxiety disorders is neither adequately diagnosed, nor appropriately informed on available treatments. Day-to-day care lags behind scientific evidence, and while knowledge is growing, the gap between theory and practice grows at a still faster rate.

More and better continuing medical education programmes will help. Nevertheless, fast-changing times call for stronger links between research and clinical work.

We need a new generation of research-minded clinicians, who have been prepared to use sharp, critical appraisal skills in order to stay up to date and implement therapeutic advances as soon as they may be of benefit to the patients. As decision making for treatment of any disorder becomes more complex, a sound insight of the underlying mechanisms will be essential. Hence, the good therapist should have an appropriate knowledge of basic neurosciences. That is the way towards reconciliation between theory and practice, research and clinic.

www.eurocertificate.org

With the above ideas in mind, a group of experts in the field of anxiety disorders decided in the late 1980s to set up an international collaborative course for physicians, residents in psychiatry, psychologists and related professionals. The primary aim was to offer a short, though intensive, teaching programme at the cutting edge of research. In a time of emerging globalization, it was obviously necessary to think of the project both as a transuniversity and transeuropean event. Accordingly the course was designed as an encounter between trainees from all over Europe and an invited panel of worldwide leading experts. Two one-week residential seminars took place for the first time in 1989. The course was one of the first instances of a formal transeuropean interuniversity project in the field of medicine, and was launched under the auspices of the European Community Erasmus Programme. The initiative enjoyed considerable success and courses have been repeated each year since 1989. In 1995 the board of directors decided to extend the scope of the programme to the field of mood disorders.

"The European Certificate in Anxiety and Mood Disorders" has been a pioneering transnational teaching initiative in the field of mental health. The practice of psychiatry is still predominantly driven by opinion rather than by evidence. It is therefore interesting to see researchers and clinicians from various countries, with diverse cultural backgrounds and practicing in different health care systems, gathering together and confronting their current habits and knowledge with the best available evidence. All of them are sharing the critical mindset that underlines evidence-based medicine. They take advantage of the unique opportunity provided by the certificate to challenge taken-for-granted ideas and procedures. The certificate has become the place to be for those wanting to meet active investigators belonging to the best groups in their field. However, the trainees themselves, reporting on their daily work and their ongoing research, contribute largely to the richness and interest of the programme.

Relying increasingly on the application of new communication technologies for distance teaching, the Certificate is now evolving as a complete two-year interuniversity educative programme officially endorsed by participating institutions and organizations. Although the content of such a course is by definition a dynamic process deemed to be updated year after year, the knowledge transfer has been organized around a basic scheme. The present book represents the core of the programme

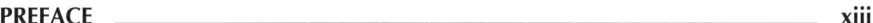

pertaining to anxiety disorders, as members of the faculty have developed it over the last few years. In the future, the board of directors intends to go on inviting leading experts to share their latest findings with the trainees. The European Certificate in Anxiety and Mood Disorders should stay in tune with the best evidence.

Eric J.L. Griez
Chairman of the Board of Directors

Introduction

Donald F. Klein

New York State Psychiatry Institute, New York

Introducing an up-to-date book covering a broad range of anxiety-related topics presents a problem. It seems in the nature of scientific activity that investment in one's conclusions may lead to a less than balanced consideration or relevant evidence and analyses. Of course, this truism applies to our views of this controversial area. We hope to contribute to this dialectical process so that those who remain open-minded may arrive at their conclusions reflectively. I will emphasize issues about the anxiety disorders that seem salient to me and promising with regard to research and treatment, however, space limitations force neglect of many real advances.

THE CURRENT STATE OF PSYCHIATRIC UNDERSTANDING

The state of patient-orientated research in psychiatry is affected by several problematic facts. Psychiatric diagnosis is almost entirely at a descriptive syndromal level. Objective, specific, diagnostic tests are not available for almost all psychiatric diseases. Therefore, our syndromal categories probably include many phenocopies comprising diverse etiologies, pathophysiologies, and moderating variables. This may account for the current wide range of treatment outcomes and our imprecise prognoses.

Both our pathophysiological and psychosocial theories have a bad historical record since few have survived pointed tests. Basic research beneficially critiqued simplistic pathophysiological notions that emphasize crucial single neurotransmitters. Although we talk about noradrenergic, serotonergic and dopaminergic systems, their functions are still obscure. Except for crude beginnings, simple rheostat models are used, positing that too much or too little neurotransmitter has some unequivocal implication concerning the direction and utility of some function. The strange fact of neuropeptide co-transmission and the multiplicity of excitatory and inhibitory pre- and post-synaptic receptors indicate the crudeness of such notions. Basic neurophysiological disease models are almost entirely speculative.

The hopes that molecular genetic research will sharply delineate psychiatric diseases have floundered amidst complex genetics, polygenic determinants and multiple phenocopies. Genomic linkage research requires careful, still quite obscure, distinctions among phenocopies or one is swamped by false positives.

The hope that molecular biology will provide specific remedies remains unfulfilled. Even though a specific chromosomal defect in the classic autosomal dominant in Huntington's Disease was isolated 15 years ago, and although the aberrant protein in question has been determined, translation into therapeutic interventions has not, as yet, occurred. This is probably due to the tremendous, still largely unknown, epigenetic, environmentally molded, cascade between gene, gene product and clinical pathophysiology. Serendipity still rules for pharmacotherapeutics, although the clinical context fostering serendipity has shrunk (Klein and Smith, 1999).

THE GROWTH OF THE CLINICAL PHYSIOLOGICAL LABORATORY

One clear advance has been the increase in direct, physiologically sophisticated investigations of real anxious patients (rather than surrogate sophomores) compared with each other and with normals. The past 20 years have demonstrated that systematic perturbations (challenges) provide fascinating data indicating, at physiological and genetic levels, that the anxiety disorders are distinct from each other and normal controls. Splitting rather than lumping seems to pay off.

Cognitive theorists deny that spontaneous panics are qualitatively unique. They posit that people with enduring catastrophizing attitudes misconstrue harmless endogenous sensations as dangerous, eliciting fear-associated autonomic responses which then increases these sensations. This confirms the erroneous cognition of imminent peril, sparking a psychophysiological vicious circle that culminates in panic, i.e., the apprehension of immediate total disaster.

This view seems contradicted by a range of data, including the antipanic effects of imipramine which does not dampen ordinary fear, while incurring unpleasant side effects resembling fear, such as tachycardia, sweating, dry mouth, and tremors (Klein, 1994; Klein, 1995).

An outstanding puzzling aspect of spontaneous panic attacks is the lack of HPA activation during the panic characteristic of panic disorder, which is also inconsistent with fear equivalence. A number of investigations of the HPA axis in panic disorder agree with this finding but have fairly inconsistent results concerning other aspects of HPA dysregulation. The limited evidence for chronic hypercortisolemia seems related more to anticipatory anxiety than to the panic state. Reports of blunted responses to CRH have primarily occurred in panic patients with elevated baseline cortisols. The belief that the absence of HPA axis activation in panic disorder might be due to chronic repeated stresses was challenged by several anecdotal reports of first panics occurring in normals, without HPA activation. It is also unclear if repeated stresses would not sensitize rather than blunt HPA responsiveness. It seems good scientific strategy, to me, to focus on such counter-intuitive findings since they are likely to lead to real novelties.

DYSPNEA

The other aspect of the spontaneous panic attack that differentiates it from fear is the common feeling of shortness of breath or dyspnea accompanying the attack. Although commonly attributed to hyperventilation, the weight of the evidence is that neither hyperventilation nor acute fear produces acute dyspnea. My suggestions with regard to a suffocation false alarm theory of panic have had the gratifying effect of eliciting much discussion and even a number of studies.

EXCITING NEW DEVELOPMENTS

That separation anxiety is a common antecedent of panic disorder has been noted. The recent work by Jerome Kagan and associates indicates the frequency of behavioral inhibition in children of patients with anxiety disorders and the possibility that behavioral inhibition may be a precursor of social anxiety disorders. This emphasizes the importance of continuity of adult with childhood anxiety disorders. Investigation of childhood disorders clearly has many technical and ethical problems, but they afford a close look at the early phases of a pathogenic process before it is obscured by multiple secondary reactions and adaptations.

The work of Dan Pine et al. (1998), who demonstrated carbon dioxide sensitivity, paralleling adult panic patients, in anxious children, and more particularly differential CO_2 sensitivity between separation anxious and socially anxious children, opens up an entire new field of investigation. Further, the attempt to find a common pathophysiology that underlines both carbon dioxide/lactate hypersensitivity and separation anxiety brings us to the question of endorphinergic regulation since endorphines regulate both of these processes.

That normals have so little effect from lactate and carbon dioxide speaks to the possibility of some protective mechanism that has been impaired in panic patients. A recent pilot study by Smit Sinha et al. (submitted manuscript) showed that the infusion of naloxone prior to lactate infusion led to marked hyperventilation and symptomatic complaint with salient dyspnea, resembling the clinical appearance of the so-called non-fearful panic. It is often not recognized that the definition of panic disorder had changed to include states of acute transient distress that are not accompanied by fearful emotions since such patients commonly exist in medical facilities, where they may undergo negative cardiac catheterizations.

One approach to the phenocopy problem is to subdivide patients with apparently common syndromes by their physiological reactivity. The work of the teams led by Griez in Maastricht and by Bellodi in Milan suggests that the pathophysiology underlying carbon dioxide hypersensitivity is closely tied to a specific genetic causal process. Griez cautiously points out that there may be specific, genetic, cognitive factors, such as anxiety sensitivity, that participate in this process. Studies of CO_2 hypersensitivity during sleep, with a view to showing that panic patients are hypersensitive to endogenous carbon dioxide fluctuations, might prove a useful strategy in achieving a homogeneous pathophysiological state.

CATEGORIES PLUS DIMENSIONS

There is still much abstract (and, I think, pointless) debate about the relative merits of dimensional rather than categorical description. Torgerson (1967) argued that there are two major mathematical approaches: those which seek to identify classes (or clusters) with a data matrix and those which seek to identify dimensions of variation (or factors) within the data. Each approach has underlying assumptions that increase the likelihood of detecting patterns conforming to the method. For example, assuming a set of variables measured in a sample of patients with anxiety disorders, both dimensional factors and clusters could be imposed on even random data by the assumptions of the particular analytic procedure used. Further, multiple discrete neurobiologic abnormalities might produce a continuum of behavioral manifestations. Thus, mathematical detection of dimensions of pathology does not rule out the presence of discrete pathophysiology.

A more inclusive model of the anxiety disorders involves a mix of both concepts: "a set of classes (either exclusive or nonexclusive) representing specific disorders, with one or more quantitative dimensions superimposed" (Torgerson, 1967). The overall objective is to determine the model best suited to the purposes for which the nosology is intended, but that depends on substantive, testable hypotheses. These are in short supply.

This heated disagreement about abstractions is probably secondary to opposing etiological frameworks. Those who believe in major determining variables underlying discrete syndromes are largely of a neurobiological frame of mind and emphasize categories. Those who believe that multiple mislearnings are essential for psychopathology emphasize continuity with normality and differences of degree across multiple dimensions.

COMORBIDITY

An extremely confusing area is the intricate relationship between the anxieties and the depressions. I emphasize the plural since it seems clear that there are multiple discrete anxiety disorders as well as several different depressed states, which coexist in multiple combinations. This is often referred to as comorbidity, but since these so-called comorbidities are so common, that the symptomatic mix is actually due to the evolution of complex syndromes seems likely. If that were true, one would expect that the relatives of "comorbid" patients would be more likely to have symptomatically mixed conditions than simple anxious or depressive states. The literature is contradictory and the question remains unresolved (Mannuzza et al., 1994/5). Again, phenocopies blur attempts to delineate genetically homogeneous, complex, classes.

That anxiety disorders often precede depressive disorders and respond to (some) antidepressants seems to support the idea that they are often a type of masked depression, but this is contradicted by the regularly poor results of ECT in anxious patients (although not in agitated depressions). Further, social phobia and the frequently comorbid atypical depression are both MAO inhibitor responsive, but only slightly tricyclic responsive. This gets even more confusing with regard to therapeutic mechanism, given the recent reports of the utility of SSRIs in social phobia. In general, pharmacological dissection fosters useful syndromal distinctions but pharmacological amalgamation is not helpful. Studies that incorporate the range of both syndromes and their complications are needed.

THE MEASUREMENT OF THERAPIES

A stimulating therapeutic development is the complex study of panic disorder by the team of Barlow, Gorman, Shear and Woods (2000) comparing cognitive-behavioral treatment versus imipramine and their combination with placebo in panic disorder. This is, by far, the best controlled study in this area, although, unfortunately, the sample was limited to panic patients with minimal or no agoraphobia, who have the best prognosis in any case.

Using a Clinical Global Improvement Scale, cognitive-behavioral therapy did as well as imipramine, but within these responders imipramine was superior, with regard to degree of symptomatic remission. It follows that if response had been defined by a cutting level on this symptom scale, there would have been more responders on imipramine.

This difficulty in estimating meaningful clinical therapeutic response was paralleled by the other first-rate placebo-controlled comparison of cognitive behavioral group therapy versus phenelzine for social phobia, co-sponsored by R.G. Heimberg and M.R. Liebowitz (1998). Here too a Clinical Global Improvement Scale indicated equivalent effectiveness for pharmacotherapy and psychotherapy but on analysis of symptomatic scales specifically relevant to social phobia, the superiority of phenelzine became plain.

Another example of difficulty in clinically meaningful description of therapeutic response was pointed out by Rappaport et al. (2000). This study had shown sertraline to be superior to placebo in the treatment of panic disorder. Nevertheless many patients on placebo had done well with regard to symptomatic ratings. However, the authors then looked, within the responders, at a patient self-rating of Quality of Life Enjoyment and Satisfaction. They found that despite equivalent initial demographic and clinical characteristics, sertraline responders were substantially superior to placebo responders on the total Quality of Life score. Such a self-rating is clearly a step in the right direction. Objective life functioning measures would be desirable.

LONG-TERM BENEFITS OF PSYCHOTHERAPY AND THE DIFFERENTIAL SIEVE

One of the charms of psychotherapy is the frequent claim for permanent benefit since the pathogenic process has been quelled. Both Barlow et al. and Heimberg et al. indicate that the benefits of psychotherapy are better maintained than those of pharmacotherapy after treatment discontinuation. This implies a prophylactic lasting benefit. However, this may not be the case as indicated by Hollon et al. (1991) who states:

> It remains possible that cognitive therapy's apparent preventive effect represents the consequences of differential retention rather than any bona fide treatment effect. The typical follow-up study focuses on patients who both complete and respond to the respective modalities. Given the 20–40% attrition rates and 60–75% response rates associated with the respective interventions, this means that the samples entering follow-up might constitute only 35–60% of the sample initially assigned. If different types of patients are likely to either complete or respond to the respective modalities, the acute treatment period could act like a *differential sieve*, producing systematic differences in the sets of patients entering the follow-up from the different modalities. It is conceivable that the differences observed to date result not from any preventive effect attributable to cognitive therapy but rather from a greater propensity for patients at risk for relapse . . . to successfully complete pharmacotherapy than cognitive therapy.

Furthermore, studies often only superficially report longitudinal data. Brown and Barlow (1995) illustrate the difference between simple cross-sectional and longitudinal evaluations of fluctuating conditions. While cross-sectional data indicate that many subjects had improved during the follow-up period, the fact that some responders relapsed and other nonresponders improved was obscured until the data was analyzed longitudinally. This fluctuating pattern indicated that substantially fewer patients had a maintained high end state functioning.

THE NEED FOR COLLABORATION

One of the major problems in therapeutic research has gone by the euphemistic label of "allegiance effect" (Klein, 1999). It has been shown repeatedly that supposed differences in therapeutic benefit and data interpretation are closely related to the antecedent beliefs of the investigators. Comparative studies of treatment or, even supposedly more objective physiological investigations, carried out by single-minded enthusiasts are inferior to collaborations between scientists with opposing views who are willing to put them to the test.

The studies by Heimberg et al. and Barlow et al. are sterling examples of how scientists with differing views can develop and pursue such a fruitful collaboration. There is no doubt that this is difficult, both administratively and financially. It would require a determined effort on the part of funding agencies to foster such work. It would also probably require a very determined effort on the part of scientists to convince funding agencies that this is worthwhile, if not positively necessary.

CONCLUSION

Clinicians should be pleased by recent progress in the treatment of anxiety disorders. A wide range of pharmacological and psychological interventions have been shown effective in controlled objective studies. Such studies afford a solid basis for evidence based practice.

Nonetheless, many of these studies have not been directed at the complex comorbid patients often seen in the community. Nor has there been sufficient attention to the combination of therapies in terms of both acute and maintenance treatments.

As for our theoretical grasp of the anxiety disorders in terms of etiology, psychogenesis and pathophysiology, it is clear that we are only in the initial phases of understanding. The combination of molecular biology and brain imaging has led to a great deal of justified enthusiasm, especially with regard to the possibility of tracking normal brain function in living detail. The translation of these findings to psychopathology remains problematic.

REFERENCES

Barlow DH, Gorman JM, Shear MK, Woods SW (2000) Cognitive-behavioral therapy, imipramine, or their combination for panic disorder: A randomized controlled trial. *JAMA* **283**(19): 2529–2536.

Bellodi L, Perna G, Caldirola D, Arancio C, Bertani A, Di Bella D (1998) CO_2-induced panic attacks: A twin study. *Am J Psychiatry* **155**: 1184–1188.

Brown TA, Barlow DH (1995) Long-term outcome and cognitive-behavioral treatment of panic disorder: Clinical predictors and alternative strategies for assessment. *J Consult Clin Psychol* **63**: 754–765.

Griez E, Verburg C (1995) *Angst, Paniek en Ademhaling.* Utrecht: De Tijdstroom.

Heimberg RG, Liebowitz MR, Schneier FR, Hope DA, Holt CS, Welkowitz LA, Juster HR, Campeas R, Bruch MA, Cloitre M, Fallon B, Klein DF (1998) Cognitive-behavioral group therapy vs phenelzine therapy for social phobia: 12-week outcome. *Arch Gen Psychiatry* **55**(12): 1133–1141.

Hollon SD, Shelton RC, Loosen PT (1991) Cognitive therapy and pharmacotherapy for depression. *J Consult Clin Psychol* **59**: 88–99.

Klein DF (1994) Testing the suffocation false alarm theory of panic disorder. *Anxiety* **1**: 1–7.

Klein DF (1995) Response to critique of suffocation alarm theory. *Anxiety* **1**(3): 145–148.

Klein DF (1999) Dealing with the effects of therapy allegiances. *Clin Psychol: Sci & Practice* **6**: 124–126.

Klein DF, Smith, LB (1999) Organizational requirements for effective clinical effectiveness studies. *Prevention and Treatment* http://journals.apa.org/prevention/volume2/pre0020002a.html, posted 21 March 1999.

Mannuzza S, Chapman TF, Klein DF, Fyer AJ (1994/1995) Familial transmission of panic disorder: Effect of major depression comorbidity *Anxiety* **1**: 180–185.

Pine DS, Coplan JD, Papp LA, Klein RG, Martinez JM, Kovalenko P, Tancer N, Moreau D,

Dummit ES, Shaffer D, Klein DF, Gorman JM (1998) Ventilatory physiology of children and adolescents with anxiety disorders. *Arch Gen Psychiatry* **55**(2): 130–136.

Rappaport MH, Pollack M, Wolkow R, Mardekian J, Clary C (2000) Is placebo response the same as drug response in panic disorder? *Am J Psychiatry* **157**(6), 1014–1016.

Sinha SS, Goetz R, Klein DF (2001) Non-fearful panic induction in normals with naloxone pretreatment of lactate infusion. Submitted. *Neuropsychopharmacology*.

Torgerson WA (1967) Multidimensional representation of similarity structures. In Katz MM, Cole JO and Barton WE (eds) *Methodology of Classification in Psychiatry and Psychopathology*. Washington, DC: US Department of Health, Education, and Welfare, pp. 212–220.

van Beek N, Griez E (2000) Reactivity to a 35% CO_2 challenge in healthy first-degree relatives of patients with panic disorder. *Biol Psychiatry* **47**: 830–835.

Epidemiology and Genetics

Epidemiology of Anxiety Disorders

T. Overbeek, E. Vermetten, and E.J.L. Griez

Maastricht University, Maastricht, The Netherlands

INTRODUCTION

Anxiety disorders have a high impact on daily life (illness intrusiveness) and cause a great deal of suffering for the individual patient (Antony et al., 1998). They also have a substantial impact economically and incur a great deal of expenditure by society as a whole. Greenberg et al. (1999) report a total of $42.3 billion per year as direct and indirect expenses in the USA and there are no obvious reasons to assume that the picture for European countries would be very different (Costa, 1998; Martin, 1998).

In the last decades some large epidemiological studies have provided much information about the occurrence of psychiatric disorders in general and anxiety disorders in particular. The Epidemiologic Catchment Area study (NIMH) and the National Comorbidity Survey (NCS) in the USA and the Munich Follow-up study in Europe are examples of landmark studies in this field (Regier et al., 1990b; Kessler et al., 1994; Wittchen et al., 1992). The WHO Study on Psychological Problems in General Health Care can be considered an intermediate stage between epidemiological and clinical study, and provides information on prevalence rates of mental disorders in primary care in 14 different countries world-wide (Sartorius et al.,1996). Many other clinical studies of specific target populations have yielded much information. Clinical studies often reveal different prevalence rates and comorbidity figures from population-based surveys and this is partly due to selection bias and severity of symptoms, and diagnostic criteria and instruments used. Therefore, Angst et al. (1997) advocate using sub-threshold syndromes to enhance further the validity of diagnostic systems. They state that if sub-threshold syndromes (especially concerning depression and anxiety) were included in diagnostic systems, the coverage of treated cases would be improved by nearly a third.

All excellent existing studies notwithstanding, there are still many reasons to be careful in making clear statements about the prevalence of mental disorders. We are facing different studies conducted in different countries in various settings: findings cannot be easily compared or generalised. Epidemiological studies have often used different diagnostic instruments, different sampling procedures, different case

Anxiety Disorders: An Introduction to Clinical Management and Research. Edited by E. J. L. Griez, C. Faravelli, D. Nutt and J. Zohar. © 2001 John Wiley & Sons, Ltd.

definitions, different time frames for the diagnoses (e.g. lifetime, six-month prevalence or current diagnoses) and different severity ratings for diagnostic decisions (Wittchen et al., 1992). The above reservations show the need for caution when interpreting the results.

Knowledge about prevalence rates of mental disorder does not automatically imply what needs to be done. There is a discrepancy between the real occurrence of disorders and the need for treatment or the possibility of finding the most adequate treatment for a diagnosed condition. Some filters can be taken into consideration. The first filter is recognition and correct diagnosis by the general practitioner. It is estimated that about 50% of cases do not pass this filter. The second filter is the most adequate treatment of the diagnosed disease, again, which only half of the patients pass. When these two filters are taken together, only roughly about 25% of disordered subjects finally receive adequate treatment. In addition, for some disorders patients do not really need treatment, e.g. most specific phobias can be adequately dealt with by means of avoidance. This means that although specific phobias are much more prevalent than, for example, obsessive-compulsive disorder (11% and 2–3% respectively), the obsessive-compulsive disorder should have preponderance.

Anxiety disorders are by far the most common psychiatric disorders (25%), followed by major depression (17%) (Kessler et al., 1994). Lifetime prevalence rates for all anxiety disorders lumped together as found in the NCS are 19.2% for men, 30.5% for women (Kessler et al., 1994). There is a strong correlation between socio-economic status and anxiety disorders. The one-year prevalence as based on ECA data is 12.6% for all types of anxiety disorders, compared with 14.6% lifetime (Regier et al., 1998).

A final important introductory caveat is the issue of comorbidity. Comorbidity between disorders quite dramatically complicates the interpretation of many studies. Even apart from the considerable comorbidity figures between the anxiety disorders themselves, comorbidity rates between anxiety disorders and depressive disorders are very high (especially panic disorder with agoraphobia, social phobia and obsessive-compulsive disorder), ranging from 30% for co-existing in time to 60% lifetime. Comorbidity rates between, for example, generalised anxiety disorder (GAD) or post-traumatic stress disorder (PTSD) and other psychiatric disorders are even higher, about 80% for GAD and 90% for PTSD lifetime figures.

In general practice the comorbidity of anxiety disorders and depressive disorders is common, with the happy consequence that the chance of recognition and the likelihood of receiving treatment are increased (Sartorius et al., 1996). However, to complicate this further for the epidemiologist, there is also a substantial comorbidity between several medical conditions (e.g. cardial, pulmonary, cerebrovascular, gastrointestinal, diabetes and dermatological diseases) and anxiety disorders (especially panic disorder, GAD and agoraphobia) (Stoudemire, 1996).

In this chapter the epidemiological findings from some large population-based surveys and some smaller but relevant clinical studies will be reviewed, all DSM-IV anxiety disorders arranged by diagnostic category.

PANIC DISORDER AND AGORAPHOBIA

According to DSM-IV (APA, 1994) panic attacks are defined as sudden spells of unidentified feelings consisting of at least four out of 13 symptoms as palpitations, chest strains, sweating, shortness of breath, feelings of choking, trembling, nausea, dizziness, paresthesias, chills or hot flushes, depersonalisation or derealisation, fear of dying or losing control. Although having panic attacks does not imply that the diagnosis of panic disorder can be made and isolated panic attacks are not diagnosed as a disorder, they are often associated with substantial morbidity and do have some clinical significance (Klerman et al., 1991).

In order to make a diagnosis of panic disorder, additional criteria are that these attacks at least once have been unexpected, followed by at least one month of fearful expectation or concern about the consequences of an attack. In the DSM-IV criteria as to the frequency of the attacks (in DSM-III-R, APA 1987, three attacks in a period of three weeks) are abandoned.

Panic disorder is frequently followed (or accompanied) by agoraphobia. Agoraphobia in DSM-IV is defined as (a) fear of being in places or situations from which escape might be difficult or help might not be available; (b) these situations are avoided or endured with marked distress or the patient needs a companion; and (c) the fear is not better explained by another mental disorder.

As such, isolated panic attacks (as defined above) are quite frequent, estimated at 7–9% for lifetime prevalence rates, although rather heterogeneous figures come from different countries (Pélissolo and Lépine, 1998). The ECA study on panic by Eaton reports 15% of all respondents have had a panic attack in a lifetime, 3% in the past month, while 1% of the subjects meet criteria for panic disorder in the past month (Eaton et al., 1994). In a survey among 1035 adolescents in Bremen, Germany, 18% of participants reported having had at least one panic attack (in a lifetime), with 0.5% of them meeting DSM-IV criteria for panic disorder (Essau et al., 1999). The prevalence of panic disorder, assessed with diagnostic criteria and structured interviews, has been found in the majority of surveys to have lifetime rates between 1.5% and 2.5%. Twelve-month prevalence rates are generally about 1% (Pélissolo and Lépine, 1998).

Although panic disorder can be diagnosed apart from agoraphobia, in clinical practice it is rare to find a patient suffering from panic disorder who did not develop agoraphobia to a certain extent. This, however, is in contrast to the results from the NCS study, where it was found that 50% of panic disorder patients report no agoraphobia (Eaton et al., 1994). Either way, it is infrequent to find an agoraphobic without a history of a panic attack. Horwath et al. (1993) have shown that epidemiological studies that used the Diagnostic Interview Schedule and lay interviewers, such as the ECA study, may have over-estimated the prevalence of agoraphobia without panic. The investigators took a sample of 22 ECA subjects diagnosed as having agoraphobia without panic attacks, and had them blindly re-interviewed. Re-analysis showed that only one of these subjects was left with the original diagnosis, one was assigned to having panic disorder with agoraphobia, one had agoraphobia with limited symptom attacks, and the vast majority were re-appraised as specific phobias (Horwath et al., 1993).

In addition, a recent study by Wittchen et al. (1998) in a community sample of 3021 young subjects (14 to 24 years old) in Munich, Germany, addresses the relationship between panic disorder and agoraphobia. They found that lifetime prevalence of panic disorder with agoraphobia was as high as for panic disorder without agoraphobia, both being 0.8%. *Post hoc* clinical review of the CIDI-positive agoraphobics revealed that many respondents did not have agoraphobia, but actually suffered from specific phobia, e.g. situational phobias. This resulted in a corrected agoraphobia prevalence of 3.5% instead of the original 8.5%. However, even after this correction, the majority of respondents with confirmed agoraphobia were found not to have a prior history of panic. However, in the NCS where agoraphobia was a separate diagnosis, it was found to have a lifetime prevalence rate of 6.7%, and a one-month prevalence of 2.3% (Magee et al., 1996).

Demographics and Risk Factors

Most studies reporting on panic disorder or panic attacks consistently show higher rates for women than for men. Panic attacks are almost twice as common in women, where panic disorder ranges from 1.5 to twice as much. The age at onset of panic disorder in general lies in the mid-twenties, with hazard rates for women ranging from 25 to 35 years, for men between 30 and 45 years (Wittchen and Essau, 1993). Marital status is a significant risk factor for panic disorder: the highest lifetime prevalence rates are found in widowed, separated or divorced subjects (Wittchen and Essau, 1993). On educational level and risk of developing panic disorder there are no consistent findings, Eaton et al. (1994) report from the NCS data a tenfold higher risk for persons with less than 12 years of education. Several studies have suggested that life events such as early parental loss or childhood abuse may enhance the risk of panic disorder, but there appears to be no specificity since this also applies to other psychiatric disorders as post-traumatic stress disorder and affective disorders.

Other supposed risk factors are smoking habits, although there is no consensus about causality or just correlation because all psychiatric patients smoke more than the general population. Breslau and Klein (1999) find evidence for smoking leading to panic disorder. Others also indicate a role for smoking in developing panic disorder (Pohl et al., 1992; Amering et al., 1999; Biber and Alkin, 1999). Another factor associated with panic disorder is the existence of pulmonary disease. All conditions that have symptoms of shortness of breath can lead to anxiety in general and panic disorder in particular (Smoller et al., 1999). It is shown that respiratory disease in childhood (especially bronchitis and asthma) predisposes to panic disorder in later life (Zandbergen et al., 1991; Verburg et al., 1995; Perna et al., 1997). In addition, chronic obstructive pulmonary disorders can lead to panic disorder in primarily lung patients (Wingate and Hansen-Flaschen, 1997), although the role of psychological factors, such as cognitive misinterpretation of bodily symptoms (shortness of breath) must be taken into account (Moore and Zebb, 1999).

Natural Course

Panic disorder and agoraphobia seem to be a chronic condition (Pollack and Smoller, 1995; Hirschfeld, 1996; Liebowitz, 1997), mostly with a fluctuating course with periods of waxing and waning (Liebowitz, 1997; Pollack and Otto, 1997). In some studies longitudinal aspects have been addressed, e.g. in a three-year follow-up only 10% were shown to be symptom-free (Noyes et al., 1990). Faravelli et al. (1995) found that only 12% of panic disorder patients after five years were in full remission. Panic disorder can be a very disabling disorder with high impact on daily life and social, personal and professional functioning and can put a great strain on quality of life (Candilis and Pollack, 1997; Candilis et al., 1999).

Comorbidity

Comorbidity of panic disorder and agoraphobia is very common, as the panic attacks are often viewed as the precipitating cause for agoraphobia to develop (Klein and Klein, 1989). From this perspective, it is unnecessary to speak of true comorbidity, because the panic disorder with agoraphobia can be considered one disease entity. The comorbidity of panic disorder with agoraphobia is reported as ranging from 29.5% to 58.2%. In the NCS (Eaton et al., 1994) 50% of the panic disorder patients had comorbid agoraphobia. Also, findings from the study of Wittchen et al. (1998), cited above, indicate that half of patients with panic disorder also developed agora-phobic avoidance. There is also a high degree of comorbidity with other anxiety disorders, such as social phobia (20–75%, see Pélissolo and Lépine, 1998) and generalised anxiety disorder (20%), 14% for obsessive-compulsive disorder and 6% for post-traumatic stress disorder (Goisman et al., 1994).

The Munich Follow-up Study (Wittchen and Essau, 1993) also stresses the risk for panic disorder patients of developing comorbid other psychiatric disorders. In more than half of the cases, some comorbid disorder will develop over time. Major depression (Merikangas et al., 1996) is the most frequent comorbid diagnosis, 30–60% of panic disorder patients suffer from a depressive disorder (Weissman et al., 1997). Most studies report a concurrent prevalence rate of about 30%, with lifetime prevalence of depression occurring in about 60% (Wetzler and Sanderson, 1995). Also, the NCS data have shown a lifetime prevalence of depression in panic disorder patients of 55.6% (Kessler et al., 1998a). There are divergent views about the order of onset in comorbid panic disorder and depression. In the ECA analysis it is shown that onset of panic is first in about 30% of cases, onset of depression precedes in another 30%, and simultaneous onset occurs in 40% (Regier et al., 1998). Also, some clinical studies have shown similar figures on the order of onset in comorbid panic disorder and depression (Lydiard, 1991; Stein et al., 1990). Other clinical studies report that the onset of panic disorder was first in about two-thirds of comorbid cases (Hunt and Andrews, 1995). The clinical significance of comorbidity lies in the severity of symptoms at the outset (Andrade et al., 1994).

Substance abuse (alcohol, drugs and medication) is also a common comorbid disorder, in 36% of cases, according to ECA data (Regier et al., 1990a). Most frequently, these abuse disorders are supposed to be secondary to the panic disorder, and can be interpreted as self-medication (Marshall, 1997; Swendsen et al., 1998; Merikangas et al., 1998). Some authors, however, dispute this; Katerndahl and Realini (1999), for example, found that the majority of drug and alcohol abusers report that the abuse started before the onset of the panic attacks.

The comorbidity of panic disorder with other general medical conditions is described in a review by Zaubler and Katon (1998). It is shown that panic disorder is common in cardiac, gastrointestinal, respiratory and neurologic disorders.

SPECIFIC PHOBIAS

Specific phobias are the second most common anxiety disorder, after social phobia. They are, however, less impressive because they are mostly less incapacitating than other anxiety disorders. A specific phobia is defined as a circumscribed, persistent, and unreasonable fear of a particular object or situation. Exposure to this phobic stimulus is associated with an acute and severe anxiety reaction. Although individuals with specific phobias recognise their fear is unrealistic, most adjust their lifestyle so that they can completely avoid or at least minimise this contact (Fyer, 1998). Within the specific phobia category there is considerable heterogeneity. In the DSM-IV, four subtypes are defined, and animal phobias, situational phobias, blood-injury phobia, and nature-environment phobia are distinguished. The first three have been differentiated on the basis of a combination of factors including age at onset, symptom response, heritability and biological challenges (Fyer, 1998; Verburg et al., 1994). On the separate position of the nature-environment phobia there is less consensus (Fyer, 1998).

Prevalence

The NCS rates for one-month and lifetime specific phobia are 5.5% and 11.3%, respectively (Magee et al., 1996). Among women, fear of animals is most frequent; fear of heights is most prevalent in men (Curtis et al., 1998). In a study addressing blood-injury phobia a lifetime prevalence of 3.5% was found, and a mean age at onset was 5.5 years. Also noteworthy is that none of the subjects had ever sought professional treatment (Bienvenu and Eaton, 1998).

Demographics and Risk Factors

Female to male ratio for specific phobia is 2.3:1. In the NCS females had a lifetime prevalence of 15.7% and men 6.7% (Kessler et al., 1994).

Natural Course

Simple phobia appeared in a study by Goisman et al. (1998) to be a chronic illness of moderate severity for which behavioural treatment methods of recognised efficacy were infrequently being used. The number of fears, independent of type, predicts impairment and professional help-seeking (Chapman et al., 1993; Curtis et al., 1998).

Comorbidity

Simple phobia is highly comorbid with other disorders; 83.4% of persons with simple phobia reported at least one lifetime comorbid disorder (Magee et al., 1996). The other anxiety disorders and major depression are most frequent. Also, specific phobia is frequently diagnosed as a comorbid disorder in other anxiety disorders (Goisman et al., 1998).

SOCIAL PHOBIAS

In recent years social phobia has gained more professional and public interest and increasingly is being recognised as a real anxiety disorder for which treatment can offer an improvement of the patient's quality of life (Kasper, 1998). Social phobia (social anxiety disorder) usually is rather disabling, characterised by marked fear of performance, excessive fear of scrutiny, and fear of acting in a way that may be embarrassing. Most patients are over-sensitive to the assumed opinion of others and have a low self-esteem, although they feel their fears are exaggerated and out of proportion. Going through the feared situations, or even anticipating them, most people suffer from physical symptoms like sweating, trembling or blushing, and these symptoms can become a trigger on their own to worry about social consequences. This all can lead to avoidance of many social situations, or they endure these situations with extreme anxiety or distress (Liebowitz, 1999). As in all cases of phobias, the individual recognises that his or her fears are unreasonable.

Social phobia can be divided in two subtypes. The first is generalised social phobia (or complex social phobia), patients being anxious in most situations concerning performance and interactional situations. The patient with non-generalised social anxiety disorder is scared of only one or two (usual performance-related) social situations, such as public speaking, or other public performance, such as writing or eating in front of others (Moutier and Stein, 1999; Stein and Chavira, 1998). Both types, however, tend to be underdiagnosed and undertreated (Stein and Chavira, 1998). There are some differences between the subgroups, the generalised type has even less chance of spontaneous recovery than the non-generalised. In the generalised subtype there is a stronger genetic factor (Kessler et al., 1998b). The generalised subtype is usually more invalidating and carries a higher risk of comorbidity. Age of onset does not differ between the subtypes.

Differential diagnoses for social anxiety disorder are: major depression with social withdrawal, panic disorder with social avoidance, agoraphobia, GAD, OCD, and body dysmorphic disorder. Another important disorder to differentiate from social phobia is the DSM-IV axis II avoidant personality disorder. Although often seen as a comorbid disorder, it is becoming increasingly clear that much avoidant personality disorder as defined by DSM-IV merely denotes a subgroup of patients with axis I generalised social phobia (Moutier and Stein, 1999).

Prevalence

Among the anxiety disorders social phobia nowadays is considered the third most common psychiatric disorder (13.3%), exceeded in lifetime prevalence only by major depression (17.1%) and alcohol dependence (14.1%) (Kessler et al., 1994), at least in the United States according to the NCS data. Prevalence rates for social phobia have increased in last decades. Earlier surveys, based on DIS and DSM-III criteria gave figures ranging from 2% to 4% (Pélissolo and Lépine, 1998). The ECA survey, for example, found one-month prevalence of 1.3%, a six-month prevalence of 1.5% and a lifetime prevalence of 2.8% (Schneier et al., 1992). Subsequent studies, based on DSM-III-R criteria and CIDI interviews which explore more abundant and diversified social situations, reveal higher lifetime prevalences for social phobia, between 4.1% and 16%. The NCS study found a one-month prevalence of 4.5% and a lifetime prevalence of 13.3% (Magee et al., 1996).

A study by Weiller and others (1996) conducted in a general health care setting revealed a one-month prevalence of 4.9%, and a lifetime prevalence of 14.4%. They also stress that social phobia is underdiagnosed by general practitioners, in only 24.2% of the social phobics a diagnosis of anxiety disorder was made. When occurring with a comorbid depression, even fewer patients were diagnosed as having a social phobia, although the presence of a comorbid depression increased the chance of diagnosing a psychological disorder. Nevertheless, it should be noted that in some epidemiological studies conducted in the Far East much lower lifetime prevalences are found, about 0.5% (Lépine and Lellouch, 1995). It is unclear whether this occurs on account of a cultural bias of response or because of true psychopathological cross-cultural differences.

Demographics and Risk Factors

Most surveys mention a slight preponderance of women in social phobia (1.5 times as many as men). The NCS reports lifetime prevalence for women of 15.5% and for men 11.1% (Magee et al., 1996). In a study specifically addressing gender differences in social anxiety disorder (Weinstock, 1999), the authors state that although women are more likely to have social phobia, men are more likely to seek treatment, possibly explained by differences in gender roles and social expectations. There seems to be a difference in feared items between men and women: concerns about eating in restaurants and writing in public were more common in men, problems with using public restrooms and speaking in public were more common in women.

Social phobia is more frequently found at a younger age (18 to 29 years), among the less educated, the single, and the lower socio-economic classes (Schneier et al., 1992). The Weiller et al. study (1996) showed an unemployment rate of 9.3%, compared with 1.3% for the control group. Employment status was also poor in the ECA study, social phobics changed their jobs more often and showed more absenteeism (Davidson et al., 1993).

Natural Course

Typically social phobia has an onset in puberty and is often preceded by general shyness in early youth (Liebowitz, 1999). The natural course tends to be chronic, unremitting and in course of time increasingly complicated by comorbid disorders. Because of the early age of onset, the disorder strongly influences further psychological development, formation of relationships, educational choices and career perspectives (Davidson et al., 1993).

Comorbidity

As is the case for panic disorder, in social phobia as well, the comorbidity rate is high. Around 80% of social phobia co-exists with other disorders (Lépine and Pelissolo, 1996; Montgomery, 1998). In particular, lifetime depression is high, about 70%, as well as other anxiety disorders. Panic disorder was diagnosed in 49%, GAD in 32% and OCD in 11% of social phobics (Van Ameringen et al., 1991). However, this study only comprised 57 subjects. Analysis of a part of ECA data with 123 social phobics revealed that 11.6% of them had lifetime panic disorder, 45% had comorbid agoraphobia, 60.8% had specific phobia, and 26.9% had GAD (Davidson et al., 1993). The data from the NCS showed a comorbidity with panic disorder in 10.9% of cases, with agoraphobia in 23.3%, GAD in 13.3% and specific phobia in 37.6% (Magee et al., 1996). Because of the early onset of social phobia, most often (in 70% of cases) the comorbid disorders appear secondary to the social phobia (Schneier et al., 1992).

The relationship between social phobia and alcoholism is a complex one. Reported prevalence rates vary widely, due to differing definitions, and methodological differences (Lépine and Pelissolo, 1998). Most studies looking for social phobia in patients with alcohol problems, abuse or dependence report prevalences of about 10% to 20%. Studies addressing social phobic patients report alcoholism in about 14% to 40% of cases. The social phobia most often predates the onset of alcohol problems. Although many social phobia sufferers use alcohol in an attempt to self-medicate their distressing anxiety symptoms, it appears that alcohol can actually increase anxiety, and a cycle may develop in which the sufferer drinks in order to relieve increasing levels of anxiety (Lépine and Pelissolo, 1998).

OBSESSIVE-COMPULSIVE DISORDER (OCD)

Obsessive-compulsive disorder is defined as the presence of recurrent obsessions (persistent thoughts, impulses, or images) or compulsions (repetitive behaviour or thought patterns induced in an attempt to prevent anxiety) that are excessively time-consuming (taking more than an hour a day) or cause marked distress or significant impairment. The subject recognises that these patterns are excessive.

Differential diagnosis of obsessive-compulsive disorder includes generalised anxiety disorder, panic disorder, phobias, compulsive personality disorder, and hypochondriasis. While many of these syndromes are characterised by intrusive thoughts, few have associated rituals. The complex tics seen in some patients with Tourette's syndrome may be difficult to distinguish from the compulsions seen in obsessive-compulsive disorder, and, in fact, there is significant overlap in symptoms between the two disorders (Rasmussen and Eisen, 1992).

Although the phenomenology of obsessive-compulsive disorder appears to be quite diverse, with many distinct kinds of obsessions and compulsions, there are three important core features: abnormal risk assessment, pathologic doubt, and incompleteness. These features cut across phenomenological subtypes and may be useful in defining homogeneous subgroups with distinct treatment outcomes (Rasmussen and Eisen, 1992). Pigott (1998) also describes core features of OCD and subdivides them in two categories: altered risk appraisal versus need for completeness/symmetry.

Prevalence

For OCD, prevalence figures have been gradually growing over the years, as is the case for social phobia. Formerly OCD was thought to be quite rare, as people did not easily request treatment due to fear or shame (Rasmussen and Eisen, 1992). Recent epidemiological studies have shown a six-month prevalence rate of obsessive-compulsive disorder of approximately 1% (Bebbington, 1998), to a lifetime prevalence rate of 2–3% (Hollander, 1997; Sasson et al., 1997), which means that OCD is much more common than previously suggested. Hollander (1997) calls OCD "the hidden epidemic", where social phobia has been called "the neglected anxiety disorder" (Liebowitz, 1999). An earlier cross-national study by Weissman et al. (1994), using DSM-III criteria, reports annual prevalence rates ranging from 1.1/100 in Korea and New Zealand to 1.8/100 in Puerto Rico. The only exception was Taiwan (0.4/100), which has the lowest prevalence rates for all psychiatric disorders. Unfortunately, one of the best epidemiological studies in the USA, the NCS, did not address OCD because the diagnostic instrument used (the CIDI) excluded these cases (Bebbington, 1998).

Demographics and Risk Factors

The cross-national collaborative study examined OCD in seven different countries and found rather consistent figures. Age of onset was mid-to-late twenties. Female to male ratio ranged from 1.2 to 3.8 (Weissman et al., 1994), but earlier studies (among which was the ECA) report an equal sex distribution. In a study that specifically addressed gender differences in a clinical sample of OCD patients, Castle et al. (1995) found a male to female ratio of 1 : 1.35. Mean age of onset for men was 22 years, for women 26 years. Mean age at assessment did not differ significantly, 32.8 years for men and 34.6 years for women.

Natural Course

Obsessive-compulsive disorder has a chronic course, and few patients achieve true remission. Although symptoms may fluctuate over time, the disorder rarely is resolved spontaneously without appropriate treatment (Goodman, 1999). Full remission of OCD symptoms is rare, but episodic improvement in OCD symptoms is not uncommon (Pigott, 1998). In a 40-year follow-up of 122 OCD patients, Skoog and Skoog (1999) substantiated these generalities: 20% achieved complete recovery, 28% recovery with subclinical symptoms, another 35% still had clinical symptoms but did improve. Some 48% had had obsessive-compulsive disorder for more than 30 years.

Comorbidity

Depression is the most frequent complication of OCD, as reported in several studies (Black and Noyes, 1990). Comorbidity rates in reported studies vary widely, from 19% to 90% (Milanfranchi et al., 1995). Within this wide range, however, most epidemiological studies show that about one-third of OCD patients suffer from a lifetime depressive episode. In clinical populations, comorbidity rates are increasing to about two-thirds (Crino and Andrews, 1996). Rasmussen found that one-third of OCD patients suffer from concurrent depression at referral, and two-thirds suffer from lifetime depression (Rasmussen and Eisen, 1994), a similar finding as in panic disorder. One explanation of the discrepancy between clinical and non-clinical studies could be that many OCD patients only seek help when depressed, as suggested by Black and Noyes (1990). As to chronology, it is found that most often the onset of OCD is before the depression (38%); transition from depression to OCD occurs in only 11% of case studies (Black and Noyes, 1990).

Personality disorders are frequently diagnosed in OCD, but may remit with effective anti-obsessional treatment (Pigott, 1998). This questions the validity of the axis II diagnosis at the outset. Also, a study by Ricciardi et al. (1992) showed that among 17 patients with OCD and concomitant personality disorder, after treatment nine out of ten responders no longer met the personality disorder criteria. OCD also co-exists with a number of other axis I disorders including panic disorder (54%, Crino and Andrews, 1996), social phobia (42%, Crino and Andrews, 1996), eating disorders (17%, Rasmussen and Eisen, 1994), and Tourette's disorder (5%, Black and Noyes, 1990). Crino and Andrews (1996) remark that the high comorbidity of panic disorder and social phobia in OCD is in contrast to the low comorbidity of OCD in primary panic disorder or social phobic patients. However, they did not find any different rate of comorbid depression among the anxiety disorders.

GENERALISED ANXIETY DISORDER (GAD)

The concept of generalised anxiety disorder is subject to discussion. Although the disorder is regarded as prevalent in primary care as well as in specialised settings, because of the high comorbidity rates associated with GAD the controversy is about whether to consider GAD an independent disorder or as a residual or prodrome of other disorders (Wittchen et al., 1994). The diagnostic category of GAD has changed a lot in the past two decades (Brawman-Mintzer and Lydiard, 1996). The shifting diagnostic criteria, the relative low diagnostic reliability, and questions regarding the diagnostic validity probably contributed to the relative little attention that has been paid to the investigation of GAD compared with most other anxiety disorders.

Prevalence

The most recent epidemiological study using DSM-III-R criteria is the NCS in the United States. The prevalence rate for current GAD was 1.6%, 12-month prevalence was 3.1% and lifetime prevalence was 5.1% (Wittchen et al., 1994). These figures make GAD more common than panic disorder in the NCS. It is shown that GAD is more common in primary care, and one of the least common anxiety disorders in mental health centres (Brawman-Mintzer and Lydiard, 1996).

Demographics and Risk Factors

Generalised anxiety disorder is twice as common among women as among men. In the age group 25–35 years the prevalence is highest (Wittchen et al., 1994). Risk factors for GAD are being separated, widowed or divorced (the same risk factors as for panic disorder), and unemployment or being a homemaker is a significant correlate of GAD. However, another recent study (Bienvenu et al., 1998) suggests that being widowed is not a risk factor.

Natural Course

Generalised anxiety disorder appears to have a chronic course. Woodman et al. (1999) conducted a five-year follow-up study comparing primary GAD patients to panic disorder patients. At baseline the GAD subjects were significantly older, had a higher level of education and occupational class, earlier age of onset and longer illness duration. At follow-up, significantly more GAD patients continued to meet full criteria for the baseline disorder, and fewer were in partial or complete remission or had fluctuations. Although global severity, measured by clinical global impression (CGI), was less at baseline, at follow-up the improvement on the CGI was significantly less for the GAD patient compared with the panic disorder patients. Findings from this study support the validity of the GAD concept, in view of the diagnostic stability and different natural course (Woodman et al., 1999).

Comorbidity

Lifetime comorbidity for GAD is very high, 90.4% of cases (Wittchen et al., 1994). The strongest comorbidities are with affective disorders (mania 10.5%, major depression 62.4%, dysthymia 39.5%). Comorbidity figures with other anxiety disorders are 23.5% for panic disorder, 25.7% for agoraphobia, 35.1% for simple phobia and 34.4% for social phobia. Alcohol abuse and dependence were seen in 37.6% of cases and drugs in 27.6%. Another study by Brawman-Mintzer et al. (1993) report comorbid social phobia in 23% and simple phobia in 21% of cases as the most frequent, after excluding lifetime depression from their study. The high comorbidity figures have led to disagreement concerning the existence of GAD as an independent diagnostic entity, and to assumptions that GAD is a prodrome or residual of other disorders (Brawman-Mintzer and Lydiard, 1996). Also, at least partly the same genetic factors contribute to major depression and GAD, as shown by Kendler (1996). However, in the NCS it is shown that at least 30% of current GAD patients had neither current nor recent (but only lifetime) comorbid disorders. This is put forward by the authors as supporting the validity of GAD as an independent diagnosis (Wittchen et al., 1994), although this does not preclude GAD from being a prodrome of any other disorder.

Generalised anxiety disorder is frequently seen in primary health care, and especially in patients with medically unexplained somatic complaints such as chest pain and irritable bowel symptoms (Roy-Byrne, 1996). As such, it is also associated with somatisation disorder and chronic fatigue syndrome (Fischler et al., 1997). Comorbidity with axis-II disorders is also high, reported up to 49% (Sanderson et al., 1994).

POST-TRAUMATIC STRESS DISORDER (PTSD)

The DSM-IV definition for PTSD contains criteria for (a) the traumatic experience;

(b) re-experiencing; (c) avoidance of associated stimuli and numbing; and (d) increased arousal. Duration of symptoms should be at least one month (e); and (f) distress or impairment in functioning is required (APA, 1994). When PTSD was first defined in DSM-III (APA, 1980), the original stressor criterion characterised traumatic experiences as being outside the range of human experience. However, when the prevalence of such events was systematically examined, it became apparent that trauma is surprisingly commonplace. Several studies have investigated the overall prevalence of traumatic events in the general population, looking both at community-based populations and populations of individuals at high risk of trauma or exposed to events such as natural disasters (Acierno et al., 1999). The nature of the trauma can be very diverse, such as childhood abuse, traffic accidents, fires, violent assault, robberies and floods or earthquakes.

Prevalence

Prevalence rates have increased from DSM-III to DSM-III-R and DSM-IV. Also, in some telephone interview surveys prevalence is much higher, and in studies among young persons where recall bias may be minimal. Kessler et al. (1995) reported on the National Comorbidity Survey of 5877 persons, aged 15 to 54 years. The estimated lifetime prevalence of PTSD was found to be 7.8%.

In routine clinical practice, PTSD is often underdiagnosed if the PTSD is not the presenting complaint but an additional diagnosis (Zimmerman and Mattia, 1999). The same comment, however, can be made for other anxiety disorders, as social phobia (Kessler et al., 1999). Reasons for misdiagnosis of PTSD include a high rate of comorbidity, patient denial or minimisation, overly high diagnostic thresholds set by clinicians, or failure to take a trauma history (Davidson and Connor, 1999). In a cohort study of 185 persons involved in a traffic accident and a hotel fire, Maes et al. (1998) found after seven to nine months a prevalence of DSM-III-R PTSD of 23%. Almost 50% of them had symptoms the first day, and about 70% developed PTSD symptoms during the first week after the event.

In one study, victims of substantiated child abuse and neglect were assessed and compared with a group of matched non-abused and non-neglected children and followed into adulthood. Victims of child abuse (sexual and physical) and neglect were found to be at increased risk of developing PTSD. More than a third of the childhood victims of sexual abuse (37.5%), 32.7% of those physically abused, and 30.6% of victims of childhood neglect, met DSM-III-R criteria for lifetime PTSD. Childhood victimisation, however, is not a sufficient condition for developing PTSD, also family, individual, and lifestyle variables place individuals at risk and contributed to the symptoms of PTSD (Widom, 1999).

North et al. (1999) report on a follow-up on the terrorist Oklahoma City bombing in 1995 where a bomb blast killed 168 people. In their sample of 182 participating adults, 45% had a post-disaster psychiatric disorder and 34.3% had PTSD. The onset of PTSD was swift, with 76% reporting same-day onset. The relatively uncommon avoidance and numbing symptoms virtually dictated the diagnosis of PTSD (94% meeting avoidance and numbing criteria had full PTSD diagnosis) and were further associated with psychiatric comorbidity, functional impairment, and treatment received. Intrusive re-experiencing and hyperarousal symptoms were nearly universal, but by themselves were generally unassociated with other psychopathology or impairment in functioning (North et al., 1999).

Demographics and Risk Factors

NCS data showed that prevalence was higher among women and the widowed, separated or divorced. The traumas most commonly associated with PTSD were combat exposure and witnessing violence among men and rape and sexual molestation among women. A variety of factors influence response to trauma and development of PTSD. They include characteristics of the stressor and exposure to it (e.g. repeated trauma increases the risk); individual factors such as gender (females are at higher risk), age and developmental level (the younger are at higher risk), and psychiatric history, family characteristics, and cultural factors (Pfefferbaum, 1997).

Natural Course

In the NCS survival analysis showed that more than one-third of people with an index episode of PTSD failed to recover even after many years (Kessler et al., 1995). Among the subjects who had ever sought professional help (58% of affected respondents), the median time to remission was 36 months, among those who did not seek help the median time to remission was 64 months. A study of 61 Vietnam combat veterans with PTSD showed that onset of symptoms typically occurred at the time of exposure to combat trauma in Vietnam and increased rapidly during the first few years after the war. Symptoms plateaued within a few years after the war, following which the disorder became chronic and unremitting. Hyperarousal symptoms developed first, followed by avoidant symptoms, and finally by symptoms from the intrusive cluster. The onset of alcohol and substance abuse was associated with the onset of PTSD symptoms, and the increase in use paralleled the increase of symptoms (Bremner et al., 1996). Another recent study of Gulf War veterans showed that PTSD increases over time, two years after the war 8% of 2949 veterans had developed a PTSD, compared with 3% immediately following the war (Wolfe et al., 1999).

Comorbidity

Post-traumatic stress disorder in the NCS findings was strongly comorbid with other lifetime DSM-III-R disorders. A lifetime history of at least one disorder was present in

88.3% of men, and 79% of women with lifetime PTSD (Kessler et al., 1995). Frequent comorbid diagnoses are: affective disorders (almost 50% of cases for major depression, 20% for dysthymia), other anxiety disorders (16% GAD, 9% panic disorder, 30% specific phobia, 28% social phobia, 19% agoraphobia, substance use disorders (52% alcohol and 34% drugs in men, 28% alcohol and 27% drugs in women) and conduct disorder (43% in men and 15% in women) (Kessler et al., 1995), and somatisation (McCauley et al., 1997).

CONCLUSION

The authors would like to end by the beginning, referring to the caveats in the introduction of the present chapter. There are still other matters of concern: the frequent use of lay interviewers in major surveys, recall bias in interviews over lifetime span, the key issue of defining a threshold for clinical significancy, just to name a few. It follows that in spite of the apparent evidence, extreme caution should be exercised when interpreting the epidemiology of anxiety.

REFERENCES

Acierno R, Kilpatrick DG, Resnick HS (1999) Posttraumatic stress disorder in adults relative to criminal victimization: Prevalence, risk factors, and comorbidity. In Saigh PA, Bremner JD et al. (eds) *Posttraumatic Stress Disorder: A Comprehensive Text*. Boston: Allyn & Bacon, Inc., pp. 44–68.

American Psychiatric Association (1980) *Diagnostic and Statistical Manual of Mental Disorders* 3rd edition. Washington, DC: American Psychiatric Press.

American Psychiatric Association (1987) *Diagnostic and Statistical Manual of Mental Disorders* 3rd revised edition. Washington, DC: American Psychiatric Press.

American Psychiatric Association (1994) *Diagnostic and Statistical Manual of Mental Disorders* 4th edition. Washington, DC: American Psychiatric Press.

Amering M, Bankier B, Berger P, Griengl H, Windhaber J, Katschnig H (1999) Panic disorder and cigarette smoking behaviour. *Compr Psychiatry* **40**: 35–38.

Andrade L, Eaton WW, Chilcoat H (1994) Lifetime comorbidity of panic attacks and major depression in a population-based study: Symptom profiles. *Br J Psychiatry* **165**: 363–369.

Angst J, Merikangas KR, Preisig M (1997) Subthreshold syndromes of depression and anxiety in the community. *J Clin Psychiatry* **58** Suppl 8: 6–10.

Antony MM, Roth D, Swinson RP, Huta V, Devins GM (1998) Illness intrusiveness in individuals with panic disorder, obsessive-compulsive disorder, or social phobia. *J Nerv Ment Dis* **186**: 311–315.

Bebbington PE (1998) Epidemiology of obsessive-compulsive disorder. *Br J Psychiatry Suppl* 1998; **35**: 2–6.

Biber B, Alkin T (1999) Panic disorder subtypes: differential responses to CO_2 challenge. *Am J Psychiatry* **156**: 739–744.

Bienvenu OJ and Eaton WW (1998) The epidemiology of blood-injection-injury phobia. *Psychol Med* **28**: 1129–1136.

Bienvenu OJ, Nestadt G, Eaton WW (1998) Characterising generalised anxiety: Temporal and symptomatic thresholds. *J Nerv Ment Dis* **186**: 51–56.

Black DW, Noyes R (1990) Comorbidity and obsessive-compulsive disorder. In Maser JD, Cloninger CR (eds) *Comorbidity of Mood and Anxiety Disorders*. Washington, DC: American Psychiatric Press, Inc., pp. 305–316.

Brawman-Mintzer O, Lydiard RB (1996) Generalised anxiety disorder: Issues in epidemiology. *J Clin Psychiatry* **57** Suppl 7: 3–8.

Brawman-Mintzer O, Lydiard RB, Naresh E, Payeur R, Johnson M, Roberts J, Jarrell MP, Ballenger JC (1993) Psychiatric comorbidity in patients with generalized anxiety disorder. *Am J Psychiatry* **150**: 1216–1218.

Bremner JD, Southwick SM, Darnell A, Charney DS (1996) Chronic PTSD in Vietnam combat veterans: course of illness and substance abuse. *Am J Psychiatry* **153**: 369–375.

Breslau N, Klein DF (1999) Smoking and panic attacks: An epidemiological investigation. *Arch Gen Psychiatry* **56**: 1141–1147.

Candilis PJ, McLean RY, Otto MW, Manfro GG, Worthington JJ 3rd, Penava SJ, Marzol PC, Pollack MH (1999) Quality of life in patients with panic disorder. *J Nerv Ment Dis* **187**: 429–434.

Candilis PJ, Pollack MH (1997) The hidden costs of untreated anxiety disorders. *Harv Rev Psychiatry* **5**: 40–42.

Castle DJ, Deale A, Marks IM (1995) Gender differences in obsessive-compulsive disorder. *Aust N Z J Psychiatry* **29**: 114–117.

Chapman TF, Fyer AJ, Mannuzza S, Klein DF (1993) A comparison of treated and untreated simple phobia. *Am J Psychiatry* **150**: 816–818.

Costa E, Silva JA (1998) The public health impact of anxiety disorders: A WHO perspective. *Acta Psychiatr Scand Suppl* **393**: 2–5.

Crino R, Andrews G (1996) Obsessive-compulsive disorder and axis I comorbidity. *J Anx Dis* **10**: 37–46.

Curtis GC, Magee WJ, Eaton WW, Wittchen HU, Kessler RC (1998) Specific fears and phobias: Epidemiology and classification. *Br J Psychiatry* **173**: 212–217.

Davidson JR, Connor KM (1999) Management of posttraumatic stress disorder: Diagnostic and therapeutic issues. *J Clin Psychiatry* **60** Suppl 18: 33–38.

Davidson JR, Hughes DL, George LK, Blazer DG (1993) The epidemiology of social phobia: Findings from the Duke Epidemiological Catchment Area Study. *Psychol Med* **23**: 709–718.

Eaton WW, Kessler RC, Wittchen HU, Magee WJ (1994) Panic and panic disorder in the United States. *Am J Psychiatry* **151**: 413–420.

Essau CA, Conradt J, Petermann F (1999) Frequency of panic attacks and panic disorder in adolescents. *Depress Anxiety* **9**: 19–26.

Faravelli C, Paterniti S, Scarpato A (1995) 5-year prospective, naturalistic follow-up study of panic disorder. *Compr Psychiatry* **36**: 271–277.

Fischler B, Cluydts R, De Gucht Y, Kaufman L, De Meirleir K (1997) Generalised anxiety disorder in chronic fatigue syndrome. *Acta Psychiatr Scand* **95**: 405–413.

Fyer, A.J. (1998) Current approaches to aetiology and pathophysiology of specific phobia. *Biol Psychiatry* **44**: 1295–1304.

Goisman RM, Allsworth J, Rogers MP, Warshaw MG, Goldenberg I, Vasile RG, Rodriguez-Villa F, Mallya G, Keller MB (1998) Simple phobia as a comorbid anxiety disorder. *Depress Anxiety* **7**: 105–112.

Goisman RM, Warshaw MG, Peterson LG, Rogers MP, Cuneo P, Hunt MF, Tomlin-Albanese JM, Kazim A, Gollan JK, Epstein-Kaye T et al. (1994) Panic, agoraphobia, and panic disorder with agoraphobia: Data from a multicentre anxiety disorders study. *J Nerv Ment Dis* **182**: 72–79.

Goodman WK (1999) Obsessive-compulsive disorder: diagnosis and treatment. *J Clin Psychiatry* **60** Suppl 18: 27–32.

Greenberg PE, Sisitsky T, Kessler RC, Finkelstein SN, Berndt ER, Davidson JR, Ballenger JC,

Fyer AJ (1999) The economic burden of anxiety disorders in the 1990s. *J Clin Psychiatry* **60**: 427–435.

Hirschfeld RM (1996) Panic disorder: Diagnosis, epidemiology, and clinical course. *J Clin Psychiatry* **57** Suppl 10: 3–8; discussion 9–10.

Hollander E (1997) Obsessive-compulsive disorder: The hidden epidemic. *J Clin Psychiatry* **58** Suppl 12: 3–6.

Horwath E, Lish JD, Johnson J, Hornig CD, Weissman MM (1993) Agoraphobia without panic: clinical reappraisal of an epidemiological finding. *Am J Psychiatry* **150**: 1496–1501.

Hunt C, Andrews G (1995) Comorbidity in the anxiety disorders: The use of a life-chart approach. *J Psychiatr Res* **29**: 467–480.

Kasper S (1998) Social phobia: The nature of the disorder. *J Affect Disord* **50** Suppl 1: S3–9.

Katerndahl DA, Realini JP (1999) Relationship between substance abuse and panic attacks. *Addict Behav* **24**: 731–736.

Kendler KS (1996) Major depression and generalised anxiety disorder: Same genes, (partly) different environments-revisited. *Br J Psychiatry* Suppl 1996; (30): 68–75.

Kessler RC, McGonagle KA, Zhao S, Nelson CB, Hughes M, Eshleman S, Wittchen HU, Kendler KS (1994) Lifetime and 12-month prevalence of DSM-III-R psychiatric disorders in the United States: Results from the National Comorbidity Survey. *Arch Gen Psychiatry* **51**: 8–19.

Kessler RC, Sonnega A, Bromet E, Hughes M, Nelson CB (1995) Posttraumatic stress disorder in the National Comorbidity Survey. *Arch Gen Psychiatry* **52**: 1048–1060.

Kessler RC, Stang P, Wittchen HU, Stein M, Walters, EE (1999) Lifetime comorbidities between social phobia and mood disorders in the US National Comorbidity Survey. *Psychol Med* **29**: 555–567.

Kessler RC, Stang PE, Wittchen HU, Ustun TB, Roy-Burne PP, Walters EE (1998a) Lifetime panic-depression comorbidity in the National Comorbidity Survey. *Arch Gen Psychiatry* **55**: 801–808.

Kessler RC, Stein MB, Berglund P (1998b) Social phobia subtypes in the National Comorbidity Survey. *Am J Psychiatry* **55**: 613–619.

Klein DF, Klein HM (1989) The utility of the panic disorder concept. *Eur Arch Psychiatry Neurol Sci* **238**: 268–279.

Klerman GL, Weissman MM, Ouellette R, Johnson J, Greenwald S (1991) Panic attacks in the community: Social morbidity and health care utilisation. *JAMA* **265**(6): 742–746.

Lépine JP, Lellouch J (1995) Classification and epidemiology of social phobia. *Eur Arch Psychiatry Clin Neurosci* **244**: 290–296.

Lépine JP, Pélissolo A (1996) Comorbidity and social phobia: Clinical and epidemiological issues. *Int Clin Psychopharmacol* **11** Suppl 3: 35–41.

Lépine JP, Pélissolo A (1998) Social phobia and alcoholism: A complex relationship. *J Affect Disord* **50** Suppl 1: S23–28.

Liebowitz MR (1997) Panic disorder as a chronic illness. *J Clin Psychiatry* **58** Suppl 13: 5–8.

Liebowitz MR (1999) Update on the diagnosis and treatment of social anxiety disorder. *J Clin Psychiatry* **60** Suppl 18: 22–26.

Lydiard RB (1991) Coexisting depression and anxiety: Special diagnostic and treatment issues. *J Clin Psychiatry* **52** Suppl: 48–54.

Maes M, Delmeire L, Schotte C, Janca A, Creten T, Mylle J, Struyf A, Pison, G, Rousseeuw PJ (1998) Epidemiologic and phenomenological aspects of post-traumatic stress disorder: DSM-III-R diagnosis and diagnostic criteria not validated. *Psychiatry Res* **81**: 179–193.

Magee WJ, Eaton WW, Wittchen HU, McGonagle KA, Kessler RC (1996) Agoraphobia, simple phobia, and social phobia in the National Comorbidity Survey. *Arch Gen Psychiatry* **53**: 159–168.

Marshall JR (1997) Alcohol and substance abuse in panic disorder. *J Clin Psychiatry* **58** Suppl 2: 46–49; discussion 49–50.

Martin P (1998) Medico-socio-economic impact of anxiety disorders. *Encephale* **24**: 280–296.

McCauley J, Kern DE, Kolodner K, Dill L, Schroeder AF, DeChant HK, Ryden J, Derogatis LR, Bass EB (1997) Clinical characteristics of women with a history of childhood abuse: unhealed wounds. *JAMA* **277**(17): 1362–1368.

Merikangas KR, Angst J, Eaton W, Canino G, Rubio-Stipec M, Wacker H, Wittchen HU, Andrade L, Essau C, Whitaker A, Kraemer H, Robins LN, Kupfer DJ (1996) Comorbidity and boundaries of affective disorders with anxiety disorders and substance misuse: Results of an international task force. *Br J Psychiatry* **30** Suppl: 58–67.

Merikangas KR, Mehta RL, Molnar BE, Walters EE, Swendsen JD, Aguilar-Gaziola S, Bijl R, Borges G, Caraveo-Anduaga JJ, DeWit DJ, Kolody B, Vega WA, Wittchen HU, Kessler RC (1998) Comorbidity of substance use disorders with mood and anxiety disorders: Results of the International Consortium in Psychiatric Epidemiology. *Addict Behav* **23**: 893–907.

Milanfranchi A, Marazziti D, Pfanner C, Presta S, Lensi P, Ravagli S, Cassano GB (1995) Comorbidity in obsessive-compulsive disorder: Focus on depression. *Eur Psychiatry* **10**: 379–382.

Montgomery SA (1998) Implications of the severity of social phobia. *J Affect Disord* **50** Suppl 1: S17–22.

Moore MC, Zebb BJ (1999) The catastrophic misinterpretation of physiological distress. *Behav Res Ther* **37**: 1105–1118.

Moutier CY, Stein MB (1999) The history, epidemiology, and differential diagnosis of social anxiety disorder. *J Clin Psychiatry* **60** Suppl 9: 4–8.

North CS, Nixon SJ, Shariat S, Mallonee S, McMillen JC, Spitznagel EL, Smith EM (1999) Psychiatric disorders among survivors of the Oklahoma City bombing. *JAMA* **282**: 755–762.

Noyes R Jr, Reich J, Christiansen J, Suelzer M, Pfohl B, Coryell WA (1990) Outcome of panic disorder: Relationship to diagnostic subtypes and comorbidity. *Arch Gen Psychiatry* **47**: 809–818.

Pélissolo A, Lépine JP (1998) Epidemiology of depression and anxiety disorders. In Montgomery SA, Den Boer JA (eds) *SSRIs in Depression and Anxiety* (pp 1–21). Chichester: John Wiley & Sons Ltd.

Perna G, Bertani A, Politi E, Colombo G, Bellodi L (1997) Asthma and panic attacks. *Biol Psychiatry* **42**: 625–630.

Pfefferbaum B (1997) Posttraumatic stress disorder in children: a review of the past 10 years. *J Am Acad Child Adolesc Psychiatry* **36**: 1503–1511.

Pigott TA (1998) Obsessive-compulsive disorder: Symptom overview and epidemiology. *Bull Menninger Clin* **62**: A4–32.

Pohl R, Yeragani VK, Balon R, Lycaki H, McBride R (1992) Smoking in patients with panic disorder. *Psychiatry Res* **43**: 253–262.

Pollack MH, Otto MW (1997) Long-term course and outcome of panic disorder. *J Clin Psychiatry* **58** Suppl 2: 57–60.

Pollack MH, Smoller JW (1995) The longitudinal course and outcome of panic disorder. *Psychiatr Clin North Am* **18**: 785–801.

Rasmussen SA, Eisen JL (1992) The epidemiology and differential diagnosis of obsessive compulsive disorder. *J Clin Psychiatry* **53** Suppl: 4–10.

Rasmussen SA, Eisen JL (1994) The epidemiology and differential diagnosis of obsessive compulsive disorder. *J Clin Psychiatry* **55** Suppl: 5–10.

Regier DA, Farmer ME, Rae DS, Locke BZ, Keith SJ, Judd LL, Goodwin FK (1990a) Comorbidity of mental disorders with alcohol and other drug abuse: Results from the Epidemiologic Catchment Area (ECA) Study. *JAMA* **264**: 2511–2518.

Regier DA, Narrow WE, Rae DS (1990b) The epidemiology of anxiety disorders: The Epidemiologic Catchment Area (ECA) experience. *J Psychiatr Res* **24** Suppl 2: 3–14.

Regier, DA, Rae DS, Narrow WE, Kaelber CT, Schatzberg AF (1998) Prevalence of anxiety disorders and their comorbidity with mood and addictive disorders. *Br J Psychiatry* **34** Suppl: 24–28.

Ricciardi JN, Baer L, Jenike MA, Fischer SC, Sholtz D, Buttolph ML (1992) Changes in DSM-III-R axis II diagnoses following treatment of obsessive-compulsive disorder. *Am J Psychiatry* **149**: 829–831.

Roy-Byrne PP (1996) Generalized anxiety and mixed anxiety-depression: Association with disability and health care utilisation. *J Clin Psychiatry* **57** Suppl 7: 86–91.

Sanderson WC, Wetzler S, Beck AT, Betz F (1994) Prevalence of personality disorders among patients with anxiety disorders. *Psychiatry Res* **51**: 167–174.

Sartorius N, Ustun TB, Lecrubier Y, Wittchen HU (1996) Depression comorbid with anxiety: Results from the WHO study on psychological disorders in primary health care. *Br J Psychiatry* **30** Suppl: 38–43.

Sasson Y, Zohar J, Chopra M, Lustig M, Iancu I, Hendler T (1997) Epidemiology of obsessive-compulsive disorder: A world view. *J Clin Psychiatry* **58** Suppl 12: 7–10.

Schneier FR, Johnson J, Hornig CD, Liebowitz MR, Weissman MM (1992) Social phobia: Comorbidity and morbidity in an epidemiological sample. *Arch Gen Psychiatry* **49**: 282–288.

Skoog G, Skoog I (1999) A 40-year follow-up of patients with obsessive-compulsive disorder. *Arch Gen Psychiatry* **56**: 121–127.

Smoller JW, Simon NM, Pollack MH, Kradin R, Stern T (1999) Anxiety in patients with pulmonary disease: Comorbidity and treatment. *Semin Clin Neuropsychiatry* **4**: 84–97.

Stein MB, Chavira DA (1998) Subtypes of social phobia and comorbidity with depression and other anxiety disorders. *J Affect Disord* **50** Suppl 1: S11–16.

Stein MB, Tancer ME, Uhde TW (1990) Major depression in patients with panic disorder: Factors associated with course and recurrence. *J Affect Disord* **19**: 287–296.

Stoudemire A (1996) Epidemiology and psychopharmacology of anxiety in medical patients. *J Clin Psychiatry* **57** Suppl 7: 64–72, 73–75.

Swendsen JD, Merikangas KR, Canino GJ, Kessler RC, Rubio-Stipec M, Angst J (1998) The comorbidity of alcoholism with anxiety and depressive disorders in four geographic communities. *Compr Psychiatry* **39**: 176–184.

Van Ameringen M, Mancini C, Styan G, Donison D (1991) Relationship of social phobia with other psychiatric illness. *J Affect Disord* **21**: 93–99.

Verburg C, Griez E, Meijer J (1994) A 35% carbon dioxide challenge in simple phobias. *Acta Psychiatr Scand* **90**: 420–423.

Verburg K, Griez E, Meijer J, Pols H (1995) Respiratory disorders as a possible predisposing factor for panic disorder. *J Affect Disord* **33**: 129–134.

Weiller E, Bisserbe JC, Boyer P, Lépine JP, Lecrubier Y (1996) Social phobia in general health care: An unrecognised undertreated disabling disorder. *Br J Psychiatry* **168**: 169–174.

Weinstock LS (1999) Gender differences in the presentation and management of social anxiety disorder. *J Clin Psychiatry* **60** Suppl 9: 9–13.

Weissman MM, Bland RC, Canino GJ, Faravelli C, Greenwald S, Hwu HG, Joyce PR, Karam EG, Lee CK, Lellouch J, Lépine JP, Newman SC, Oakley-Browne MA, Rubio-Stipec M, Wells JE, Wickramaratne PJ, Wittchen HU, Yeh EK (1997) The cross-national epidemiology of panic disorder. *Arch Gen Psychiatry* **54**: 305–309.

Weissman MM, Bland RC, Canino GJ, Greenwald S, Hwu HG, Lee CK, Newman SC, Oakley-Browne MA, Rubio-Stipec M, Wickramaratne PJ et al. (1994) The cross national epidemiology of obsessive-compulsive disorder: The Cross National Collaborative Group. *J Clin Psychiatry* **55** Suppl: 5–10.

Wetzler S, Sanderson W (1995) Comorbidity of panic disorder. In Asnis G, van Praag H (eds) *Panic Disorder: Clinical, Biological and Treatment Aspects.* New York: Wiley, pp. 80–98.

Widom CS (1999) Posttraumatic stress disorder in abused and neglected children grown up. *Am J Psychiatry* **156**: 1223–1229.

Wingate BJ, Hansen-Flaschen J (1997) Anxiety and depression in advanced lung disease. *Clin Chest Med* **18**: 495–505.

Wittchen HU, Essau CA (1993) Epidemiology of panic disorder: Progress and unresolved issues. *J Psychiatr Res* **27** Suppl 1: 47–68.

Wittchen HU, Essau CA, Von Zerssen D, Krieg JC, Zaudig M (1992) Lifetime and six-month prevalence of mental disorders in the Munich Follow-Up Study. *Eur Arch Psychiatry Clin Neurosci* **241**: 247–258.

Wittchen HU, Reed V, Kessler RC (1998) The relationship of agoraphobia and panic in a community sample of adolescents and young adults. *Arch Gen Psychiatry* **55**: 1017–1024.

Wittchen HU, Zhao S, Kessler RC, Eaton WW (1994) DSM-III-R generalised anxiety disorder in the National Comorbidity Survey. *Arch Gen Psychiatry* **51**: 355–364.

Wolfe J, Erickson DJ, Sharkansky EJ, King DW, King, LA (1999) Course and predictors of posttraumatic stress disorder among Gulf War veterans: A prospective analysis. *J Consult Clin Psychol* **67**: 520–528.

Woodman CL, Noyes R Jr, Black DW, Schlosser S, Yagla SJ (1999) A 5-year follow-up study of generalised anxiety disorder and panic disorder. *J Nerv Ment Dis* **187**: 3–9.

Zandbergen J, Bright M, Pols H, Fernandez I, De Loof C, Griez EJ (1991) Higher lifetime prevalence of respiratory diseases in panic disorder? *Am J Psychiatry* **148**: 1583–1585.

Zaubler TS, Katon W (1998) Panic disorder in the general medical setting. *J Psychosom Res* **44**: 25–42.

Zimmerman M, Mattia JI (1999) Is posttraumatic stress disorder underdiagnosed in routine clinical settings? *J Nerv Ment Dis* **187**: 420–428.

2

Genetics of Anxiety Disorders: Part I

M.C. Cavallini and L. Bellodi

Fondazione Centro San Raffaele del Monte Tabor, Milan, Italy

INTRODUCTION

Anxiety disorders are a heterogeneous group of psychiatric disorders with no clear knowledge of their aetiology and pathogenesis. Several familial, biological, and genetic risk factors have been invoked for the obsessive-compulsive disorder (OCD) or the panic disorder (PD), but to date none has shown a main role in their aetiology. The observation that some pharmacological treatments substantially modify the prognosis of affected patients may be one of the main proofs of the role of biological factors in the development of these illnesses. Additional support for the biological hypothesis derives from neuroradiological images (NMR), PET allowed physicians to isolate specific anomalies in some OCD patients (Calabrese et al., 1993; Perani et al., 1995; Saxena et al., 1998) and PD patients (Dager et al., 1996). Furthermore, the presence of secondary cases in families of probands affected with anxiety disorders suggests the existence of a familial component and probably a genetically transmissible basis for specific liabilities. The genetic basis of anxiety disorders may be further confirmed by studies of twins. Moreover, molecular biology today allows testing specific genetic hypotheses derived from clinical or neuro-imaging fields. With the aim of presenting a detailed and clear over-view of the genetic components of anxiety disorders and potential development of this idea we will discuss different anxiety disorders and their genetic background.

OBSESSIVE-COMPULSIVE DISORDER (OCD)

The evidence of the existence of a genetic component in obsessive-compulsive disorder (OCD) is derived mainly from twin and familial studies. However, the fact that patients with Tourette's Syndrome (TS) frequently have an OCD co-diagnosis, and their relatives show significantly increased morbidity risk for OCD, suggested that OCD belongs to TS spectrum (Pauls et al., 1986; Pitman et al., 1987; Grad et al.,

Anxiety Disorders: An Introduction to Clinical Management and Research. Edited by E.J.L. Griez, C. Faravelli, D. Nutt and J. Zohar. © 2001 John Wiley & Sons, Ltd.

1989). Genetic background of TS is well defined by several familial and segregation studies although to date no specific genomic region seems to be strongly associated with the disorder. However, the relationship between TS and OCD has heavily influenced the genetic research on OCD, as discussed later in this chapter.

Twin and Familial Studies

From a methodological point of view twin and familial studies are powerful tools for defining the presence of genetic component in a disorder. Twin studies on OCD produced contrasting results. The majority of the twin case reports and studies come from the Maudsley Hospital Twin Registry, which gives reliable zygosity diagnosis through blood grouping. McGuffin and Mawson (1980) reported two concordant monozygotic twin pairs from the Maudsley Registry. Carey and Gottesman, in 1981, studied a cohort of 30 twin pairs, equally subdivided in monozygotic (MZ) and dizygotic (DZ); 87% of the MZ co-twins had obsessive symptoms, versus 47% of the DZ co-twins. This concordance supports the hypothesis of the genetic basis for OCD, although the fact that the MZ concordance is lower than 100% indicates the presence of no genetic factors in OCD aetiology. A subsequent study by Torgersen, from the Norwegian Twin Registry, investigated three MZ and nine DZ twin pairs, with at least one of the two having OCD. He found none of the pairs to be concordant for OCD (Torgersen, 1983).

The familial epidemiology of OCD has been studied since 1942 (Brown, 1942); results indicated that the disease clusters in the families of the index cases, and therefore familial or genetic components seem to influence the expression of the disorder. Early studies of children and adolescents (Swedo et al., 1989; Lenane, 1990) found high rates of affected relatives, ranging between 20 and 25%; this over-estimate is most probably due to a sampling bias depending on the young age of the probands. In fact, it is known that the early onset conditions have a higher penetrance and a greater familial loading. Following studies conducted on adult clinical samples lowered this estimate; McKeon and Murray (1987), studying a sample of 50 OCD patients compared to a control group, found no significant increase in secondary OCD cases, but a significant excess of other anxiety and mood disorders in the relatives. This result is consistent with data from work by Black et al. (1992); the conclusions suggested that a "neurotic" predisposition may be transmitted and the expression of OCD would require additional factors (biological or psychosocial). Bellodi et al. (1992) studied an Italian sample of 92 OCD patients, calculating a morbidity risk for OCD equal to 3.4%, slightly higher than the expected prevalence in the general population. In the same study, the morbidity risk was evaluated for the early onset patients (onset < 14 years); the rates of illness among their relatives were significantly higher than those of the later onset probands' relatives (8.8% versus 3.4%). The most up-to-date work on OCD epidemiology is the one by Pauls on 100 families of OCD probands (versus a sample of 100 families of control probands); the inclusion of full and sub-threshold secondary OCD cases yielded a morbidity risk of

18.2, providing evidence that some forms of OCD are familial and that the condition is heterogeneous (Pauls et al., 1995). Table 2.1 briefly summarises these familial studies on OCD.

The variability of results in familial studies is caused by different sampling techniques and nosological criteria, making comparison between studies difficult. Sometimes these studies are not controlled. However, the observations that in some studies OCD recurrence is increased in families of OCD probands suggest that a familial component, and probably a genetic one, may be present in such families. Positive familiarity for OCD may identify a specific subtype of OCD patients: in fact, Pauls et al. (1995) subdivided OCD patients into at least three groups: those with OCD familiarity; those without positive OCD familiarity; and those with tics. Each group might have different aetiologies.

Twin and familial studies suggest that a transmissible component is implicated in the aetiology of OCD. However, twin and familial/segregation studies are the preliminary stages when evaluating the role of a genetic component in a disorder. The next task is the detailed definition of this familial component and whether it is due to a major gene effect. Segregation studies investigate and discover whether a major, potentially autosomal, gene can account for the transmission of OCD and allow for a more specific definition of its parameters (gene frequency, genotypic penetrances, Mendelian probabilities of transmission).

We introduced the problem of the Tourette Syndrome/OCD relationship. There is compelling evidence, from family and segregation studies of probands with Tourette's Syndrome (TS), of a relationship between this syndrome and OCD (Pauls et al., 1986; Pitman et al., 1987; Grad et al., 1989). The reported rates for OCD among first-degree relatives of TS are 26% (Pauls et al., 1986), 7% (Pitman et al., 1987), and 6% (Eapen et al., 1993), higher rates than those calculated for control groups. The mode of transmission of TS and Chronic Motor Tics (CMT) is consistent with Autosomal Dominant inheritance with incomplete penetrance and sex-influenced expression (Eapen et al., 1993; Pauls et al., 1986). The inclusion of OCD or obsessive-compulsive behaviour as a part of the TS spectrum enhances the best fit for the major gene in segregation studies of TS. By contrast, several studies revealed a

TABLE 2.1 Familial studies on obsessive-compulsive disorder

Studies	Affected relatives
McKeon and Murray, 1987	No differences between relatives of OCD and controls
Swedo et al., 1989	25% of first-degree relatives of OCD are affected with OCD
Lenane et al., 1990	35% of first-degree relatives are affected with OCD or subthreshold OCD
Black et al., 1992	First-degree relatives are affected with a neurotic predisposition
Bellodi et al., 1992	Morbid Risk (MR) = 3.4.% for first-degree relatives, MR = 8.8% if the onset of probands is lower than 14
Pauls et al., 1995	18.2% of first-degree relatives are OCD (10.3% full OCD + 7.9% sub-threshold OCD)

higher rate of TS and CMT among relatives of OCD as compared with the general population (Leonard et al., 1992; Pauls et al., 1995). Recently the hypothesis has been advanced that the transmission of TS and related behaviours may be more complex and should include the assortative mating effect and should analyse larger samples (Hasstedt et al., 1995; Walkup et al., 1996; Seuchter et al., 2000).

Although there are several differences in the manifestations, the course and the current treatment of the two diseases, we might hypothesise that a common aetiologic background exists and, consequently, that the same gene/genes control their expression. Nicolini et al. (1991) investigated the segregation of OCD in a familial sample of 24 OCD/Tourette probands. They found that a Mendelian model may account for OCD transmission in OCD families, but the small size of the recruited sample did not allow a definite choice between Recessive or Dominant models. Cavallini et al. (1999) recruited 107 families of probands affected with OCD or OCD/tic. Probands with other co-diagnosis have been excluded from the analysis. In this case, the best fit was for a Mendelian Dominant model of transmission with a gene frequency of 0.01 and penetrances for homozygotes AA and for heterozygotes Aa = 8%. Females have higher penetrances than males (8.47% versus 7.9%). Enlarging the phenotypic boundaries to include TS and tic disorder, the best fit was for a non-Mendelian model of transmission. The results of these two studies suggest that a relatively simple genetic model may explain the inheritance pattern. Although the diagnosis of OCD is standardised across studies (DSM criteria), phenotypic and aetiologic heterogeneity confounds most studies of complex psychiatric disorders.

Recently, Alsobrook et al. (1999) proposed a different approach to the phenotype problem. Analysing the overall sample of OCD patients, the best model of transmission is a non-Mendelian model of transmission. Sub-dividing OCD patients according to positive family history for OCD, the best model of transmission is represented by a mixed model of transmission, that is a Single Major Locus (SML) plus a multifactorial background. Applying factor analysis to the OC contents of these patients they identified a four factor solution (Leckman et al., 1997), and on the basis of factor scores all the patients have been reclassified. In families of patients with a high score on the "third" factor characterised by symmetry/ordering contents, the polygenic model of transmission was rejected and an SML of transmission obtained the best fit.

Segregation studies support the existence of an SML, at least for some subgroups of OCD patients: these findings allow us to look for a specific aetiologic gene. Nevertheless, definite hypotheses need to search for these genes, which might involve starting from other research areas.

Molecular Genetics

Findings in neuroscience are not conclusive, due to the complexity of the research field, but in some cases they do allow us to formulate specific aetiologic hypotheses. Molecular biology is a powerful tool to test them. In the case of OCD, the observation that Serotonin Re-uptake Inhibitors (SRI) are effective in the reduction of symptoms and selective agonists of serotonergic receptors (such as Methyl Chloro Phenyl Piperazine: mCPP) enhance the OC symptoms, allows us to consider that dysfunction in serotonergic pathways might influence OCD development. For this reason, genes coding for serotonergic structures may be appropriate candidate genes, playing the main aetiologic role in OCD. Nevertheless, case control studies on specific genotypes or alleles of functional polymorphisms for serotonergic receptors 5HT2c (109 OCD patients versus 107 healthy controls) (Cavallini et al., 1998a) and 5HT2a (67 OCD patients and 54 healthy controls) (Nicolini et al., 1996) exclude for the available clinical populations a major or slight effect of these elements in the OCD development. These results are very far from findings in eating disorders (ED), which are frequently described as part of the clinical OCD spectrum (Kaye et al., 1993).

Recently, a positive association of a functional polymorphism in the promoter region of the 5HT2a-receptor gene with ED (Collier et al., 1997; Enoch et al., 1998; Sorbi et al., 1998) has been described. Also, the gene for the serotonin transporter, that re-uptakes serotonin in the intersynaptic cleft, thus a probable action site of SRI, may be a candidate gene in OCD. A mutation screening study performed in 1996 (Altemus et al., 1996) did not highlight specific variations in the sequence of serotonin transporter gene of 22 OCD patients compared with control individuals. Then Heils et al. (1996) detected a mutation in the promoter region of the serotonin transporter gene (5HTTLPR): the absence of 44 bp sequence determines a reduction in the transcription activity of the gene (Lesch et al., 1996). Billett et al. (1997) tested a sample of Canadian OCD patients for this polymorphism and did not find any association with the disorder. Exploring the association between the described polymorphism and the response to drug treatment as phenotype, the authors did not find any association, even though the definition of drug response used in this study was not standardised. Our group replicated the negative finding of Canadian group, analysing a sample of 124 Italian OCD patients (Bellodi et al., 1998a) and comparing them with a control group.

Considering the co-morbidity of OCD with TS and the potential involvement of dopaminergic mechanisms in TS, the hypothesis of a dopaminergic dysfunction was extended also to OCD aetiology. However, to date no positive findings are available for association studies with dopaminergic receptors genes, that is with DRD2 (Novelli et al., 1994), DRD3 (Catalano et al., 1994), even though the seven-repeat variant of the dopamine D4 receptor seems to be significantly increased in OCD patients with tics (Cruz et al., 1997). Karayiorgou et al. found and replicated a positive association between a functional polymorphism of Catechol-O-Methyl-Transferase (COMT) enzyme gene on chromosome 22q and male OCD patients (Karayiorgou et al., 1997; Karayiorgou et al., 1999). COMT is an enzyme implicated in the inactivation of catecholamines (adrenaline, noradrenaline, dopamine). A common functional allele of this gene, which results in a three- to four-fold reduction in enzyme activity, is associated with OCD diagnosis in male subjects. The mechanism underlying this sex-selective association remains to be defined and may include a sexual dimorphism in COMT activity.

Observing the efficacy of SRI, we started from the assumption that serotonergic pathways have an aetiologic role in the expression of OCD. Nevertheless, the alterations of serotonergic structures may be a consequence of a more complex dysfunction starting or involving additional neurotransmitters. For example, given the evidence of an over-activity of the cholinergic system in TS and the exacerbation of TS symptoms after administration of drugs which stimulate cholinergic receptors, (Sandyk, 1995), muscarinic receptors genes could be candidate genes in OCD/TS aetiology.

Karayiorgou et al. (1999) analysed 110 nuclear OCD families for the inheritance of functional variants of monamine oxidase-A (Mao-A): a sexually dimorphic association between OCD and an allele of the Mao-A gene, previously linked to high Mao-A enzymatic activity, is evident. In agreement with the well-established action of Mao-A inhibitors as antidepressants, this association is marked among male OCD probands with co-morbid MDD. In a previous study, increased frequency of a low activity-related allele of the Mao-A was found in female OCD subjects (Camarena et al., 1998). A rare silent mutation detected by SSCP in the coding region of Tryptophane Hydroxylase (TPH) (Han et al., 1999) is not significantly increased in OCD patients when compared with other diagnostic groups.

Recent methodologies of analysis permit us to overcome the straight definition of mode of transmission of disorders and to test the association with interesting genes directly. Nevertheless, a central question remains unsolved, that is the correct definition of the affected phenotype. We have already cited the hypothesis of the existence of at least three subtypes of OCD patients. Furthermore, is OCD a definite phenotype or an element of a wide aetiologic/genetic spectrum? Some evidence exists of a link between TS and tic disorder, but from a clinical point of view other disorders might belong on this spectrum, on the basis of clinical and familial observations (i.e. eating disorders, dysmorphophobic disorder, impulsive disorders, autism). Obviously, if the spectrum concept has some validity, it is important to include these phenotypes in familial/ genetic studies to better define the genetic nature of pathologies. Therefore, we can suppose that the absence of strong positive results may also be caused by the approximate phenotype definition.

PANIC DISORDER (PD)

For panic disorder (PD) aetiology, we observed a condition similar to that presented for obsessive-compulsive disorder. There is some evidence favouring the existence of a biological basis for PD, nevertheless the definition of genetic components involved in this disorder is not yet well established.

Twin and Familial Studies

As in the case of OCD, familial and twin studies support the existence of heredity of the disorder. In Table 2.2 the main familial studies are summarised: the familial risks

TABLE 2.2 Familial studies on panic disorders

Authors		Results
Crowe et al., 1983 Noyes et al., 1986 Weissman et al., 1993 Mendlewicz et al., 1993	First-degree relatives of PD	MR is in a range from 8% to 17%
Maier et al., 1993 Heun and Maier, 1995	First-degree relatives of PD	MR is in a range from 3.4% to 14.7%
Hopper et al., 1987	First-degree relatives of PD probands	Family history of 12%
Moran et al., 1985	First-degree relatives of PD probands	Family history of 12.5%
Battaglia et al., 1995	First-degree relatives of PD probands	Family history of 8%
Perna et al., 1996	First-degree relatives of 203 PD probands	Patients with positive response to 35% CO_2 challenge have a genetic risk for PD (MR = 14.4%), significantly higher than that for patients with a negative response to 35% CO_2 challenge (MR = 3.9%)
Goldstein et al., 1997	First-degree relatives of PD with onset before and after 20 years	MR for PD probands with onset before 20 yrs: 22% and MR for PD with onset after 20 yrs: 8%

range from 3.4% to 17%. In the two more recent studies, reclassifying PD patients on the basis of CO_2 response (Perna et al., 1996) or on the basis of age at onset (Goldstein et al., 1997), a significant variability of morbidity risk among first-degree relatives was observed. The higher risk of PD in relatives of probands with panic disorder onset at or before 20 years of age suggests that age at onset may differentiate familial subtypes of panic disorder (Goldstein et al., 1997). Furthermore, it has been observed that a positive family history for PD with agoraphobia influenced age at onset of panic disorder (Battaglia et al., 1995).

To date, twin studies on concordance for PD are few, even if generally they confirm a higher concordance in MZ twin pairs than in DZ twin pairs (Torgersen, 1983; Torgersen, 1990; Perna et al., 1997). The largest twin study (Kendler et al., 1993) reported MZ versus DZ proband-wise concordance rates of 24:11, with respective heritability estimates of 35% and 46% for a narrow phenotype and a multiple threshold model. Furthermore, in 1995 Kendler and colleagues completed a complex multivariate analysis on a sample of 1033 female twin pairs, to define the genetic and environmental risk factors for different psychiatric disorders, including PD (Kendler et al., 1995). They found two factors which best explained genetic influences on these disorders, the first of which heavily emphasised phobia, panic disorder, and bulimia nervosa, and the second, major depression and generalised anxiety disorder.

Segregation studies revealed a Mendelian mode of transmission for PD. Pauls et al. (1980) were unable to reject a Dominant model of transmission in 19 pedigrees. Extending this sample to 41 pedigrees, an SML with a polygenic background provided the best fit for these data (Crowe et al., 1983). In two more recent studies, Vieland and colleages found that if PD is genetic, a Mendelian model of transmission better explains its transmission in their pedigrees, even though there was little evidence to support a Dominant over a Recessive model, possibly because of the lack of power of the selected samples (Vieland and Hodge, 1995; Vieland et al., 1996). The main differences among cited studies could be represented by a potential heterogeneity of probands: indeed, probands recruited in the Pauls et al. (1980) study may have a co-diagnosis of affective disorders. In their first segregation study, Vieland and Hodge selected 30, two- and three-generations pedigrees without affective disorder co-diagnosis, while in the second one Vieland et al. (1996) studied 126 nuclear pedigrees with or without affective disorder. In this study, families were subdivided according to the presence of comorbid major depression (MD) in PD patients: the effect of restricting the analysis to families of probands without any lifetime history of MD was examined. Apparently, MD co-diagnosis does not influence the PD transmission. In a sample of 165 Italian pedigrees, PD segregates following an Additive Mendelian model of transmission (Cavallini et al., 1999). PD genetic transmission may be a complex phenomenon and additional genetic mechanisms may contribute or interfere, confounding classical Mendelian paradigms. Battaglia et al. (1998) observed a significant decrease in the time before the first episode of panic and onset of panic disorder from the older to the younger generation in 38 unilineal PD families. In this set of families the presence of anticipation is supported and, if it is confirmed by other studies, from a molecular genetic point of view, a role for trinucleotide repeat sequences could be considered to account for the familial aggregation of PD.

Molecular Genetics

Available molecular studies on PD are disappointing and contrasting. After the test for linkage between PD and a battery of 29 genetic markers, only locus for alpha-haptoglobin (chromosome 16q22) was suggestive of linkage in 26 families (Lod score = 2.27) (Crowe et al., 1987; Crowe, 1990). A linkage study on 23 families of PD probands analysing a set of genetic markers covering all the autosomic chromosomes did not highlight positive linkage (Lod score > 3) for any of the analysed markers (Knowles et al., 1998). Recent reports suggest an association between the 5-HTT polymorphism and anxiety-related traits, as measured by personality assessment. A linkage study performed on 45 PD families for the polymorhism in the promoter region of serotonin transporter gene (see Chapter on OCD) (Heils et al., 1996) produced negative results. A case control study on 158 PD patients and 169 healthy controls (Deckert et al., 1997) and an association study performed using a family-based design (74 parents/probands families) confirmed the absence of genetic association (Hamilton et al., 1999) for this polymorphism. These results provide evidence that the genetic basis of panic disorder may be distinct from anxiety-related traits assessed by personality inventories in normal populations.

There is also evidence for the role of the cholecystokinin (CCK) neurotransmitter system in the neurobiology of PD. The CCK receptor agonist, CCK-tetrapeptide (CCK-4) fulfils criteria for a panicogenic agent and there is evidence that PD might be associated with an abnormal function of the CCK system. The CCK receptors have been classified into two subtypes: CCK-A and CCK-B, with different brain distribution. After a mutational screening of promoter region of CCK gene, Wang et al. (1998) detected statistically significant transmission disequilibrium of a polymorphism (CCK-36CT) ($\chi^2 = 4.00$, $P < 0.05$) when panic disorder or attacks were considered as affected. Furthermore, from a biochemical point of view Garvey et al. (1998) found that PD subjects carrying the CCK mutation have higher levels of the enzyme N-acetyl-beta-glucosaminidase than PD patients without CCK mutation. For a CCK-B receptor gene polymorphism in the coding region, PD patients showed a significant association (Kennedy et al., 1999), suggesting that CCK-B receptor gene variation may contribute to neurobiology of PD. Deckert et al. (1998) hypothesised that variation in A2a adenosine receptor gene modifies genetic susceptibility to panic disorder. They found a positive association between PD patients and a 1083C/T allelic variant.

The serotonergic hypothesis has built in an observing therapeutic effect of SRI on panic symptoms, but inhibition of monoamine oxidase A (Mao-A) is clinically effective in the treatment of PD. It has been described as a polymorphism of Mao-A promoter gene determining a variation of enzymatic activity. In a sample of female patients with PD there is a significant excess of the allelic variant of the Mao-A promoter gene, conditioning high enzymatic activity (Deckert et al., 1999). These findings suggest that increased Mao-A activity may be a risk factor for PD in female patients. Also, Gamma-Aminobutyric acid type A (GABAA) receptor subunit genes may be candidate genes for PD. Benzodiazepine agonists acting at this receptor can suppress panic attacks, and both inverse agonists and antagonists can precipitate them. The human GABAA receptor subtypes are composed of various combinations of 13 subunits, each encoded by one gene. No linkage between panic disorder/agoraphobia and the GABAA beta 1 locus, located on chromosome 4p13-p12, was found in five Icelandic pedigrees (Schmidt et al., 1993). Crowe et al. (1997) tested eight GABAA subunits in a candidate gene linkage study of PD, but they failed to find any positive result.

The noradrenergic neurotransmitter system may be involved in the pathogenesis of PD. Since a mutation in a gene coding for one of the adrenergic receptors could account for both the familial nature and the autonomic dysfunction of PD, Wang et al. (1992) performed analyses of the linkage between 14 multiplex PD families and five adrenergic receptor loci. Lod scores less than -2.0 were found at all five receptor loci. The involvement of tyrosine hydroxylase gene in the aetiology of PD was excluded in 14 PD families (Mutchler et al., 1990).

We already stated that in psychiatric disorders, diagnostic definitions sometimes are not completely reliable. From a genetic perspective, there are not even fully reliable markers to define clinical groups suitable for genetic studies. The responses to challenge tests (35% CO_2 inhalation test, lactate infusion, colecystochinine injection, etc.) could help in the definition of PD biological determinants. To date, the 35% CO_2 challenge test is not only a specific and reliable clinical test for PD (Battaglia et al., 1995; Verburg et al., 1998; Coryell and Arndt, 1999), but a positive response in PD probands is associated with a higher familial risk for PD (14.4% versus 3.9%) (Perna et al., 1996), than in families of probands with a negative response. The 35% CO_2 hypersensitivity is present in 75% of clinical samples and this challenge could be proposed as a good dissection tool in the understanding of different subtypes of panic disorder (respiratory versus and non-respiratory PD) (Biber and Alkin, 1999). Familial data on 35% CO_2 response are confirmed also by twin data: in a sample of 20 MZ twin pairs and 25 DZ twin pairs there is a concordance rate for the response with a panic attack to the CO_2 challenge test respectively of 55.6% versus 12.5% (Bellodi et al., 1998b). These findings suggest that the response to 35% CO_2 inhalation may be controlled by genetic factors, even though the MZ twin concordance of 55.6% indicates the additional effect of no genetic factors. We performed a complex segregation analysis on 134 families of probands with a positive response to 35% CO_2 response (Cavallini et al., 1998b; Cavallini et al., 1999): a single major gene accounts for the distribution of PD and agoraphobia in families of these patients. A dominant Mendelian model of transmission has the best fit, while in 31 families of probands with a negative response to CO_2 inhalation, genetic transmission has been rejected. Further development of this study is the evaluation of co-segregation of 35% CO_2 response and PD in first-degree relatives of PD probands (Cavallini et al., 1998b), to establish if CO_2 response mechanisms and PD genetic liability share a common genetic basis. Additional endophenotypes are under study in order to improve the phenotype definition of PD.

A case control study conducted of a sample of 99 PD patients versus 64 medical patients showed that joint hypermobility syndrome (JHS) is more frequent in patients with PD (67.7%) than in controls (12.5%) (Martin-Santos et al., 1998). This finding suggests that JHS may reflect a constitutional disposition to suffer from anxiety. Weissman et al. (2000) proposed the existence of "chromosome 13 syndrome", which includes panic disorder, kidney or bladder problems, serious headaches, thyroid problems (usually hypothyroid), and/or mitral valve prolapse (MPV). Families where any individual with any one of the "syndrome" conditions as affected show a linkage with one marker (D13S779) on chromosome 13.

POST-TRAUMATIC STRESS DISORDER (PTSD)

Acute traumatic stress may lead to post-traumatic stress disorder (PTSD), which is characterised by delayed neuropsychiatric symptoms including depression, irritability, and impaired cognitive performance. There is evidence that familial factors serve as determinants of risk for PTSD, especially familial anxiety. It has also been suggested that PTSD following rape is associated with familial vulnerability to major depression, which may thus serve as a risk factor for developing PTSD. On this hypothesis PTSD may on occasion represent a form of depression that is induced and/or modified neurobiologically and phenomenologically by extreme stress (Davidson et al., 1998).

Genetic component might not directly influence the development of PTSD, apart from the probability of exposure to specific traumatic environment, which predisposes to PTSD. Data from 4029 twin pairs who served in the US military during the Vietnam era (1965–75) were used to examine genetic and non-genetic factors that influence wartime exposure to traumatic events. The correlation for self-reported combat experiences is 0.53 and 0.30 of MZ and DZ twins respectively. Heritability estimates ranged from 35% to 47% (Lyons et al., 1993). A genetic association study on subjects who had been exposed to severe combat conditions in Vietnam and suffer from PTSD shows linkage disequilibrium with an allelic variant of DRD2 receptor gene (D2A1). This DRD2 variant confers an increased risk to PTSD, while the absence of the variant confers a relative resistance to PTSD (Comings et al., 1996).

CONCLUSION

Findings in genetics of anxiety disorders are to date limited by the lack of strong hypotheses on the aetiology of these disorders. Several elements contribute to the limitation of our knowledge.

1. Diagnostic and consequently phenotypic boundaries are not completely defined, compelling the research to work with heterogeneous samples.
2. We analyse genetic data assuming over-simplified models: multiple studies suggest that probably a Single Major Locus does not account for these disorders. Additional sources of variability have to be included in our models. These sources may be due to genes with small effects, which may be detected by collecting and analysing large samples of patients.
3. The environment could interact with gene expression and modify it. Kendler and Eaves (1986) proposed at least three different ways to solve the gene–environment interaction: we can hypothesise additive effects of genotype and environment; genetic control of sensitivity to the environment; and genetic control of exposure to the environment. However, these theoretical models represent a simplification of the true gene–environment relationship.
4. Statistical techniques available to date show some limitations. Traditional case control studies have to deal with stratification problems, linkage analysis does not allow a search for minor effect genes: all these aspects complicate our effort to circumscribe the genetic basis of anxiety disorders.

REFERENCES

Alsobrook II JP, Leckman JF, Goodman WK, Rasmussen SA, Pauls DL (1999) Segregation analysis of obsessive-compulsive disorder using symptom-based factor scores. *Am J Med Genet* **88**(6): 669–675.

Altemus M, Murphy DL, Greenberg B, Lesch KP (1996) Intact coding region of the serotonin transporter gene in obsessive-compulsive disorder. *Am J Med Genet* **26**, 67(4): 409–411.

Battaglia M, Perna G (1995) The 35% CO_2 challenge in panic disorder: Optimization by receiver operating characteristic (ROC) analysis. *J Psychiatr Res* **29**(2): 111–119.

Battaglia M, Bertella S, Bajo S, Binaghi F, Bellodi L (1998) Anticipation of age at onset in panic disorder. *Am J Psychiatry* **155**(5): 590–595.

Battaglia M, Bertella S, Politi E, Bernardeschi L, Perna G, Gabriele A, Bellodi L (1995) Age of onset of panic disorder: The influence of familial liability to the disease and of childhood separation anxiety disorder. *Am J Psychiatry* **152**: 1362–1364.

Bellodi L, Di Bella D, Cavallini MC, Catalano M (1998a) Genetic basis of obsessive-compulsive disorder and related conditions (i.e. Tourette's Syndrome) in the Italian population. Proceedings of Telethon, scientific convention, 1998.

Bellodi L, Perna G, Caldirola D, Arancio C, Bertani A, Di Bella D (1998b) CO_2-induced panic attacks: A twin study. *Am J Psychiatry* **155**(9): 1184–1188.

Bellodi L, Sciuto G, Diaferia G, Ronchi P, Smeraldi E (1992) Psychiatric disorders in the families of patients with obsessive compulsive disorder. *Psychiatry Res* **42**: 111–120.

Biber B, Alkin T (1999) Panic disorder subtypes: differential responses to CO_2 challenge. *Am J Psychiatry* **156**(5): 739–744.

Billett EA, Richter MA, King N, Heils A, Lesch KP, Kennedy JL (1997) Obsessive compulsive disorder, response to serotonin reuptake inhibitors and the serotonin transporter gene. *Mol Psychiatry* **2**(5): 403–406.

Black DW, Noyes R, Goldstein RB, Blum NA. (1992) A family study of obsessive compulsive disorder. *Arch Gen Psychiatry* **49**: 362–368.

Brown FW (1942) Heredity in the psychoneurosis. *Proceedings of the Royal Society of Medicine* **35**: 785–790.

Calabrese G, Colombo C, Bonfanti A, Scotti G, Scarone S (1993) Caudate nucleus abnormalities in obsessive-compulsive disorder: Measurements of MRI signal intensity. *Psychiatry Res* **50**(2): 89–92.

Caldirola D, Perna G, Arancio C, Bertani A, Bellodi L (1997) The 35% CO_2 challenge test in patients with social phobia. *Psychiatry Res* **71**(1): 41–48.

Camarena B, Cruz C, de la Fuente JR, Nicolini H (1998) A higher frequency of a low activity-related allele of the MAO-A gene in females with obsessive-compulsive disorder. *Psychiatr Genet* **8**(4): 255–257.

Carey G, Gottesman II (1981) Twin and family studies of anxiety, phobic and obsessive disorders. In Klein, DF, Rabkin, J (eds) *Anxiety: New Research and Changing Concepts*. New York: Raven Press.

Catalano M, Sciuto G, Di Bella D, Novelli E, Nobile M, Bellodi L (1994) Lack of association between obsessive-compulsive disorder and the dopamine D3 receptor gene: some preliminary considerations. *Am J Med Genet* **54**(3): 253–255.

Cavallini MC, Di Bella D, Pasquale L, Henin M, Bellodi L (1998a) 5HT2C CYS23/SER23 polymorphism is not associated with obsessive-compulsive disorder. *Psychiatry Res* **9**; 77(2): 97–104.

Cavallini MC, Perna GP, Caldirola D, Bellodi L (1999) A segregation of panic disorder in families of panic patients responsive to 35% CO_2 challenge. *Biol Psychiatry* **46**: 815–820.

Cavallini MC, Perna GP, Caldirola D, Di Bella D, Bellodi L (1998) Segregation analysis of panic disorder and 35% CO_2 response in Italian pedigrees. In Bellodi L, Perna GP (eds) *The Panic Respiration Connection*. Milan: MDM Medical Media.

Collier DA, Arranz MJ, Li T, Mupita D, Brown N, Treasure J (1997) Association between 5-HT2A gene promoter polymorphism and anorexia nervosa. *Lancet* **350** (9075): 412.

Comings DE, Muhleman D, Gysin R (1996) Dopamine D2 receptor (DRD2) gene and susceptibility to posttraumatic stress disorder: A study and replication. *Biol Psychiatry* **40**(5): 368–372.

Coryell W, Arndt S (1999) The 35% CO_2 inhalation procedure: Test-retest reliability. *Biol Psychiatry* **45**(7): 923–927.

Crowe RR (1990) Panic disorder: Genetic considerations. *J Psychiatr Res* **24** Suppl 2: 129–134.

Crowe RR, Noyes R Jr, Pauls DL, Slyman DJ (1983) A family study of panic disorder. *Arch Gen Psychiatry* **40**: 1065–1069.

Crowe RR, Noyes R Jr, Wilson AF, Elston RC, Ward LJ (1987) A linkage study of panic disorder. *Arch Gen Psychiatry* **44**(11): 933–937.

Crowe RR, Wang Z, Noyes R Jr, Albrecht BE, Darlison MG, Bailey ME, Johnson KJ, Zoega T (1997) Candidate gene study of eight GABAA receptor subunits in panic disorder. *Am J Psychiatry* **154**(8): 1096–1100.

Cruz C, Camarena B, King N, Paez F, Sidenberg D, de la Fuente JR, Nicolini H (1997) Increased prevalence of the seven-repeat variant of the dopamine D4 receptor gene in patients with obsessive-compulsive disorder with tics. *Neurosci Lett* **231**(1): 1–4.

Dager SR, Layton M, Richards T (1996) Neuroimaging findings in anxiety disorders. *Semin Clin Neuropsychiatry* **1**(1): 48–60.

Davidson JR, Tupler LA, Wilson WH, Connor KM (1998) A family study of chronic post-traumatic stress disorder following rape trauma. *J Psychiatr Res* **32**(5): 301–309.

Deckert J, Catalano M, Heils A, Di Bella D, Friess F, Politi E, Franke P, Nothen MM, Maier W, Bellodi L, Lesch KP (1997) Functional promoter polymorphism of the human serotonin transporter: lack of association with panic disorder. *Psychiatr Genet* **7**(1): 45–47.

Deckert J, Catalano M, Syagailo YV, Bosi M, Okladnova O, Di Bella D, Nothen MM, Maffei P, Franke P, Fritze J, Maier W, Propping P, Beckmann H, Bellodi L, Lesch KP (1999) Excess of high activity monoamine oxidase A gene promoter alleles in female patients with panic disorder. *Hum Mol Genet* **8**(4): 621–624.

Deckert J, Nothen MM, Franke P, Delmo C, Fritze J, Knapp M, Maier W, Beckmann H, Propping P (1998) Systematic mutation screening and association study of the A1 and A2a adenosine receptor genes in panic disorder suggest a contribution of the A2a gene to the development of disease. *Mol Psychiatry* **3**(1): 81–85.

Eapen V, Pauls DL, Robertson MM (1993) Evidence for autosomal dominant transmission in Tourette's syndrome: A United Kingdom cohort study. *Br J Psychiatry* **162**: 593–596.

Enoch MA, Kaye WH, Rotondo A, Greenberg BD, Murphy DL, Goldman D (1998) 5-HT2A promoter polymorphism -1438G/A, anorexia nervosa, and obsessive-compulsive disorder. *Lancet* **351**(9118): 1785–1786.

Garvey MJ, Crowe RR, Wang Z (1998) An association of NAG levels and a mutation of the CCK gene in panic disorder patients. *Psychiatry Res* **80**(2): 149–153.

Goldstein RB, Wickramaratne PJ, Horwath E, Weissman MM (1997) Familial aggregation and phenomenology of "early"-onset (at or before age 20 years) panic disorder. *Arch Gen Psychiatry* **54**(3): 271–278.

Grad LR, Pelcovitz D, Olson M, Matthews M, Grad JL (1989) Obsessive-compulsive symptomatology in children with Tourette's syndrome. *J Am Acad Child Adolesc Psychiatry* **26**: 69–73.

Hamilton SP, Heiman GA, Haghighi F, Mick S, Klein DF, Hodge SE, Weissman MM, Fyer AJ, Knowles JA (1999) Lack of genetic linkage or association between a functional serotonin transporter polymorphism and panic disorder. *Psychiatr Genet* **9**(1): 1–6.

Han L, Nielsen DA, Rosenthal NE, Jefferson K, Kaye W, Murphy D, Altemus M, Humphries J, Cassano G, Rotondo A, Virkkunen M, Linnoila M, Goldman D (1999) No coding variant of the tryptophan hydroxylase gene detected in seasonal affective disorder, obsessive-compulsive disorder, anorexia nervosa, and alcoholism. *Biol Psychiatry* **45**(5): 615–619.

Hasstedt SJ, Leppert M, Filloux F, van de Wetering BJ, McMahon WM (1995) Intermediate inheritance of Tourette syndrome, assuming assortative mating. *Am J Hum Genet* **57**(3): 682–689.

Heils A, Teufel A, Petri S, Stober G, Riederer P, Bengel D, Lesch KP (1996) Allelic variation of human serotonin transporter gene expression. *J Neurochem* **66**(6): 2621–2624.

Heun R, Maier W (1995) Relation of schizophrenia and panic disorder: Evidence from a controlled family study. *Am J Med Genet* **60**(2): 127–132.

Hopper JL, Judd FK, Derrick PL, Burrows GD (1987) A family study of panic disorder. *Genet Epidemiol* **4**(1): 33–41.

Karayiorgou M, Altemus M, Galke BL, Goldman D, Murphy DL, Ott J, Gogos JA (1997) Genotype determining low catechol-O-methyltransferase activity as a risk factor for obsessive-compulsive disorder. *Proc Natl Acad Sci USA* **94**(9): 4572–4575.

Karayiorgou M, Sobin C, Blundell ML, Galke BL, Malinova L, Goldberg P, Ott J, Gogos JA (1999) Family-based association studies support a sexually dimorphic effect of COMT and MAOA on genetic susceptibility to obsessive-compulsive disorder. *Biol Psychiatry* **45**(9): 1178–1189.

Kaye WH, Weltzin T, Hsu LKG (1993) Anorexia nervosa. In Hollander E (ed.) *Obsessive-compulsive Related Disorders*. Washington, DC: American Psychiatric Press.

Kendler KS, Eaves LJ (1986) Models for the joint effect of genotype and environment on liability to psychiatric illness. *Am J Psychiatry* **143**(3): 279–289.

Kendler KS, Neale MC, Kessler RC, Heath AC, Eaves LJ, (1993) Panic disorder in women: A population based twin study. *Psychol Med* **23**: 397–406.

Kendler KS, Walters EE, Neale MC, Kessler RC, Heath AC, Eaves LJ (1995) The structure of the genetic and environmental risk factors for six major psychiatric disorders in women: Phobia, generalized anxiety disorder, panic disorder, bulimia, major depression, and alcoholism. *Arch General Psychiatry* **52**(5): 374–383.

Kennedy JL, Bradwejn J, Koszycki D, King N, Crowe R, Vincent J, Fourie O (1999) Investigation of cholecystokinin system genes in panic disorder. *Mol Psychiatry* **4**(3): 284–285.

Knowles JA, Fyer AJ, Vieland VJ, Weissman MM, Hodge SE, Heiman GA, Haghighi F, de Jesus GM, Rassnick H, Preud'homme-Rivelli X, Austin T, Cunjak J, Mick S, Fine LD, Woodley KA, Das K, Maier W, Adams PB, Freimer NB, Klein DF, Gilliam TC (1998) Results of a genome-wide genetic screen for panic disorder. *Am J Med Genet* **81**(2): 139–147.

Leckman JF, Grice DE, Boardman J, Zhang H, Vitale A, Bondi C, Alsobrook J, Peterson BS, Cohen DJ, Rasmussen SA, Goodman WK, McDougle CJ, Pauls DJ (1997) Symptoms of obsessive compulsive disorder. *Am J Psychiatry* **154**: 911–917.

Lenane M, Swedo SE, Leonard M, Pauls DL, Scheery W, Rapoport JL (1990) Psychiatric disorders in first degree relatives of children and adolescents with obsessive compulsive disorder. *J Am Acad Child Adolesc Psychiatry* **29**: 407–412.

Leonard HL, Lenane MC, Swedo SE, Rettew DC, Gershon ES, Rapaport JL (1992) Tics and Tourette's disorder: A 2 to 7 years follow-up of 54 obsessive-compulsive children. *Am J Psychiatry* **149**: 1244–1251.

Lesch KP, Bengel D, Heils A, Sabol SZ, Greenberg BD, Petri S, Benjamin J, Muller CR, Hamer DH, Murphy DL (1996) Association of anxiety-related traits with a polymorphism in the serotonin transporter gene regulatory region. *Science* **274**(5292): 1527–1531.

Lyons MJ, Goldberg J, Eisen SA, True W, Tsuang MT, Meyer JM, Henderson WG (1993) Do genes influence exposure to trauma? A twin study of combat. *Am J Med Genet* **1**; 48(1): 22–27.

Maier W, Lichtermann D, Minges J, Oehrlein A, Franke P (1993) A controlled family study in panic disorder. *J Psychiatr Res* **27** Suppl 1: 79–87.

Martin-Santos R, Bulbena A, Porta M, Gago J, Molina L, Duro JC (1998) Association between joint hypermobility syndrome and panic disorder. *Am J Psychiatry* **155**(11): 1578–1583.

McGuffin P, Mawson D (1980) Obsessive compulsive neurosis: Two identical twin pairs. *Br J Psychiatry* **137**: 285–287.

McKeon P, Murray R (1987) Familial aspect of obsessive-compulsive neurosis. *Br J Psychiatry* **151**: 528–534.

Mendlewicz J, Papadimitriou G, Wilmotte J (1993) Family study of panic disorder: comparison with generalised anxiety disorder, major depression and normal subjects. *Psychiatr Gen* **3**: 73–78.

Moran C, Andrews G (1985) The familial occurrence of agoraphobia. *Br J Psychiatry* **146**: 262–267.

Mutchler K, Crowe RR, Noyes R Jr, Wesner RW (1990) Exclusion of the tyrosine hydroxylase gene in 14 panic disorder pedigrees. *Am J Psychiatry* **147**(10): 1367–1369.

Nicolini H, Cruz C, Camarena B, Orozco B, Kennedy JL, King N, Weissbecker K, de la Fuente JR, Sidenberg D (1996) DRD2, DRD3 and 5HT2A receptor genes polymorphisms in obsessive-compulsive disorder. *Mol Psychiatry* **1**(6): 461–465.

Nicolini H, Hanna G, Baxter L, Schwartz J, Weissbacker K, Spence MA (1991) Segregation analysis of obsessive compulsive disorders: Preliminary results. *Ursus Medicus* **1**: 25–28.

Noyes R Jr, Clarkson C, Crowe RR, Yates WR, McChesney CM (1987) A family study of generalized anxiety disorder. *Am J Psychiatry* **144**(8): 1019–1024.

Noyes R Jr, Crowe RR, Harris EL, Hamra BJ, McChesney CM, Chaudhry DR (1986) Relationship between panic disorder and agoraphobia: A family study. *Arch Gen Psychiatry* **43**(3): 227–232.

Novelli E, Nobile M, Diaferia G, Sciuto G, Catalano M (1994) A molecular investigation suggests no relationship between obsessive-compulsive disorder and the dopamine D2 receptor. *Neuropsychobiology* **29**(2): 61–63.

Pauls DL, Alsobrook JP II, Goodman W, Rasmussen S, Leckman JF (1995) A family study of obsessive-compulsive disorder. *Am J Psychiatry* **152**: 76–84.

Pauls DL, Bucher KD, Crowe RR, Noyes R Jr. (1980) A genetic study of panic disorder pedigrees. *Am J Hum Genet* **32**: 639–644.

Pauls DL, Leckman JF (1986) The inheritance of Gilles de la Tourette's Syndrome and associated behaviors. *N Engl J Med* **315**: 993–997.

Pauls DL, Towbin KE, Leckman JF, Zahner GEP, Cohen DJ (1986) Gilles de la Tourette's syndrome and obsessive-compulsive disorder. *Arch Gen Psychiatry* **43**: 1180–1182.

Perani D, Colombo C, Bressi S, Bonfanti A, Grassi F, Scarone S, Bellodi L, Smeraldi E, Fazio F (1995) [^{18}F]FDG PET study in obsessive-compulsive disorder: A clinical/metabolic correlation study after treatment. *Br J Psychiatry* **166**(2): 244–250.

Perna G, Bertani A, Caldirola D, Bellodi L (1996) Family history of panic disorder and hypersensitivity to CO_2 in patients with panic disorder. *Am J Psychiatry* **153**(8): 1060–1064.

Perna GP, Caldirola D, Arancio C, Bellodi L (1997) Panic attacks: A twin study. *Psychiatry Res* **66**: 69–71.

Pitman RK, Green RC, Jenike MA, Mesulam MM (1987) Clinical comparison of Tourette's disorder and obsessive-compulsive disorder. *Am J Psychiatry* **144**: 1166–1171.

Sandyk R (1995) Cholinergic mechanisms in Gilles de la Tourette's Syndrome. *Intern J Neurosc* **81**(1–2): 95–100.

Saxena S, Brody AL, Schwartz JM, Baxter LR (1998) Neuroimaging and frontal-subcortical circuitry in obsessive-compulsive disorder. *Br J Psychiatry* Suppl **35**: 26–37.

Schmidt SM, Zoega T, Crowe RR (1993) Excluding linkage between panic disorder and the gamma-aminobutyric acid beta 1 receptor locus in five Icelandic pedigrees. *Acta Psychiatr Scand* **88**(4): 225–228.

Seuchter SA, Hebebrand J, Klug B, Knapp M, Lehmkuhl G, Poustka F, Schmidt M, Remschmidt H, Baur MP (2000) Complex segregation analysis of families ascertained through Gilles de la Tourette syndrome. *Genet Epidemiol* **18**(1): 33–47.

Sorbi S, Nacmias B, Tedde A, Ricca V, Mezzani B, Rotella CM (1998) 5-HT2A promoter polymorphism in anorexia nervosa. *Lancet* **351**(9118): 1785.

Swedo SE, Rapoport JL, Leonard HL, Cheslow DL (1989) Obsessive-compulsive disorder in children and adolescents. *Arch Gen Psychiatry* **46**: 335–341.

Torgersen S (1983) Genetic factors in anxiety disorders. *Arch Gen Psychiatry* **40**: 1085–1089.

Torgersen S (1990) Comorbidity of major depression and anxiety disorders in twin pairs. *Am J Psychiatry* **147**: 1199–1202.

Verburg K, Pols H, de Leeuw M, Griez E (1998) Reliability of the 35% carbon dioxide panic provocation challenge. *Psychiatry Res* **78**(3): 207–214.

Vieland VJ, Goodman DW, Chapman T, Fyer AJ (1996) New segregation analysis of panic disorder. *Am J Med Genet* **67**: 147–153.

Vieland VJ, Hodge SE (1995) Inherent intractability of the ascertainment problem for the pedigree data: A general likelihood framework. *Am J Hum Genet* **56**(1): 33–43.

Walkup JT, LaBuda MC, Singer HS, Brown J, Riddle MA, Hurko O (1996) Family study and segregation analysis of Tourette syndrome: Evidence for a mixed model of inheritance. *Am J Hum Genet* **59**(3): 684–693.

Wang ZW, Crowe RR, Noyes R Jr (1992) Adrenergic receptor genes as candidate genes for panic disorder: A linkage study. *Am J Psychiatry* **149**(4): 470–474.

Wang Z, Valdes J, Noyes R, Zoega T, Crowe RR (1998) Possible association of a cholecystokinin promotor polymorphism (CCK-36CT) with panic disorder. *Am J Med Genet* **8**; 81(3): 228–234.

Weissman MM, Fyer AJ, Haghighi F, Heiman G, Deng Z, Hen R, Hodge SE, Knowles JA (2000) Potential panic disorder syndrome: Clinical and genetic linkage evidence. *Am J Med Genet* **96**(1): 24–35.

Weissman MM, Wickramaratne P, Adams PB, Lish JD, Horwarth E, Charne D, Woods SW, Leeman E, Frosh E (1993) The relationship between panic disorder and major depression: A new family study. *Arch Gen Psychiatry* **50**: 767–780.

Genetics of Anxiety Disorders: Part II

B. de Brettes and J.P. Lépine

Hôpital Fernand Widal, Paris, France

INTRODUCTION

Due to the extremely fast development of molecular genetic methods in the past 10 years, more and more studies have been and are being currently carried out on the genetic factors of schizophrenia, bipolar disorder and Alzheimer's disease. However, in connection with environmental factors, genetic vulnerabilities are suspected in many other psychiatric disorders such as alcoholism and other addictive disorders, autism, eating disorders, and also anxiety disorders. Indeed, familial aggregation of anxiety disorders has been repeatedly reported, but this phenomenon may be explained by various aetiologic factors, namely familial environment and genes.

Early theories, as developed by Darwin, suggested that through natural selection humans have evolved an inherited tendency to anxiety and phobic reaction to certain stimuli (Kendler et al., 1992c). More recently, family and twin studies, as well as linkage and association studies have been conducted on the various nosological categories of anxiety disorders, with conflicting but in some cases positive results. Since the majority of genetic studies in anxiety disorders have been carried out with a categorical approach, we will present the main results obtained syndrome by syndrome. However, it is worth noting, in order to understand discrepancies between studies, that complex disorders like anxiety disorder pose numerous challenges for genetic research. Indeed, most cases are the result of the interaction of environmental effects with a set of genes and each accounts only for a small part in the liability of the disorder, with the possibility, as not fully studied, of gene–gene interactions (epistasis). Furthermore, genetic complexity is compounded by the complexity of the psychiatric phenotype. Where available, after a review of the results for generalised anxiety disorder and phobias in terms of family, twins, linkage and genetic association studies, the methods and results for refining phenotypes to improve future research will be discussed.

Anxiety Disorders: An Introduction to Clinical Management and Research. Edited by E. J. L. Griez, C. Faravelli, D. Nutt and J. Zohar. © 2001 John Wiley & Sons, Ltd.

GENERALISED ANXIETY DISORDER (GAD)

Genetics studies of generalised anxiety disorder (GAD) were especially influenced by the progressive modifications of the diagnostic systems. Indeed, GAD as defined in DSM-III bears at least only partial resemblance to the GAD described by the DSM-III-R criteria, in which the core symptom for GAD is chronic worry, with excessive or unrealistic worries involving two or more life circumstances. The increasingly restrictive criteria for GAD, from RDC, DSM-III, DSM-III-R to current DSM-IV, obviously sought more reliability and to reduce clinic heterogeneity, although it remains unclear and controversial whether the more stringent criteria have improved this syndromal validity. This results, however, in a more independent familial transmission of GAD from other anxiety disorders or depressive disorders (Wolk et al., 1996), but on the other hand, few studies exploring GAD, genetics or pharmacologicals are able to respect those stringent criteria (Swinson et al., 1993).

Familial Aggregation Studies

Three studies focused clearly on GAD familial transmission (Cloninger et al., 1981; Noyes et al., 1987; Reich, 1995). First, among the first degree relatives of anxious subjects with a GAD-like syndrome in fact classified as "other anxiety neurosis", there was no significant excess of anxiety disorders compared with control probands (Cloninger et al., 1981).

Second, with DSM-III criteria (Noyes et al., 1987), rates of GAD appeared significantly higher among 123 relatives of "pure GAD" (without panic disorder or panic attack) probands compared to relatives of non-psychiatry ill subjects (19.5% vs. 3.5%, $P < 0.001$). Relatives of probands with GAD who shared the same disorder were at the onset of illness significantly older than the probands. More had remissions and seemed stress-related and fewer reported secondary depression and abnormal personality traits. Therefore, the familial risk for GAD appears specific for the disorder: the frequency of GAD appeared no higher among relatives of GAD probands versus relatives of panic (5.4%, $N = 40$) or agoraphobic probands (3.9%, $N = 40$) and rates of major depressive disorder among relatives of GAD probands were similar compared to controls (7.3% vs. 7.1%).

A third study (Reich, 1995) confirmed the family predisposition, in a male population only, using family history methods. The prevalence of GAD among relatives of GAD probands (12.7%) was significantly higher compared with relatives of subjects with major depressive disorder (6.8%), GAD with major depressive disorder (4.2%), or control subject (1.9%).

Twin Studies

Three studies used the conservative, purely descriptive, κ statistical measure of twin concordance to analyse the familial heredity of GAD (Table 3.1). All studies found no

TABLE 3.1 Twin studies of concordance for GAD

	Diagnostic criteria	Concordance for MZ twins	Concordance for DZ twins	Relative risk
Torgersen, 1983	DSM-III	0% (0/12)	5% (1/12)	0
Andrews et al., 1990	DSM-III	20.6%	13.6%	1.5
Skre et al., 1993	DSM-III-R	60% (3/5)	14% (1/7)	4.3

significant difference between monozygotic (MZ) and dizygotic (DZ) twins: these studies were Torgersen (1983) in a sample of 159 pair of psychiatric ill twins (32 MZ and 53 DZ with anxiety disorder; GAD probands with major depressive disorder were excluded); Andrews et al. (1990) among 446 pairs of twins in the general population, with no diagnostic hierarchy for GAD (186 MZ and 260 DZ); and Skre et al. (1993) in a total sample of 81 same-sex twin-pairs mainly hospitalised, where all cases of GAD had, however, a lifetime history of mood disorder.

Kendler et al. (1992a), using another approach and statistical measure of the twin concordance, the tetrachoric correlation coefficient (TCC), tried to determine the relative support for a genetic or environmental influences, or both influences, in the explanation of the familial resemblance for GAD. However, this method is currently under discussion (Kraemer, 1997; Lyons et al., 1997). In fact, tetrachoric correlation coefficient analysis is based on the hypothesis that there is a latent trait, often unknown in psychiatric diseases, that is unidimensional with a standard normal distribution on which the diagnosis are based.

In a first study on 2163 female twins (Kendler et al., 1992a), the twin correlation was investigated for different definitions of GAD: GAD with and without panic disorder and major depressive disorder (MDD), and with one-month or six-month duration of GAD. The prevalence of GAD with a six-month duration was 5.9%, and 5.7% if subjects presenting a PD co-occurring with GAD are excluded, and 3.6% if subjects presenting MDD co-occurring with GAD are excluded. Tetrachoric correlation coefficient for one-month GAD diagnosed without hierarchy were $+0.35 \pm 0.07$ among MZ and $+0.12 \pm 0.08$ among DZ twins, arguing for a genetic susceptibility of GAD. Hierarchical conditions do not modify these results significantly. For GAD six-month without hierarchy, the correlation presented quite the same value among MZ and DZ (0.28 ± 0.15 and 0.28 ± 0.14). In this study, GAD correlation within twins seems to be only due to genetics factors (best fitting model from nine tested); however, the estimated liability of heredity of GAD appeared moderate, ranging from 19% to 30% for different definitions (one- or six-month duration, diagnostic hierarchy, models with threshold). In addition, the remainder of the variance in liability seems to result from individual–specific environmental experiences, probably critical for the emergence of GAD, and not from familial environmental factors. Duration of the episode does not seem to affect this heritability, quite the same with one-month or six-month definitions of GAD. For the authors, there was a modest decline in the estimated heritability of GAD when exclusion of the probands who concurrently had GAD and MDD was applied. However, it should be outlined that comorbidity in this report was in fact restricted to the co-occurrence of two disorders, so uncertainty remains about the impact of the comorbidity between GAD and MDD in the familial/genetic transmission of GAD.

In the same sample of female twins (Kendler et al., 1992b), the correlation in one twin between MDD and GAD one-month was systematically higher than any of the cross-twin cross-disorder correlation, suggesting that subject-specific experiences contribute to the GAD/MDD correlation. Furthermore, they indicated that cross-twin MDD/GAD one-month correlation was found more than twice as often in MZ vs. DZ (+0.37 and +0.13, respective means), suggesting that genetic factors contribute to the correlation. However, a possible causality between these disorders cannot be evaluated: MDD may cause GAD, or the inverse. They suggested at least that genetic factors influencing the two disorders are highly correlated in women, and that GAD and MDD could be the different manifestations of the same underlying transmissible factors.

Roy et al. (1995), in a study of male and female twins combining clinically ascertained and general population samples, tried to replicate these findings concerning the aetiologic determinants of comorbidity. For GAD (with modifications of criteria: one-month duration and a single area of worry were sufficient, no hierarchy with MDD), the familial aggregation of GAD could be fully accounted for by genetic factors, but as in the Virginian sample of Kendler, heritability remains moderate (49.0% in the best fitting model using broad definitions of GAD, to 14.3% with narrower definitions). In contrast, estimations for the heritability of MDD were systematically higher (62.1% and 50.9% with respectively broad or narrow definitions of MDD).

Finally, it seems that genetic factors could play a role in the aetiology of GAD. However, last reports suggest that heredity, if it exists, is moderate. In addition, despite the family predisposition indicated for GAD by familial aggregation studies, classical twins studies (Torgersen 1983; Andrews et al., 1990; Skre et al., 1993) report no significant differences between MZ and DZ twins, although with small sample size. What is noteworthy, in the various studies exploring genetic factors in GAD, is that inclusion or exclusion of cases of GAD with a mood disorder co-occurring or comorbid seems to have a major influence on the results and on the interpretation. Thus, there currently remain doubts about the heredity of "pure" GAD, and some authors suggest that GAD is hereditary only when there is a comorbid history of MDD (Skre et al., 1993). Comorbidity and co-segregation for GAD and MDD could also be understood as alternative expressions of the same aetiologic factors. Otherwise, the hypothesis that genes may act mainly by a predisposition to a general distress, rather than specific symptom or disorder was also suggested by some family studies that suggested that GAD and MDD co-segregate within families (Weissman et al., 1984; Angst et al., 1990).

PHOBIAS

All phobias show an irrational and fearful avoidance of objects or situations that are not explained as a function of the threat, truly posed therewith. However, they seriously differ in terms of age at onset (Ost, 1987), patterns of comorbidity (Boyd et al., 1984), and type of phobic stimulus, which is well circumscribed for specific phobia or relatively diffuse for agoraphobia and social phobia. Consequently, an important question for phobias investigates whether each of them is familial and has a specific familial aggregation: are the subtypes of phobias distinct, unrelated syndromes, or do subtypes of phobias represent minor variations of a single disorder?

Social Phobia

The familial transmission of social phobia (SP) was mainly investigated by the Study Group of Columbia. Restricting the probands to individuals who have only one of the three phobic disorders (simple, social or agoraphobia), and with their largest social phobia sample (Fyer et al., 1995), they found that DSM-III-R Social Phobia is associated with a significant but moderate familial risk (relative risk: 2.5 (CI: 1.2–5)). Rates of DSM-III-R anxiety disorders other than SP did not differ significantly among the relatives of SP probands as compared with those of controls who were not ill (15% vs. 8%, $P \leq 0.01$). Otherwise, the two other phobic disorders are not associated with increased familial risk for social phobia. Thus, the specificity of this pattern of intergenerational transmission supports the existence of an SP category that is separate from other phobic disorders, consistent with the current DSM-IV.

Homogeneity, both clinical and aetiologic, within the SP category remains, however, a subject of investigation, in terms of social phobic stimuli or in terms of generalised/not generalised criterion. For instance, rate of SP was significantly greater among relatives of 67 patients with generalised vs. relatives of 62 non-generalised SP (16% vs. 6%, $P < 0.05$), and significantly greater among relatives of patients with generalised vs. relatives of non-psychiatry ill subjects (16% vs. 6%, $P < 0.05$) (Mannuzza et al., 1995). However, there was no evidence that patients with generalised SP were more likely to transmit this form of the syndrome. Another study had replicated these results in an independent group, with a relative risk for generalised SP (and avoidant personality disorder) approximately 10 times higher among first degree relatives (N = 106) of generalised SP probands compared with first degree relatives (N = 74) of comparison subjects (Stein et al., 1998). In contrast, when the subtypes are defined as a class of speaking fears only, versus a class of a broader range of social fears, there is no difference in terms of family history of SP (and in age at onset), from the data of the National Comorbidity Survey (Kessler et al., 1998). However, maternal generalised anxiety was lower among those with pure speaking fears than among those with other social phobias ($P < 0.001$).

Furthermore, there is no evidence suggesting an exact specificity of intergenerational symptom transmission. Although within a small sample size, this issue was assessed by Fyer et al. (1993) with the 13 relatives of SP probands who also received a DSM-III-R SP diagnosis: none had exactly the same types and number of social phobias than the probands to whom they were related, but in 10 cases, there was a partial intergenerational overlap of social phobias types. Otherwise, it seems that irrational social fears that occur in individuals who do not also have SP are neither familial nor associated with an increased familial risk for SP (Fyer et al., 1993). The rate of threshold social fears, that do not meet the DSM-III-R impairment/distress criterion, among relatives of probands with social fears only, was not significantly different from that among relatives of probands with no fears and no phobias (46% vs. 52%). Rates of DSM-III-R SP in the relatives of these two groups also did not differ (7% vs. 4%). These result differ from twin and family studies of social fears and shyness, which have uniformly showed heritable components (Plomin and Daniels, 1986; Stevenson et al., 1992; Thapar and McGuffin, 1995). However, many subjects in those studies might have social phobia criteria, although they were not recruited from clinical settings. In another study with four probands groups (PD, SP, PD + SP, not ill controls), Fyer et al. (1996) examined the effect of comorbidity between PD and SP on familial transmission, since an unexpectedly high comorbidity has been noted in both epidemiological and clinical samples (Barlow, 1988; Stein et al., 1989; Klerman et al., 1991). Relatives of SP probands had a higher rate of SP (15%), but not of PD (2%), relatives of probands with PD only had a higher rate of PD (10%) but not of SP (9%), when compared with relatives of controls (SP: 6%, PD: 3%). Among the relatives of probands with SP + PD, familial aggregation of PD was not affected by proband social comorbidity (rate of PD: 9%). In contrast, SP among these relatives was not different when compared with relatives of controls. From a genetic point of view, this suggests that SP in individuals who have, or subsequently develop, PD differs from SP which occurs without lifetime anxiety comorbidity, and that at least some cases of SP + PD may be non-familial and/or causally related to PD.

Three twin studies have examined clinically defined phobias. First, Carey and Gottesman (1981), examining 21 twin probands hospitalised with phobia, found low and similar concordance rates in monozygotic (MZ) and dizygotic (DZ) twins. However, using a broad definition of phobic "symptoms or features", they found a much higher concordance rate in MZ (88%) than in DZ (38%) twins. In a second study among 12 twin probands with a primary diagnosis of phobia, Torgersen (1983) found that none of the co-twins were phobic. Third, with 2163 female twins from a population-based registry, Kendler et al. (1992c) showed a less than two times higher probandwise concordance for SP in MZ when compared with DZ. Nevertheless, the familial aggregation of SP appeared to result solely from genetic, and not from familial-environmental factors, with estimation of genetic heritability of liability of 30% (Kendler et al., 1992c).

Agoraphobia

Although family studies could challenge categorical distinctions between agoraphobia and panic disorder, and between agoraphobia and other phobias, few data are currently available on this topic. The risk for agoraphobia was initially noted to be significantly higher among parents and siblings of 60 agoraphobic patients than estimates of the population incidence (Moran and Andrews, 1985). A second family study, including non-anxious controls and their relatives, confirmed this familial aggregation of agoraphobia, showing that the morbidity risk for agoraphobia was significantly increased among relatives of agoraphobics but not the relatives of PD patients nor non-anxious subjects (Noyes et al., 1986). Furthermore, with 144 patients with PD and/or agoraphobia according to DSM-III, agoraphobia was strictly clustered in families of agoraphobic patients (Gruppo Italiano Disturbi d'Ansia, 1989). This familial aggregation of agoraphobia seems moderate, with a threefold increased risk for DSM-III-R PD with agoraphobia versus not ill controls (10% vs. 3%, $P < 0.001$), but with a specific familial loading for other phobias (Fyer et al., 1995). In contrast to this, Kendler et al. (1992c) found evidence of both partial distinctness and overlap with respect to the genetic contribution to the aetiology of agoraphobia, social and situational phobias. Similarly, in a second epidemiologically based twin study including panic agoraphobia and social phobia probands, no genetic contributions were specific to either phobia (Andrews et al., 1990). It is noteworthy that those two twin studies did not report separately single and comorbid cases of phobias, otherwise the two sets of findings should be consistent.

For agoraphobia, heredity of liability was 39% in a female twin population, whereas the rest of the variance in liability was due to individual–specific environmental effects. Probandwise concordance for agoraphobia was 23.2 among MZ and 15.3 among DZ twins, and tetrachoric correlation ranged from 0.41 ± 0.11 among MZ to 0.15 ± 0.13 among DZ twins (Kendler et al., 1992c).

Specific Phobias

As for other phobias, a moderate but statistically significant and specific familial aggregation was found for situational phobias, with a relative risk, as compared with not ill controls, of 3.9 (95% CI: 1.8–8.1) (Fyer et al., 1995). However, twin studies are less conclusive. Kendler et al. (1992c) failed to show a clear genetic effect for situational phobias, in contrast, they found that disease liability was solely the result of individual specific environmental effects (73% of the variance) in conjunction with familial environmental influences, although a model with additive genetic and specific environmental effects could not be rejected. Correlation in MZ twins was similar or much lower than the corresponding DZ correlation (respectively, for probandwise concordance 22.2 vs. 23.7, and for tetrachoric correlation 0.27 ± 0.10 vs. 0.27 ± 0.11). With an expanded definition of situational phobias including other simple, non-animal phobias (fear of water, of thunderstorms), tetrachoric correlations remained similar. A new sample supports this conclusion, with no significant differences between MZ and DZ co-twins (Skre et al., 1993). For isolated animal phobia (Kendler et al., 1992c), it seems that disease liability may result from additive genetic effects (32% of the variance) and individual specific, but not familial, environmental effects (68% of the variance).

Finally, family studies support the existence of a specific familial contribution to each particular phobia, with a relative risk ranging from 2.5 for social phobia to 3.9

for specific phobia, with an intermediate risk for agoraphobia. Despite its specificity, the magnitude of this increased familial risk appears only moderate, suggesting that although familial factors contribute to the aetiology of those disorders, other non-familial factors require investigation. Supporting this conclusion, twin studies indicate heritability of liability of phobias, which although significant, are substantially lower than those previously described by twin studies of bipolar illness and schizophrenia, where they have usually ranged from 60% to 90% (McGuffin and Katz, 1989; Kendler, 1983). Nevertheless, for some authors, familial aggregation of each phobia, except situational phobias, could be solely explained by additive genetic factors, with no role for familial environmental factors (Kendler et al., 1992c).

However, specific familial aggregation for each phobia does not mean aetiologic homogeneity between each group of phobia, as the high comorbidity among anxiety disorders suggests (Boyd et al., 1984; Mannuzza et al., 1990; Merikangas and Angst, 1995). Kendler's multivariate genetic model so suggested the existence of a common set of genes that predisposed to all phobias, that might have a major role in animal phobia and a least important impact for agoraphobia, and an intermediate role for social phobia. In contrast, environmental factors predisposing to all phobias would share the major loading for agoraphobia and social phobia, with a relatively unim-portant impact for specific phobias (Kendler et al., 1992c). Finally, results are midway between the two extreme hypotheses regarding the interrelationship of the subtypes of phobias, the discrete categorical or the unitary theories of anxiety, which supposed a common underlying process, despite differing symptomatic and developmental elements.

CONCLUSION

Although the evidence is fragmentary, there appears to be a general consensus that the different categories of anxiety disorders are familial and probably have a moder-ate genetic component. Currently, the greatest research activity is an attempt to apply molecular genetic designs, and indeed, identifying modifying or susceptibility genes involved in anxiety disorders could have different implications. The most important, and the most obvious, is that such information will inspire new and more effective therapies, but we could expect also that, by looking at the correlation of genetic factors risks with syndromes and/or symptoms, it should be possible to better understand heterogeneity among the anxiety disorders, or also to investigate the ways in which genes and environment interact. However, a serious lack of basic knowledge remains for most of the anxiety disorders, specially for phobias and GAD, as to whether genes do contribute in the heredity, and if so, to what extent they do so. Therefore, much work still needs to be done in exploiting classical genetic methods, that is, family, twins and adoption studies, and most energy should be focused on refining phenotypes. Otherwise it should be noted that an alternative research field, not developed here, could be promising, based on personality traits theory, investigat-ing anxiety proneness with a dimensional approach.

Indeed, numerous family, twin and adoption studies have shown that individual differences in personality traits such as neuroticism, shyness, harm avoidance or behavioural inhibition in many cases—between one third and one half—may be explained by genetic variance. In recent years, some polymorphisms in the serotonin transporter gene have been found to be associated with variance in neuroticism (Lesch et al., 1996), even if other studies failed to replicate this result. Other dimensions were described as potent vulnerability factors for anxiety disorders, such as anxiety sensitivity for panic disorder (Stein et al., 1999), and these dimensions may have a heritable component that needs in particular to be explored.

REFERENCES

Andrews G, Stewart G, Allen R, Henderson AS (1990) The genetics of six neurotic disorders: A twin study. *J Affect Disord* **19**(1): 23–29.

Angst J, Vollrath M, Merikangas K, Ernst C (1990) Comorbidity of anxiety and depression in the Zurich Cohort Study of Young Adults. In Maser JD, Cloninger CR (eds) *Comorbidity of Mood and Anxiety Disorders*. Washington, DC: American Psychiatric Press Inc., pp. 123–127.

Barlow DH (1988) *Anxiety and its Disorders*. New York: Guilford Press.

Boyd JH, Burke JD Jr, Gruenberg E, Holzer CE, Rae DS, George LK, Karno M, Stoltzman R, McEvoy L, Nestadt G (1984) Exclusion criteria of DSM-III: A study of co-occurrence of hierarchy-free syndromes. *Arch Gen Psychiatry* **41**(10): 983–989.

Carey G, Gottesman II (1981) Twin and family studies of anxiety, phobic and obsessive disorders. In Klein DF, Rabkin JG (eds) *Anxiety: New Research and Changing Concepts*. New York: Raven Press.

Cloninger CR, Martin RL, Clayton P et al. (1981) A blind follow-up and family study of anxiety neuroses: Preliminary analyses of the St Louis 500. In Klein DF, Rabkin JG (eds) *Anxiety: New Research and Changing Concepts*. New York: Raven Press.

Fyer AJ, Mannuzza S, Chapman TF, Liebowitz MR, Klein DF (1993) A direct interview family study of social phobia. *Arch Gen Psychiatry* **50**(4): 286–293.

Fyer AJ, Mannuzza S, Chapman TF, Lipsitz J, Martin LY, Klein DF (1996) Panic disorder and social phobia: Effects of comorbidity on familial transmission. *Anxiety* **2**(4): 173–178.

Fyer AJ, Mannuzza S, Chapman TF, Martin LY, Klein DF (1995) Specificity in familial aggregation of phobic disorders. *Arch Gen Psychiatry* **52**(7): 564–573.

Gruppo Italiano Disturbi d'Ansia (1989) Familial analysis of panic disorder and agoraphobia. *J Affect Disord* **17**(1): 1–8.

Kendler KS (1983) Overview: A current perspective on twin studies of schizophrenia. *Am J Psychiatry* **140**(11): 1413–1425.

Kendler KS, Neale MC, Kessler RC, Heath AC, Eaves LJ (1992a) Generalised anxiety disorder in women: A population-based twin study. *Arch Gen Psychiatry* **49**(4): 267–272.

Kendler KS, Neale MC, Kessler RC, Heath AC, Eaves LJ (1992b) Major depression and generalised anxiety disorder: Same genes, (partly) different environments? *Arch Gen Psychiatry* **49**(9): 716–722.

Kendler KS, Neale MC, Kessler RC, Heath AC, Eaves LJ (1992c) The genetic epidemiology of phobias in women: The interrelationship of agoraphobia, social phobia, situational phobia, and specific phobia. *Arch Gen Psychiatry* **49**(4): 273–281.

Kessler RC, Stein MB, Berglund P (1998) Social phobia subtypes in the National Comorbidity Survey. *Am J Psychiatry* **155**(5): 613–619.

Klerman GL, Weissman M, Quellette R, Johnson J, Greenwald MA (1991) Panic attacks in the community: Social morbidity and health care utilisation. *JAMA* **265**: 742–746.

Kraemer HC (1997) What is the "right" statistical measure of twin concordance (or diagnostic reliability and validity)? *Arch Gen Psychiatry* **54**(12): 1121–1124.

Lesch KP, Bengel D, Heils A, Sabol SZ, Greenberg BD, Petri S, Benjamin J, Muller CR, Hamer DH, Murphy DL (1996) Association of anxiety-related traits with a polymorphism in the serotonin transporter gene regulatory region. *Science* **274**(5292): 1527–1531.

Lyons MJ, Faraone SV, Tsuang MT, Goldberg J, Eaves LJ, Meyer JM, True WR, Eisen SA (1997) Another view on the "right" statistical measure of twin concordance. *Arch Gen Psychiatry* **54**(12): 1126–1128.

Mannuzza S, Fyer AJ, Liebowitz MR, Klein DF (1990) Delineating the boundaries of social phobia: Its relationship to panic disorder and agoraphobia. *J Anxiety Disord* **4**: 1–59.

Mannuzza S, Schneier FR, Chapman TF, Liebowitz MR, Klein DF, Fyer AJ (1995) Generalized social phobia: Reliability and validity. *Arch Gen Psychiatry* **52**(3): 230–237.

McGuffin P, Katz R (1989) The genetics of depression and manic-depressive disorder. *Br J Psychiatry* **155**: 294–304.

Merikangas KR, Angst J (1995) Comorbidity and social phobia: Evidence from clinical, epidemiologic, and genetic studies. *Eur Arch Psychiatry Clin Neurosci* **244**(6): 297–303.

Moran C, Andrews G (1985) The familial occurrence of agoraphobia. *Br J Psychiatry* **146**: 262–267.

Noyes R Jr, Clarkson C, Crowe RR, Yates WR, McChesney CM (1987) A family study of generalised anxiety disorder. *Am J Psychiatry* **144**(8): 1019–1024.

Noyes RJ, Crowe RR, Harris EL, Hamra BJ, McChesney CM, Chaudhry DR (1986) Relationship between panic disorder and agoraphobia: A family study. *Arch Gen Psychiatry* **43**(3): 227–232.

Ost LG (1987) Age of onset in different phobias. *J Abnorm Psychol* **97**: 223–229.

Plomin R, Daniels D (1986) Genetics and shyness. In Jones WH, Cheek JM, Briggs SR (eds) *Shyness: Perspectives on Research and Treatment.* New York: Plenum, pp. 63–90.

Reich J (1995) Family psychiatric histories in male patients with generalised anxiety disorder and major depressive disorder. *Ann Clin Psychiatry* **7**(2): 71–78.

Roy MA, Neale MC, Pedersen NL, Mathe AA, Kendler KS (1995) A twin study of generalised anxiety disorder and major depression. *Psychol Med* **25**(5): 1037–1049.

Skre I, Onstad S, Torgersen S, Lygren S, Kringlen E (1993) A twin study of DSM-III-R anxiety disorders. *Acta Psychiatr Scand* **88**(2): 85–92.

Stein MB, Chartier MJ, Hazen AL, Kozak MV, Tancer ME, Lander S, Furer P, Chubaty D, Walker JR (1998) A direct-interview family study of generalised social phobia. *Am J Psychiatry* **155**(1): 90–97.

Stein MB, Jang KL, Livesley W (1999) Heritability of anxiety sensitivity: A twin study. *Am J Psychiatry* **156**(2): 246–251.

Stein MB, Shea CA, Uhde TW (1989) Social phobic symptoms in patients with panic disorder: Practical and theoretical implications. *Am J Psychiatry* **146**: 235–238.

Stevenson J, Batten N, Cherner M (1992) Fears and fearfulness in children and adolescents: A genetic analysis of twin data. *J Child Psychol Psychiatry* **33**(6): 977–985.

Swinson RP, Cox BJ (1993) Diagnostic validity in genetics research on generalised anxiety disorder. *Arch Gen Psychiatry* **50**(11): 916–917.

Swinson RP, Cox BJ, Fergus KD (1993) Diagnostic criteria in generalised anxiety disorder treatment studies. *J Clin Psychopharmacol* **13**(6): 455.

Thapar A, McGuffin P (1995) Are anxiety symptoms in childhood heritable? *Child Psychol Psychiatry* **36**(3): 439–447.

Torgersen S (1983) Genetic factors in anxiety disorders. *Arch Gen Psychiatry* **40**(10): 1085–1089.

Weissman MM, Gershon ES, Kidd KK, Prusoff BA, Leckman JF, Dibble E, Hamovit J, Thompson D, Pauls DL, Guroff JJ (1984) Psychiatric disorders in the relatives of probands with affective disorders. *Arch Gen Psychiatry* **41**: 13–21.

Wolk SI, Horwarth E, Goldstein RB, Wickramaratne P, Weissman MM (1996) Comparison of RDC, DSM-III, DSM-III-R diagnostic criteria for Generalised Anxiety Disorder. *Anxiety* **2**: 71–79.

Nosology and Treatment of Anxiety Disorders

Panic Disorder: Clinical Course, Morbidity and Comorbidity

C. Faravelli and A. Paionni

Florence University Medical School, Florence, Italy

INTRODUCTION

With the abolition of the term "neurosis" and the consequent reclassification of anxiety states, the recurrent crises of acute anxiety (panic attacks), whether associated with agoraphobia or not, have acquired a new nosological autonomy (DSM-III: APA, 1980; DSM-III-R: APA, 1987; DSM-IV: APA, 1993). In the past two decades, the recognition of the wide prevalence of panic disorder (PD), its consequences, the discovery that panic may be induced by chemical cues, its association with cardiovascular problems, possible neuroanatomical locations and distinctive physiological concomitants have stimulated intense interest. Panic disorder has therefore received wide attention and its features have been adequately described. PD is presently seen as the most typical, and probably the core of anxiety disorders.

THE PANIC ATTACK

Panic attack is defined as a discrete period of intense fear or discomfort accompanied by somatic and psychic symptoms. The attack has a sudden onset and rapidly builds to a peak (usually in 10 minutes or less). It is accompanied by a sense of imminent danger or impending doom and an urge to escape.

A panic attack is also made up of severe, acute, systemic symptoms: cardiovascular (palpitations, pounding heart, accelerated heart rate), respiratory (dyspnea, chest pain or discomfort, sensations of shortness of breath or smothering), neurological-like (dizziness, trembling or shaking, paresthesias), sweating, nausea or abdominal distress, chills or hot flushes. Often the somatic symptoms mask or are predominant over anxiety and such patients are primarily referred to non-psychiatric physicians.

The psychic symptoms are: feelings of dizziness, unsteadiness, lightheadedness, or fainting, derealisation or depersonalisation, fear of losing control or going crazy, fear

Anxiety Disorders: An Introduction to Clinical Management and Research. Edited by E. J. L. Griez, C. Faravelli, D. Nutt and J. Zohar. © 2001 John Wiley & Sons, Ltd.

of dying. Individuals seeking help for panic attacks will usually describe the fear as intense and report that they thought they were about to die, lose control, have a heart attack or a stroke, or "go crazy". They also usually report an urgent desire to flee from wherever the attack is occurring (escape behaviour).

The attack usually lasts few minutes, but is generally followed by a sense of malaise, distress, uneasiness that may persist for several hours. The anxiety that is characteristic of a panic attack can be differentiated from generalised anxiety by its intermittent, almost paroxysmal nature and its typically greater severity. DSM-IV requires that a panic attack has an abrupt onset with a time lag to reach its peak of less than 10 minutes (APA, 1993). Scupi et al. (1997) found, however, that panickers with prolonged onset do not differ significantly from rapid onset panickers on any clinical features. DSM-IV lists 13 symptoms, four of which are necessary in order to satisfy the criteria of panic attack. ICD-10 considers approximately the same set of symptoms.

The symptoms of panic may be present in a variety of situations: physical effort, use or withdrawal from drugs, medical conditions such as hyperthyroidism, pulmonary embolism, hypoglycaemia, hyperparathyroidism, pheochromocytoma, vestibular dysfunction, seizure disorders, cardiac conditions (arrhythmia, supraventricular tachycardia). Generally, all the acute cardiopulmonary diseases and all the situations that cause a sudden and intense activation of the sympathetic system may produce the same symptoms as panic. For this reason DSM-IV criteria for panic attack require the explicit exclusion of organic causes [Criterion C: "The panic attacks are not due to the direct physiological effects of a substance (e.g., a drug of abuse, a medication) or a general medical condition (e.g., hyperthyroidism)"]. Even in the field of mental disorders panic attacks can be found in other conditions, including all the phobic states. In determining the differential diagnostic significance of a panic attack, it is important to consider the context in which it occurs.

Basically, there are two types of panic attacks, depending on the presence or absence of situational triggers: *unexpected panic attacks*, in which the onset of the panic attack is not associated with a situational trigger (occurring spontaneously, "out of the blue"); and *situationally bound panic attacks*, in which the panic attack almost invariably occurs immediately on exposure to, or in anticipation of, a situational cue. A third variation could be that of *situationally predisposed panic attacks*, which are more likely to occur on exposure to the situational cue or trigger, but are not invariably associated with the cue and do not necessarily occur immediately after the exposure (e.g., attacks are more likely to occur while driving, but there are times when the individual drives and does not have a panic attack or times when the panic attack occurs after driving for half an hour). Unexpected panics and cued panics do not differ in terms of severity, while the relative frequency of symptoms differs according to the kind of panic. Subjects with unpredictable panic more often report symptoms such as dizziness, parasthesia, shaking, chest pain, and fear of going crazy or losing control. More than 90% of patients with unpredictable panic attacks report feelings of loss of control and dizziness, which are less common among people suffering from situationally bound panic (Barlow et al., 1985). The kind of phobic stimuli may also be associated with a different somatic symptom pattern: shortness of breath is a common symptom in panic attacks associated with agoraphobia, whereas blushing is common in panics related to social or performance anxiety (DSM-IV: APA, 1993).

As regards severity, DSM-IV differentiate "full-blown" panic attacks from "limited-symptoms" attacks. The full-blown panic attack is accompanied by at least four of the estimated 13 somatic or cognitive symptoms. Attacks that meet all the other criteria but have less than four somatic or cognitive symptoms are referred to as limited-symptom attacks and these are very common in individuals with panic (APA, 1993). Limited-symptom attacks may also occur in subjects without PD. Their lifetime prevalence has been estimated around 2% (Katerndahl and Realini, 1993) and their clinical significance remain dubious. Although this distinction is somewhat arbitrary, full-blown attacks are generally associated with a greater morbidity.

Apart from phobic states, where panic is a basic aspect of the disorder, panic attacks may be observed during the course of several other psychiatric conditions, including major depression, obsessive-compulsive disorder, borderline personality disorder, brief psychosis and others: in this case it is controversial whether the panic attack should be considered as part of the original symptomatology or rather as an independently occurring phenomenon. Classifications that privilege hierarchy tend to consider panic as secondary to the original state, whereas nosological systems that allow comorbidity enforce a double diagnosis.

The panic attack may occasionally occur in otherwise healthy people without any particular pathological consequence (so called *sporadic* or *infrequent panic attacks*). Sporadic panic has been revealed as extremely frequent, so much so as to exceed all the other types of panic that can be nosographically codified: a consistent number of cases (epidemiological figures vary from 2% up to 35%) in the population are reported to have had at least one panic attack without any further consequence. In respect to this data two possibilities can be suggested:

1. The panic attacks in themselves are not intrinsically pathological forms; in the majority of cases they do not reoccur and do not result in consequences on social adaptation or quality of life. Other factors are necessary in order to condition the frequent repetition of the crisis or/and their evolution into clearly pathological forms.
2. The second possibility is that sporadic panic attacks represent the weaker subpathological form of PD. In this case, an early recognition of this form is essential in order to prevent their evolution into disorders of increased intensity.

There are also nocturnal panic attacks, characterised by sudden awakening, terror and hyperarousal. Nearly 40% of PD patients has panic attacks during sleep (Mellman and Uhde, 1989). The electroencephalographic studies point out that those panic attacks are not in REM sleep. Klein (1993) suggested that the presence of this sleep panic attack is specific to PD.

PANIC DISORDER

Panic disorder is a pathological condition characterised by repeated panic attacks, combined with a series of long-lasting symptoms and attitudes that are present between the attacks. The DSM-IV time criterion requires an abrupt onset to panic attacks with a time to peak intensity of less than 10 minutes (APA, 1993). Scupi et al. (1997) found that prolonged onset panickers do not differ significantly from rapid onset panickers on any clinical features. The authors therefore suggest evaluating the reliability, validity and clinical relevance of the current DSM-IV time criterion in future studies.

Since, as explained above, panic attacks may be observed during the course of other psychiatric conditions as well as in healthy people, present classification criteria require either a minimum number of attacks or that the presence of unexpected panic attacks is followed by persistent concern about having another panic attack, worry about the possible implications or consequences of the panic attacks, or a significant behavioural change (usually avoidance or restrictive behaviour).

Panic disorder is characterised by recurrent panic attacks with a tendency to have a chronic course; associated common features are agoraphobia, hypochondriasis, anticipatory anxiety, demoralisation. Patients with PD have also been reported to have an increased risk of other psychiatric conditions (comorbidity) as well as of medical illnesses.

Recurrent Panic Attacks

Whereas at least two unexpected panic attacks are required for the diagnosis, most individuals have considerably more. Although at least one uncued (unexpected) panic is necessary for the diagnosis, patients with PD frequently also have situationally predisposed panic attacks; situationally bound attacks can also occur, but they are less common.

The frequency of the panic attacks varies widely: some individuals have moderately frequent attacks (e.g., once a week) that occur regularly for months at a time; others report short bursts of more frequent attack (e.g., daily for a week) separated by weeks or months without any attacks or with less frequent attacks (e.g.., one attack per month) over many years.

Both full-blown and limited-symptom attacks are usually observed during the course of PD. It is quite common to observe that the frequency of full-blown attacks tends to decrease during the course of the illness, whereas the limited-symptom attacks may persist for longer periods. The common pattern during the years in fact is a decrease in the frequency of major attacks with a persistence of the sub-threshold panics. In this case it may be difficult to distinguish PD from generalised anxiety disorder (GAD): PD patients were more likely to complain of palpitation, breathlessness, chest pain, numbness, choking sensations and especially fear of dying; GAD patients tend to complain of feeling tense, insomnia, headaches, weakness, restlessness and muscle aches.

The mechanisms by which panic attacks become recurrent in some subjects, while in others these attacks are not repeated, still appear to be very speculative. In this field, the cognitive theories have been the object of recent developments which call on notions both of hyperarousal and "locus of control perception" (Cottraux, 1987). The subject's interpretation of the indications relative to the state of peripheral and central stimulation occurring with panic attacks can play a major part in the maintenance of symptomatology. In this respect, the so-called "external" subjects, who have a tendency to perceive situations as if they were under the control of external forces, are more likely to experience recurrent attacks than the so-called "internal" subjects, who tend to perceive the situation under their own self-control. Thus, the catastrophic and inescapable interpretation of hyperarousal, whatever its cause, maintains and reinforces the patients' symptomatology of anxiety. The efficacy of cognitive therapies which aim to re-establish a more "internalised" control point in these patients and to combat the mistaken interpretation which they give to their symptoms demonstrates the probable importance of these factors in the pathogenesis of recurrent panic attacks (Hallarm, 1978).

Anticipatory Anxiety

After the first attack, most patients develop the fear that another attack may occur. During the intervals between the attacks, therefore, the level of non-panic (diffuse) anxiety increases. Anticipatory anxiety has many of the characteristics of generalised anxiety: increase of attention, apprehension, and hyperactivity. This condition can be intrusive enough to cancel the difference between panic attack and generalised anxiety. It is speculated that such a higher level of diffuse anxiety may lower the threshold for panic, thus increasing the risk of new attacks. The anticipatory anxiety leads to avoidance behaviour, so that agoraphobia ensues.

Agoraphobia

The term agoraphobia was first coined by Westphal in his description of three males who experienced intense anxiety when walking across open spaces or through empty streets (Westphal, 1871).

> The essential feature of Agoraphobia is anxiety about being in places or situations from which escape might be difficult (or embarrassing) or in which help may not be available in the event of having a Panic Attack or panic-like symptoms (e.g., fear of having a sudden attack of dizziness or a sudden attack of diarrhoea).
>
> (DSM-IV: APA, 1993)

Other defining characteristics are physiological changes associated with accompanying panic attacks. These can include palpitations, lightness in the head, weakness, atypical chest pain, and dyspnea. Most agoraphobics also express fears of losing control, going insane, embarrassing themselves and others, dying and fainting. The anxiety typically leads to a pervasive avoidance of a variety of situations that may include being alone outside the home or being home alone; being in a crowd of people, travelling in a car, train, coach or aeroplane; or being on a bridge or in a lift. The level of discomfort may range from mild uneasiness (with no avoidance) to severe distress with marked avoidance. Some individuals are able to expose themselves to the feared situations but endure these experiences with considerable dread. Usually, an individual is better able to confront a feared situation when accompanied by a companion, even if this companion is clearly unable to provide any help, such as a small child or even a dog; other forms of support such as push-chairs and walking sticks can be helpful. When agoraphobia is severe the individuals' avoidance of situations may seriously impair their ability to travel, to work, or to carry out homemaking responsibility. In its extreme form, agoraphobia is totally invalidating: the subject cannot go out of the house by any means and cannot stay at home alone either. Agoraphobia is therefore to be seen as a potentially severely disabling illness.

In psychiatric samples 75% of patients with PD present some degree of agoraphobia, whereas in epidemiological surveys agoraphobia accompanies PD in 30–50% of the cases. All the clinical descriptions agree that almost invariably panic precedes agoraphobia. The onset of agoraphobia follows the first panic attack with a time lag varying from few days to several years. As Klein points out, PD starts with the initial panic attack, which is followed by the fear of subsequent attacks (anticipatory anxiety) and then by the avoidance of situations that are believed to trigger panic attacks or result in embarrassment and/or danger in case of a new attack (Klein, 1981; Klein, 1987). However, the relationship between panic and agoraphobia is still controversial. Roth first observed that, even though the first attack of panic often develops abruptly, "more detailed investigation will usually reveal that the disorder has not emerged out of an entirely clear sky and that the complex repertoire of avoidance behaviours and helpless dependence on others were not entirely without premorbid antecedents" (Roth, 1984). Fava et al. (1988) confirm Roth's remarks: the large majority of patients (90%) suffered from mild phobic or hypochondriacal symptoms before the onset of panic attacks. Anxiety and hypochondriacal fears and beliefs were also exceedingly common. These findings are in accordance with several converging developments in agoraphobia research: it has been shown in epidemiological surveys that some individuals suffer from agoraphobia without panic attacks (Weissman and Merikangas, 1986) and some normal subjects report occasional panic attacks (Norton et al., 1985). Moreover, there is growing recognition of cognitive factors (catastrophic misinterpretations of certain bodily sensations) related to panic anxiety (Clark, 1986; Clark, 1989a). It has been hypothesised that the perception of the panic attack as a catastrophic medical problem, rather than a manifestation of anxiety, results in an exaggerated fear of having subsequent panic attacks. This unrealistic and exaggerated fear results in raised anticipatory anxiety and in a stronger tendency to avoid situations that are believed to hasten additional panic attacks.

The course of agoraphobia and its relationship to the course of panic attacks are variable. In some cases, a decrease or remission of panic attacks is followed closely by a corresponding decrease in agoraphobic avoidance and anxiety. In other cases, agoraphobics may become chronic regardless of the presence of panic attacks.

Basically, there are three positions, that gave rise to a strong debate during the 1980s:

1. The panic attack is the central and primitive feature; anticipatory anxiety and agoraphobia are the comprehensible psychological consequences of the recurrent, unpredictable panics. The panic attack is also seen as a primarily biological phenomenon, the origin of which is in some brain dysfunction. Biochemical and brain imaging studies, the possibility of inducing panic chemically, the specific response to some drugs are all in accordance with this interpretation.
2. The opposite position contends that a phobic attitude precedes the first panic and that the disorder derives from the abnormal (phobic) psychological response to an otherwise aspecific phenomenon such as the panic attack.
3. Goisman et al. (1994) argued for the construction of separate diagnoses for panic disorder and agoraphobia that could occur singly or together without presumption of any particular causal sequence.

Goisman et al. (1995) found that patients with agoraphobia without a history of panic disorder seem to be on a continuum with patients with panic disorder with agoraphobia along a number of variables; they suggest that a more sensible approach would be that of seeing agoraphobia without a history of panic disorder simply as one variation among others in the array of disorders that present in various combinations of acute bursts of anxiety combined with chronic avoidance.

Classification systems vary according to the relative prevalence of one of the previous positions. In 1980 DSM-III considered three separate categories: panic disorder, agoraphobia with PD, and agoraphobia without PD (APA, 1980). However, a number of investigators (Klein, 1981; Garvey and Tuason, 1984; Buller et al., 1986) later began to argue that agoraphobia was not a separate entity but rather a secondary response to panic disorder. They reported that agoraphobia before the onset of panic attacks was uncommon and that panic disorder and agoraphobia were similar in their clinical presentation. Studies of familial transmission of panic disorder and agoraphobia further supported the concept of agoraphobia as a more severe variant of panic disorder, rather than a separate entity (Noyes et al., 1986). Thus, consistent with this body of research, in 1987 DSM-III-R reclassified agoraphobia as mainly a sequel of panic disorder, which could present itself either with or without agoraphobia (APA, 1987) and this classification is maintained in DSM-IV (APA, 1993). Agoraphobia without panic remained in both classification systems because of the repeated reports that agoraphobia without panic, although non-existent in the clinical practice of psychiatry, had continued to be reported as a fairly common diagnosis in community surveys. DSM-III-R and DSM-IV, therefore, privilege the interpretation of panic being the central feature with agoraphobia as a complication. ICD-10, conversely, classifies the association of panic and agoraphobia among phobic disorders, thus accepting the position that the phobic attitude is the core aspect of this disorder.

Hypochondriasis

Most of the patients develop a particular attention towards their bodily sensations, with an exaggerated sensitivity for minor and normal changes. The patient at first associates a number of somatic symptoms with the subjective experience of a panic attack, these symptoms thus acting as conditional stimuli. Later on, the occurrence of these symptoms, whatever their origin, then bring on by conditioning the subjective anxiety symptoms of the attack. This mechanism, termed "interoceptive conditioning", makes some subjects avoid activities that provoke physical sensations which can be interpreted as anxiety-like (e.g. physical efforts, drinking coffee, etc.). A similar phenomenon could also explain these patients' intolerance to the side-effects of antidepressants, the frequent worsening of their anxiety symptoms during somatic affections. Many patients (around 20%) develop a true hypochondriac elaboration, during which they are seriously afraid of being ill or even persuaded they are ill. The hypochondriac worries mainly concern the fear of cardiac illness or of the cerebral ictus.

Interoceptive conditioning could account for the anxiety "crescendo" which is often described by these patients during the premonitory phase of certain attacks (Boulenger and Uhde, 1987). In fact, the sudden, brutal and unpredictable nature of the first panic attacks often disappears after a time progression of the disease, with subsequent attacks occurring when the patient is confronted with phobogenic situations or at the apex of a period of rapidly growing apprehension. These "provoked" patients often describe a "vicious circle": their apprehension brings on somatic symptoms which in turn increase their anxiety which gradually grows in intensity until the panic attack is triggered off in all its severity. Often patients are perfectly aware of this mechanism and some even describe this phenomenon as if they were capable of triggering it themselves (Boulenger and Bisserbe, 1992).

Demoralisation

Some patients with PD or PD/agoraphobia (about 30%) develop feelings of sadness, guilt, anhedonia. Generally, this state may be considered as psychological demoralisation due to the fact that their ability to live normally and to achieve social goals is seriously compromised by the disorder; in other cases, however, the possibility of a true depressive episode must be taken into account.

EPIDEMIOLOGY

The rates of panic disorders are consistent across diverse countries. The annual rate of panic disorder ranged from 1.7 per 100 in West Germany to 0.2 per 100 in Taiwan, a country that has low rates of all psychiatric disorders (Weissman et al., 1997). The lifetime ranged from 3.8 per 100 in Holland (Bijl et al., 1998) to 0.4 per 100 in Taiwan (Weissman et al., 1997). These lifetime rates are twice as high as the rate in the Epidemiologic Catchment Area (ECA) (1.7 per 100). These differences may be caused by a period effect with increasing rates between the ECA conducted in the early 1980s and this study conducted in the early 1990s. It could also be caused by differences in the DSM-III and DSM-III-R criteria for panic disorder; DSM III requires three panic attacks in a three-week period, while the DSM- III-R criteria used in the latter study are broader than DSM-III criteria because they include persistent worry about having another attack. DSM-III-R also includes an additional symptom (nausea or abdominal distress) as one of the criteria.

The lifetime prevalence of panic disorder with agoraphobia is around 1.5% (Eaton et al., 1994). Numbers of years of education produced strong and significant differences in the probability of panic attacks, panic disorder, and panic disorder with agoraphobia. Persons with less than 12 years of education were more than four times as likely to have panic attacks, more than 10 times as likely to have panic disorders, and more than seven times as likely to have panic disorder with agoraphobia versus the reference group with a college education (16 or more years). The pattern is not linear, in that those with some college education have odds similar to the odds of those who finish college, and those who do not complete high school have odds similar to the odds of those who complete high school but take no further education (Eaton et al., 1994). Therefore, the occurrence of panic might well be related to stressful situations in which the individual is at a disadvantage relative to others. On the other hand, panic might be strongly mediated by cognitive factors involving the appraisal of risk. Working people, married people, and those living with others have a generally lower estimated prevalence of panic. Those living in a city appear to have a somewhat greater prevalence of panic, but the result is not statistically significant (Eaton et al., 1994).

The estimated prevalence of panic and related experiences is very different in men and women. The preponderance of women among patients with anxiety disorders is a consistent epidemiological and clinical finding. In every category of increasing severity of panic disorder, the prevalence is slightly more than twice as great among women as among men (Eaton et al., 1994), as in the ECA results (1985): across epidemiological surveys the ratio of females to males varying from 1.3 to 5.8 (Weissman et al., 1997). Among agoraphobics women largely predominate: over three-quarters of PD patients manifesting extensive avoidance are women (Myers et al., 1984; Thyer et al., 1985; Wittchen, 1986; Barlow, 1988). Women are also more likely to develop phobic complications, to present with generalised anxiety (Aronson and Logue, 1987) and to suffer more depression (Delay et al., 1981; Buller et al., 1986). Male patients have a significantly longer duration of illness compared with females (Scheibe and Albus, 1992). Women suffer significantly more frequently from anticipatory anxiety and from current or past depressive mood. In spite of the longer duration of illness in male patients, the less frequent occurrence of concomitant phobic avoidance and depressive disorders in males indicates that men might be less severely impaired than female patients. Males also display less frequent search for help (Buller et al., 1986; Scheibe and Albus, 1992; Breier et al., 1984); the economic imperative of males to work may help reduce agoraphobia.

ONSET OF PANIC DISORDER

Age of Onset

The age of onset for PD varies considerably, but most typically is the early to mid-twenties, with later onset in West Germany (age at onset, 35.5 years) and Korea (age at onset, 32.1 years) (Weissman et al., 1997). In clinical samples the mean age of onset is around 25 years: the total estimated prevalence of panic attacks and PD is greatest in people aged 15–24 years. The association with age seems to differ by sex (Eaton et al., 1994). For men, the highest rates for both panic attacks and PD are in the lowest age group, but for women, the peak is in the age range of 35–44 for attacks. The pattern for both men and women suggests a bimodal distribution: the early mode for panic disorder is in the same age range of 15–24 for both and the later mode occurs in the age range of 45–54. A small number of cases begin during childhood. In about 15% of the patients the age of onset is after age 40 (Buller et al., 1991; Scheibe and Albus, 1992).

The strikingly higher risk of panic disorder in relatives of probands with PD onset at or before 20 years of age suggests that age at onset may be useful in differentiating familial subtypes of PD and that genetic studies of panic disorder should consider age at onset (Goldstein et al., 1997). Whereas PD without agoraphobia prevails during the late twenties, PD with agoraphobia most frequently develops during the early twenties.

Situation of Onset

With regard to the context in which the first panic attack occur, Lelliott et al. (1989) reported that 92% of their agoraphobic patients with panic experienced their first panic attack in phobogenic situations rather than at home. These sites are usually a loosely knit agoraphobic cluster of cues concerning public places, such as streets, stores, public transportation, auditoriums and crowds, and less central concerning elevators, tunnels, bridges, open spaces, and heights. These findings are consistent with those reported by Faravelli et al. (1992): they found that such an onset was significantly less common among patients with panic disorder who did not develop agoraphobia later.

The association between public onset and agoraphobia merits special interest. An interpretation could suggest that a sort of subclinical agoraphobia might pre-date clinical panic, thus supporting the previously mentioned view that some predisposition pre-dates the acute onset of PD. Lelliott et al. (1989) suggest a role for an ethological factor (an evolutionary vulnerability to extraterritoriality), in addition to the biological and learning components of the disorder. Another simpler interpretation could be taken into account. The different psychological meaning of the context in which panic occurs might explain the evolution of the disorder. Experiencing the drama of an unexpected panic attack in a setting in which, objectively, help is not available has a different psychological impact from experiencing the same symptoms in protected settings (e.g., at home). It is possible that undergoing such a stressful experience as having an attack in contexts in which one is helpless will affect the later course of the disorder. In this case the basic core of PD would be the pathological evolution of panic, rather than panic itself.

Lelliott et al. (1989) also found that, at least in Britain, the first panic attack occurred more often in late spring-summer and during warm weather than in winter and cold weather. The heat may lessen the stimulation needed to reach an intolerable degree of sweating and other autonomic discomfort that is felt to be anxiety or panic when in public places. On the other hand, good weather may simple increase the probability of being away from home.

Stressful Life Events

Uncontrolled clinical descriptions have reported that the first panic attack is often preceded by some stressful life event (Klein DF, 1964; Finlay-Jones and Brown, 1981; Raskin et al., 1982). Controlled studies generally confirm the excess of life stress prior to the onset of PD (Faravelli, 1985; Faravelli and Pallanti, 1989; Roy-Byrne et al., 1986c). It was found that panic patients experience more life events in the year before the onset of the illness than do healthy control subjects and that the highest concentration of life stress occurs in the last few months before the initial symptoms (Faravelli, 1985; Faravelli and Pallanti, 1989). However, they did not confirm the findings by Finlay-Jones and Brown (1981) who reported that danger events were significantly over-represented among patients with "anxiety", whereas loss events were more frequent among patients with "depression". This information leads us to attribute a role as precipitating factors for the onset of PD to life events, but in a rather aspecific way. The degree of association between stressful events and PD, however, is not in any case very great: the Population Attributable Risk varies in fact between 30–39% (Faravelli et al., 1992). Most PD patients described how their first panic attacks occurred *after* rather than *during* a period of their lives they considered particularly stressful, which, however, they managed to cope with quite adequately (Boulenger and Bisserbe, 1992). Apart from the obvious role of psychogenetic mechanisms in the occurrence of these symptoms, another possible interpretation is in terms of biological exhaustion or sensitisation or even in terms of an interruption of cognitive schemes (Hallarm, 1978).

Roy-Byrne et al. (1986b) examined the subsequent course of illness in patients with PD as a function of whether or not the onset of illness had been preceded by major loss or separation. Their results suggest that the occurrence of severe loss before the onset is not related to the severity of subsequent anxiety symptoms but does appear to be related to the subsequent occurrence of a major depression. Since events preceding onset of the disorder are generally assigned a causative-precipitating role, it is plausible to suggest that the same types of events would have a role in maintaining or exacerbating the disorder. This would be consistent with a study showing that agoraphobic patients who continued to experience adverse life events after behavioural treatment had a poorer outcome (Wade et al., 1993).

ANTECEDENTS

Early Life Events

It has been suggested that there may be a link between the experience of traumatic life events during childhood and adolescence and the development of anxiety disorder in adults: Raskin et al. (1982), examining developmental antecedents in a variety of types of anxiety disorder, found that 53% of panic disorder group had some record of parental separation in childhood. It was found that agoraphobic patients with panic attacks experience more traumatic life events (such as death of parents, prolonged separation from parents, divorce of parents) during childhood and adolescence compared with normal subjects (Faravelli et al., 1985; Tweed et al., 1989). Although part of the excess of these events is the result of a greater prevalence of psychiatric disorders in their families (Harris et al., 1983), this does not account entirely for the bulk of the difference, and a cause-and-effect relationship between early traumatic life events and anxiety disorders should be considered.

Almost all the studies that considered the effects of early traumata for adult psychopathology are consistent in reporting early events are associated with an increased risk for all anxiety and depressive disorders, somatization and greater comorbidity, but with little specificity for any single disorder (Kessler et al., 1997; Young et al., 1997).

On the other hand, at least restricting the field of observation to panic/agoraphobia phenomenon, the occurrence of separation events during childhood/adolescence seems to be specifically associated with later development of agoraphobia. In fact, two-thirds of patients with panic and agoraphobia showed at least one traumatic event in the first 16 years of life, compared with 22% of panic patients without agoraphobia (Faravelli et al., 1988). Early events of separation can lead to experiences of deep insecurity. These, in turn, in the absence of a protective figure, may discourage the normal exploratory behaviour. The subject, therefore, faces a world where he senses his precariousness and where several situations can be seen as dangerous. Together with the feelings of anger and desperation, which involve the vegetative system in a continuous alertness, the necessity to be independent may give rise to dysfunctional patterns of attachment (Guidano and Liotti, 1983).

Recently, there has been an increasing interest in child assaults as risk factors for the development of mental disorders. Saunders et al. (1992) report that in children physically and sexually abused before the age of five, the most common adult psychiatric disorder is agoraphobia which occurs in 44% of cases, whereas Swanston et al. (1997) found an increase of general anxiety in sexually abused children followed up for 5 years after the event. Of a sample of 59 Cambodian young adults who survived massive trauma as children, a significant number of those with PTSD (59%) had one or more additional DSM-III-R axis I disorders. Major depression and generalised anxiety disorder were the most common comorbid disorders. Also, the rate of PTSD diagnoses found in this sample 15 years after the trauma of Pol Pot shows that the effects of trauma experienced in childhood persist into early adulthood (Hubbard et al., 1995). Here again, therefore, whereas it seems that abuse in children brings an increased risk of psychopathology during adulthood, the specificity of these traumata for PD/agoraphobia is questionable.

Maternal Over-protection

It is a common clinical impression that the parents of patients with PD appear to be over-protective, stern and rigid (Errera, 1962; Marks, 1969). On empirical grounds, Terhune, Webster and Tucker all described a background of parental over-protection (especially maternal) in their agoraphobic patients. Among the controlled studies, using the Maternal Overprotection Questionnaire (Terhune, 1949; Webster, 1953; Tucker, 1956). Solyom et al. (1976) found that the mothers of agoraphobics were more protective than those of normal controls.

Parker, using the Parental Bonding Instrument (PBI), reported that patients suffering from anxiety neurosis scored both their parents as significantly less caring and more over-protective than did matched normal controls (Parker, 1979a), whereas another study by Parker found that agoraphobics differed from controls only on the scale measuring maternal care, which was reduced among patients (Parker, 1979b). Using the PBI in operationally defined panic disorder, it was found that patients affected by PD reported childhood interactions with significantly less caring and more controlling parents (Faravelli et al., 1991; Silove et al., 1991). No differences emerged between agoraphobic and non-agoraphobic patients, nor was there any correlation with the level of phobic avoidance. However, although PBI has been shown to be an acceptable measure of actual and not merely perceived parental characteristics, it is possible that the subjects with emotional pathology might search for the causes of their problems in the past: they might attribute a more negative value to their earlier interactions with parents than they in fact warrant. On other hand, as a family concentration of anxiety does exist, it is reasonable to conceive that parents with an anxious or phobic condition might have reduced capacity to care for children and might over-protect the child as they protect themselves from the feared situations. Conversely, phobic-type behaviours by children, such as those frequently reported in the past personal history of patients with PD, could induce reactions of over-protection in their parents.

Separation Anxiety

Increasing evidence points to an association between childhood anxiety and PD during adult life (Raskin et al., 1982; Crowe et al., 1983; Breier et al., 1986; Turner et al., 1987; Perugi et al., 1988; Zitrin and Ross, 1988; Klein and Klein, 1988; Klein, 1992; Klein, 1995; Pollak et al., 1990; Rosenbaum et al., 1993; Laraia et al., 1994), though some reports failed to confirm this association (Thyer et al., 1985; Thyer et al., 1986; Van der Molen et al., 1989; Lipsitz et al., 1994). Silove et al. found that early separation anxiety was associated with risk of adult PD and that subjects with a lifetime history of PD–agoraphobia had more separation anxiety symptoms than those with GAD or other phobic disorders without a history of PD (Silove and Manicavasagar, 1993; Silove et al., 1993; Silove et al., 1995). Pollak et al. (1990) reported that 55% of adult patients with PD met the criteria for childhood anxiety disorder, and found that those cases where a childhood history of anxiety was retraceable had a higher rate of comorbid anxiety disorders. Patients with a child-hood history of anxiety disorders were also characterised by greater avoidance and greater fear of anxiety symptoms, even though they did not demonstrate a greater overall severity of PD. Only one prospective study of well-diagnosed children with separation anxiety has been conducted (Klein, 1995): although panic disorder was infrequent in the cases, it was significantly higher than in the controls.

Kagan et al. (1984) reported that behavioural inhibition in childhood might be a risk factor for the later development of anxiety disorders. Rosenbaum et al. (1988) have reported a high rate of behavioural inhibition in young children of parents with panic disorder and agoraphobia. To investigate further the link between behavioural inhibition and anxiety disorders, Biederman et al. (1990) examined the psychiatric correlates of behavioural inhibition by evaluating a sample of offspring of parents with panic disorder and agoraphobia and an existing epidemiological derived sample of children, followed over a seven-year period by Reznick et al. (1986). They found that inhibited children had increased risk for multiple anxiety, over-anxious, and phobic disorders, especially social phobia.

Further evidence for the link between childhood and adult anxiety psycho-pathology comes from family studies reporting high rates of childhood anxiety difficulties in the offspring of adult patients with panic disorder (Turner et al., 1987; Weissman et al., 1984; Last et al., 1991); whether childhood anxiety predisposes the individual to adult panic disorder by influencing cognitive or behavioural reactions to symptoms, or whether it is an early manifestation of the same disorder, is still unclear.

Personality

Anecdotal reports contend that PD subjects had a normal or even sociable and outgoing nature before the onset of the disorder. Although this is true at a superficial observation, clinicians have long suspected that patients with agoraphobia have more dependent personality traits than the average person. Andrews (1996) hypothesised that dependence on others was a major coping style of agoraphobic patients. To some extent this was reported by Shafar (1970) who, using undefined ratings, concluded that dependence problems were present in 38% of her agoraphobic patients, and Buglass et al. (1977), although reporting an overall negative study, found that 27% of their patients and none of their control subjects were aware of dependence about which they were resentful. Finally, Torgersen, in his study of monozygotic twins, found that the agoraphobic twin was most likely to be dependent (Torgersen, 1979).

The personality of subjects affected by PD during a phase of remission is characterised by pessimism, excessive preoccupation with physical functions, insecurity, egocentrism, immaturity, excessive rumination, indecisiveness and excessively high standards of morality (Faravelli et al., 1987). The Maudsley Personality Inventory revealed high levels of neuroticism, and the Sensation Seeking Scale showed the wish of agoraphobic subjects to cope with those situations they do not dare confront in reality. Since all these studies have been retrospective, it is not clear whether the dependent personality traits observed are primary or secondary to the occurrence of the symptoms. On one hand, the possibility that this disorder might be a predisposing condition for the development of PD is supported by the findings of Nystrom and Lyndergard: in a prospective study of more than 3000 subjects, these authors found dependent premorbid personality traits in people who later developed anxiety disorders (Nystrom and Lyndergard, 1975). Consequently, it is reasonable to believe that personality traits or disorders can contribute to the development of an illness. On the other hand, it may be that personality disturbances are secondary to PD, especially when complicated by phobic avoidance. Some patients claim that before the onset of their phobic disorder they had been independent and self-confident, in contrast to the fearful clinging to a companion that later accompanied their illness. Their avoiding behaviour and phobic cognitive style may well have contributed to an unwelcome dependence.

Hoffart (1995), examining the relationship between psychoanalytical personality types and agoraphobia before and after the treatment, found that higher scores on the oral scale predicted poorer course of symptoms in the year immediately after treatment. Scores on the oral scale decreased with the improvements of agoraphobic and general symptoms, but did not attain a normal level. This result supported a combined predisposition-state model for the relationship between oral traits and agoraphobia. Skodol et al. (1995) examined patterns of comorbidity of DSM-III-R anxiety disorders and personality disorders. Results revealed that PD, either current or lifetime, is associated with borderline, avoidant and dependent personality disorders; anxiety disorders with personality disorders are characterised by chronicity and lower levels of functioning compared with anxiety disorders without personality disorders. The results of a study by Noyes et al. (1995) indicate that social phobia and panic disorder patients are distinguishable on the basis of personality characteristics. In particular, social phobics had more severe personality pathology, higher anxious and schizoid cluster scores and differed from panic subjects in having more avoidant personality traits; panic subjects had more dependent traits. In a recent study, Perugi et al. provide evidence that characterological and prodromal antecedents represent a putative phobic-anxious temperamental substrate occurring in at least 30% of their sample (Perugi et al., 1998); this temperament seems to be of familial origin as a result of which the illness tends to declare itself earlier.

CLINICAL COURSE

Short and Long-term Outcomes

After DSM-III reclassification of anxiety disorders, several reports focused on the long-term outcome of panic disorder. Retrospective descriptions by individuals seen in clinical settings suggest that the usual course of the illness is generally chronic, with waxing and waning. Some individuals may have episodic outbreaks with years of remission in between, and others may have continuous severe symptomatology. Specific follow-up studies confirm the general chronicity of PD, although with a variety of possible outcomes. Although the earliest studies, which included relatively brief follow-up periods, showed a relatively good prognosis, with recovery rates ranging from 25% to 72% after 1 or 2 years (Gloger et al., 1981; Faravelli and Albanesi, 1987; Maier and Buller, 1988), further studies reported less favourable outcomes (Coryell et al., 1983; Nagy et al., 1989; Noyes et al., 1990; Faravelli et al., 1995). After five years of prospective follow-up, only 10–12% of patients fully recovered (i.e. no symptoms and no treatment). Moreover, higher risks of suicide, major depressive episodes, cardiovascular diseases, as well as an increased general morbidity and mortality, have been reported in these patients (Coryell et al., 1988; Weissman et al., 1989; Lépine et al., 1993). However, since PD is frequently comorbid with other axis I and II disorders, the long-term consequences could be attributed to the comorbid condition rather than to PD itself. Recent studies seem to confirm this position: the worst consequences in terms of fatality, morbidity, and substance abuse seem to be related to the associated conditions (Wittchen and Essau, 1989; Johnson et al., 1990; Lépine et al., 1993).

Noyes et al. (1990) found that patients with extensive phobic avoidance or agoraphobia have a more severe form of PD, with a longer duration of illness, more severe symptoms and greater social maladjustment than subjects with limited or no phobic avoidance. Breier et al., Lesser et al. and Noyes et al. found that subjects with panic disorder with secondary depression (current or past) were part of a more severely ill group: they had been ill longer and had more severe anxiety symptoms, more frequent panic attacks and more extensive phobic avoidance, and they more frequently had personality disorders (Breier et al., 1984; Lesser et al., 1988; Noyes et al., 1990). There is some evidence that concomitant personality disorders influence the outcome of patients with PD: the presence of a personality disturbance predicts in fact a less favourable treatment response (Reich et al., 1987; Roy-Byrne et al., 1988; Noyes et al., 1990). When PD is the primary psychopathological condition, the rate of recovery is relatively low (12%) and that PD tends to be chronic disturbance (Faravelli et al., 1995); the long-term outcome shows a wide variability, with the intermediate outcome of neither ill nor well being the most common. Among the predictors taken into consideration, only duration of the disorder before treatment showed a close relationship to outcome: patients with a shorter duration of illness more frequently experienced a complete recovery or remission and reported fewer relapses. In this sample, the number of suicides is small.

Using data from the ECA study, Markowitz et al. (1989) reported that PD (with or without agoraphobia) was associated with a greater risk of poor physical and emotional health, alcohol and other drug abuse, suicide attempts, poorer marital functioning, and greater financial dependence. The risk for PD was even greater than for major depression for many measures, including alcohol abuse and financial dependence. ECA suicide rates for the separate diagnoses of panic disorder or major depression alone were similar and were higher than rates for the general population. Patients with PD had levels of mental health and role functioning that were substantially lower than those of patients with other major chronic medical illnesses (Sherbourne et al., 1996). PD is associated with poor quality of life (Katerndahl and Realini, 1997): comorbid depression, social support, worry and severity of chest pain predicted quality of life. Although subjects with infrequent panic attacks reported a lower quality of life than controls, subjects with PD had more panic-related disability and poorer quality of life than those with infrequent panic attacks. Predictors of work disability included panic frequency, illness attitudes and family dissatisfaction.

Coryell (1988) reviewed earlier studies from 1936 to 1986 and concluded that patients with anxiety states appeared as likely as patients with primary depression to commit suicide. Weissman et al. (1989) found a very high rate of suicide attempt and suicidal ideation in subjects suffering from PD even when controlling for lifetime major depressive episode and alcoholism. Lépine et al. (1993) found that 42% of outpatients with PD had attempted suicide at some time during their lives. In patients with PD, they found demographic determinants for suicide attempts to be similar to those of other clinical populations, such as depressed patients: the suicide attempts occur most frequently in single, divorced, or widowed women. In this study the authors found a significantly longer duration of panic disorder at the time at referral in suicide attempters. Otherwise, severity of the worst episode of PD did not differ between suicide attempters and non-attempters. They found that suicide attempt in patients with PD were often associated with a lifetime diagnosis of major depressive episode and alcohol and/or other substance abuse. Warshaw et al. (1995) found that suicidal behaviour in subjects with PD seems to be better related to factors not inherent in the PD; presence of depression, post-traumatic stress disorder, eating disorders, substance abuse/dependency or personality disorders (in particular, borderline and antisocial personality disorders) and factors related to quality of life (in fact, being married or having a child, working full-time all seemed to be protective factors).

Comorbidity

PD is often associated with other anxiety disorders and with depression. Based on lifetime rates, the odds ratios for comorbidity of PD with agoraphobia range from 7.5 in the ECA to 21.4 in Puerto Rico, and those of PD with major depression range from 3.8 in Savigny to 20.1 in Edmonton (Weissman et al., 1997). In the NCS the odds ratio is 10.6 for agoraphobia and 5.7 for major depression. The presence of agoraphobia with PD represents more severe disturbance and involves a higher likelihood of one or more comorbid diagnoses.

Goisman et al. (1995) found lifetime panic with and without agoraphobia to co-exist with at least one other anxiety disorder 37% of the time. Klerman et al. (1991) found 33% of 254 subjects with PD to have comorbid agoraphobia and 72% of these 254 to have comorbid agoraphobia, major depression, alcohol abuse, or drug abuse. Johnson et al. (1990) found more than two-thirds of ECA subjects with lifetime PD to meet criteria for more than one of 10 other axis I diagnoses. Cassano et al. (1999) found 70% of 302 patients with current DSM-III-R panic disorder to also have at least one of seven additional current syndromes of which the most common is GAD. Uncomplicated panic is most likely to exist independently, but even this disorder is found alone in less than 50% of the time (Goisman et al., 1995): GAD and social phobia were the most frequent comorbid diagnosis. Panic with agoraphobia is seen as a sole diagnosis on 40% lifetime. The comorbid diagnoses at similar rates (about 20%) are simple and social phobia and GAD. Joyce et al. (1989) found lifetime DSM-III GAD to be more frequent in subjects with a history of panic attacks with "moderate phobic avoidance" than in those with a history of panic attacks alone. Subjects with agoraphobia without a history of PD have at least two additional diagnoses at almost twice the frequency of subjects with uncomplicated PD and GAD was the disorder most frequently comorbid, followed by social phobia and simple phobia; 32% of subjects had agoraphobia without a history of PD as the sole diagnosis (Goisman et al., 1995).

A possible explanation of high comorbidity between anxiety disorders is that these disorders may share some common aetiologic pathways. Barlow (1988) notes that the experience of some symptoms of anxiety may lead to an anticipation of more anxiety: this anticipation, in fact, is itself anxiety-provoking, leading to ever-increasing expectation, pattern recognition, and further expectation. If this is the case, then it is likely that having one anxiety diagnosis should decrease the threshold for having a second. The studies indicate that this second diagnosis is often GAD (Goisman et al., 1995; Noyes et al., 1992): this argument could lead to a call to abolish GAD as a separate entity and regard it only as a somewhat inevitable non-specific by-product of having any of a number of chronic anxiety disorders. In addition, PD appears to be more likely to be preceded by another psychiatric disorder than to be a chronologically primary condition. Apart from the affective disorders, there are relatively few other psychiatric conditions appearing after the onset of PD. This finding implies that some primary disorders (e.g., simple phobia, social phobia, substance abuse) may represent a specific predisposition for the development of PD.

There are reports that 35% to 91% of patients with panic disorder also suffer from a major depressive episode during their life (Cloninger et al., 1981; Breier et al., 1985; Stein et al., 1990). Data from family and twin studies have suggested that anxiety and depression are present in pure forms in the relatives of probands, but that some degree of overlap in the transmission of these disorders occurs as well (Merikangas et al., 1990; Weissman, 1990): these data are inconclusive as to whether one condition predisposes another or whether there is common aetiology. Leckman et al. (1983) found that first-degree relatives of patients dually diagnosed with major depression and PD have markedly increased morbidity risk for depression, panic, phobias and alcoholism. In many cases, both disorders occur at the same time (Vollrath et al., 1990). In others PD occurs before the onset of depressive disorder as well as before the onset of substance abuse (Wittchen, 1988).

Breier et al. (1984) found that patients with PD and/or agoraphobia who had a current or past major depressive episode had more severe symptoms of both anxiety and depression than those who had never been depressed. In a naturalistic study, Van Valkenburg et al. (1984) reported that patients with secondary depression had an earlier age at onset of their PD but did not differ from non-depressed patients with PD in their treatment response or psychosocial outcome. While it might be reasonable to expect that patients with depression would have suffered from PD longer than those without depression, patients with and without histories of depression have had PD for similar lengths of time (Starcevic et al., 1993). Also, while it is conceivable that patients with more severe agoraphobic avoidance would be more likely to experience depression than patients with less severe avoidance, this is not supported by empirical evidence. Thus, there is little support for the hypothesis that the depression, which frequently complicates PD, is aetiologically secondary to the long-term demoralising effects of chronic agoraphobic avoidance.

The co-existence of social phobia and PD is far from rare. The patients comorbid with social phobia and PD have an earlier PD age of onset; have more obsessive compulsive disorders and more severity in the social phobia scale from the Fear Questionnaire of Marks and Mathews (Segui et al., 1995). While neither duration of PD nor agoraphobic severity was related to a history of major depression, the concomitant diagnosis of social phobia was associated with significantly greater lifetime risk for depression. The data, however, should not be used to support a casual relationship. It is possible that in making concomitant diagnoses of social phobia, we are identifying a subgroup of PD patients with a constellation of personality traits that includes low self-esteem, extreme self-consciousness, and a tendency towards negative self-appraisal. Such a subgroup could be at considerable risk from depression based on psychological, particularly cognitive, factors. Additionally, the social isolation experienced because of social avoidance could contribute to a propensity for becoming depressed. Alternatively, concomitant social phobia may merely be a marker for a more severe illness.

Since the co-occurrence of significant obsessive-compulsive symptoms has also been noted to increase the lifetime risk for depression in patients with PD, it is possible that PG complicated by the presence of any other disorder, rather than social phobia specifically, may increase the risk for depression.

Another risk factor in PD is the development of alcohol abuse, which some view as "self-medication" (Munjack and Moss, 1981). Unquestionably, intake of alcohol initially decreases anticipatory anxiety in patients with PD, but alcoholism later becomes a complication (Cox et al., 1989). Several studies (Leckman et al., 1983; Noyes et al., 1986) suggest that PD has a higher than expected prevalence among alcoholics compared with the prevalence in the general population. The question concerning primary and causal relationship between the two disorders, i.e. whether alcoholism leads to the development of anxiety disorders or vice versa, is less clear. George et al. (1990) suggest that a possible mechanism for the link between alcoholism and anxiety is a kindling process: the hyper-responsive CNS state that results from repeated alcohol withdrawal may, in susceptible individuals, give rise to a heightened state of anxiety and panic attacks even during sobriety. The model of kindling process has been proposed by Ballanger and Post. They demonstrated that the alcohol withdrawal syndrome becomes progressively more severe with increasing years of heavy daily alcohol abuse, irrespective of age. They propose that repeated episodes of withdrawal in chronic alcoholics serve as stimuli for kindling of subcortical structures, primarily limbic, hypothalamic, and thalamic nuclei. They hypothesise that the spectrum of withdrawal symptoms from mild withdrawal with tremor and autonomic symptoms to the more severe withdrawal symptoms of hallucinations, psychic symptoms, epileptic seizures, and delirium tremens are secondary to cumulative physiological changes which accompany a kindling-like process (Ballanger and Post, 1978). Malcolm et al. (1989), in a double-blind controlled study, found that carbamazepine, because of its ability both to retard the development of kindling and suppress established kindled foci, is as effective and safe as benzodiazepine treatment for alcohol withdrawal.

Marazziti et al. (1995) found that current anxiety disorders, especially panic and related conditions, are the most common psychiatric disorders associated with headache. These findings were particularly true of the subgroup of migraine with aura; in the relatively few patients with mood disorders, depression was nearly always comorbid PD and past history of depression was mainly a characteristic of the tension headache group. These data are compatible with the hypothesis that migraine, especially that with aura, PD and some forms of depressive illness are part of the same spectrum.

Irritable bowel syndrome (IBS) is fairly common in patients seeking treatment for PD: in Kaplan's study 46.3% patients with PD met the criteria for IBS (Kaplan et al., 1996). Patients with PD and IBS were more likely to report symptoms of back pain as well as personal history of bowel disease compared with patients with panic disorder but without IBS.

Otoneurological abnormalities have been reported in PD; vestibular abnormalities are most prevalent in the patients with PD with moderate to severe agoraphobia (Jacob et al., 1996). Vestibular dysfunction was associated with space and motion discomfort and with frequency of vestibular symptoms between, but not during, panic attacks. The constellation of vestibular test most specific for agoraphobia was one indicating compensated peripheral vestibular dysfunction. Therefore a subclinical vestibular dysfunction may contribute to the phenomenology of PD, particularly in the development of agoraphobia in panic disorder.

PD and subsyndromal panic are relatively common and may be unrecognised and inadequately treated in patients who present respiratory symptoms (Pollak et al., 1996). There were no significant differences between patients with and without panic in the severity of pulmonary function abnormalities or in the response to bronchodilators. However, patients with panic attacks were significantly more likely to report dyspnea at rest and irritable bowel symptoms and tended to report difficulty swallowing.

Bouwer and Stein (1997) found a specific association between PD and a history of traumatic suffocation which is significantly more frequent among the PD patients than among the comparison subjects. Within the PD group, patients with a history of traumatic suffocation were significantly more likely to exhibit predominantly respiratory symptoms and nocturnal panic attacks, while patients without such a history were significantly more likely to have predominantly cardiovascular symptoms, oculovestibular symptoms and agoraphobia.

REFERENCES

American Psychiatric Association (1980) *Diagnostic and Statistical Manual of Mental Disorders* 3rd edition. Washington, DC: American Psychiatric Association.

American Psychiatric Association (1987) *Diagnostic and Statistical Manual of Mental Disorders* 3rd revised edition. Washington, DC: American Psychiatric Association.

American Psychiatric Association (1993) *Diagnostic and Statistical Manual of Mental Disorders* 4th edition. Washington, DC: American Psychiatric Association.

Andrews JDW (1966) Psychotherapy of phobias. *Psychol Bull* **66**: 455–480.

Aronson TA, Logue CM (1987) On the longitudinal course of panic disorder: Development history and predictors of phobic complications. *Compr Psychiatry* **28**: 344–355.

Ballanger JC, Post RM, Kindling AS (1978) A model for alcohol withdrawal syndromes. *Br J Psychiatry* **133**: 1–14.

Barlow DH (1988) *Anxiety and its Disorders: The Nature and Treatment of Anxiety and Panic*. New York: Guilford Press.

Barlow DH, Vermileyea J, Blanchard EB et al. (1985) The phenomenon of panic. *Abnormal Psychol* **94**: 320–328.

Biederman J, Rosenbaum JF, Hirshfeld MA et al. (1990) Psychiatric correlates of behavioural inhibition in young children of parents with and without psychiatric disorders. *Arch Gen Psychiatry* **47**: 21–26.

Bijl RV, Ravelli A, van Zessen G (1998) Prevalence of psychiatric disorders in the general population: results from the Netherlands Mental Health Survey and Incidence Study (NEMESIS). *Soc Psychiatry Psychiatr Epidemiol* **33**: 587–595.

Boulenger JP, Bisserbe JC (1992) Clinical efficacy of selective anxiolytic compounds. *Clin Neuropsychopharmacol* **15**(1): Pt A: 529A–530A.

Boulenger JP, Uhde TW (1987) Acute anxiety attacks and phobia: Historical aspects and clinical manifestations of the agoraphobia syndrome. *Ann Med Psychol* (Paris) **145**(2): 113–131.

Bouwer C, Stein DJ (1997) Association of panic disorder with a history of traumatic suffocation. *Am J Psychiatry* **154**(11): 1566–1570.

Breier A, Charney DS, Heninger GR (1984) Major depression in patients with agoraphobia and panic disorder. *Arch Gen Psychiatry* **41**: 1129–1135.

Breier A, Charney DS, Heninger GR (1985) The diagnostic validity of anxiety disorders and their relationship to depressive illness. *Am J Psychiatry* **142**: 787–797.

Breier A, Charney D, Heninger GR (1986) Agoraphobia with panic attacks. *Arch Gen Psychiatry* **43**: 1029–1036.

Buglass D, Clarke J, Hendersen AS et al. (1977) A study of agoraphobic housewives. *Psychol Med* **7**: 73–86.

Buller R, Maier W, Benkert O (1986) Clinical subtypes in panic disorder: Their descriptive and prospective validity. *J Affect Disord* **11**: 105–114.

Buller R, Maien W, Goldenberg IM et al. (1991) Chronology of panic and avoidance, age of onset of panic disorder, and prediction of treatment response: A report from the Cross-National Collaborative Panic Study. *Eur Arch Psychiatry Clin Neurosci*: 163–168.

Cassano GB, Pini S, Saettoni M, Dell'Osso L (1999) Multiple anxiety disorder comorbidity in patients with mood spectrum disorders with psychotic features. *Am J Psychiatry* **156**: 474–476.

Clark DM (1986) A cognitive approach to panic. *Behav Res Ther* **24**: 461–467.

Clark DM (1989a) A cognitive model of panic. In Hawton K, Salkovskis P, Kirk J, Clark DM (eds) *Cognitive Behaviour Therapy for Psychiatric Problems: A Practical Guide*. Oxford: Oxford University Press.

Clark DM (1989b) Anxiety states: Panic and generalised anxiety. In Hawton K. Salkovskis P, Kirk J, Clark DM (eds) *Cognitive Behaviour Therapy for Psychiatric Problems: A Practical Guide*. Oxford: Oxford University Press.

Cloninger CR, Martin RL, Clayton P, Guze SB (1981) A blind follow-up and family study of anxiety neurosis: Preliminary results of the St Louis 500. In Klein DF, Rabtkin J (eds) *Anxiety: New Research and Changing Concepts*. New York: Raven Press.

Coryell W (1988) Panic disorder and mortality. *Psychiatr Clin North Am* **11**: 433–440.

Coryell WH, Endicott J, Andreasen NC et al. (1988) Depression and panic attacks: The significance of overlap as reflected in follow-up and family study data. *Am J Psychiatry* **145**: 293–300.

Coryell W, Noyes R, Clancy J (1983) Panic disorder and primary unipolar depression: A comparison of background and outcome. *J Affective Disord* **5**: 511–517.

Cottraux J (1987) Treatment of panic attacks and generalised anxiety. *Rev Med Suisse Romande* **107**(12): 993–999.

Cox BJ, Norton R, Dorward J, Fergusson PA (1989) The relationship between panic attacks and chemical dependencies. *Addict Behav* **14**: 53–60.

Crowe RR, Noyes R, Pauls DL, Slymen D (1983) A family study of panic disorder. *Arch Gen Psychiatry* **40**: 1065–1069.

Delay RS, Ishiki DM, Avery DM (1981) Secondary depression in anxiety disorder. *Compr Psychiatry* **22**: 612–618.

Eaton WW, Kessler RC, Wittchen HU, Magee WJ (1994) Panic and panic disorder in the United States. *Am J Psychiatry* **151**(3): 413–420.

Errera P (1962) Some historical aspects of the concept of phobia. *Psychiatr Q* **36**: 325–336.

Faravelli C (1985) Life events preceding the onset of panic disorder. *J Affective Disord* **9**: 103–105.

Faravelli C, Albanesi G (1987) Agoraphobia with panic attacks: 1-year prospective follow-up. *Compr Psychiatry* **28**: 481–487.

Faravelli C, Guerrini Degl'Innocenti B, Sessarego A et al. (1987) Personality features of patients with panic anxiety. *New Trends Exper Clin Psychiatry* **3**: 13–23.

Faravelli C, Pallanti S (1989) Recent life events and panic disorder. *Am J Psychiatry* **146**: 622–626.

Faravelli C, Pallanti S, Biondi F et al. (1992) Onset of panic disorder. *Am J Psychiatry* **149**(6): 827–828.

Faravelli C, Pallanti S, Frassine R et al. (1988) Panic attacks with and without agoraphobia: A comparison. *Psychopathol* **21**: 51–56.

Faravelli C, Panichi C, Pallanti S et al. (1991) Perception of early parenting in panic and agoraphobia. *Acta Psychiatr Scand* **84**: 6–8.

Faravelli C, Paterniti S, Scarpato A (1995) 5-year prospective, naturalistic follow-up study of panic disorder. *Compr Psychiatry* **36**: 271–277.

Faravelli C, Webb T, Ambonetti A et al. (1985) Prevalence of traumatic early life events in 31 agoraphobic patients with panic attacks. *Am J Psychiatry* **142**: 1493–1494.

Fava GA, Grandi S, Canestrari R (1988) Prodromal symptoms in panic disorder with agoraphobia. *Am J Psychiatry* **145**: 1546–1547.

Finlay-Jones R, Brown GW (1981) Types of stressful life events and the onset of anxiety and depressive disorders. *Psychol Med* **11**: 803–815.

Garvey MJ, Tuason VB (1984) The relationship of panic disorder to agoraphobia. *Compr Psychiatry* **25**(5): 529–531.

George DT, Nutt DJ, Dwier BA, Linnoila M (1990) Alcoholism and panic disorder: Is the comorbidity more than a coincidence? *Acta Psychiatr Scand* **81**: 97–107.

Goisman RM, Warshaw MJ, Peterson LG et al. (1994) Panic, agoraphobia, and panic disorder with agoraphobia. Data from a multicentre anxiety disorder study. *J Nerv Ment Dis* **182**(2): 72–79.

Goisman RM, Warshaw MJ, Steketee GS et al. (1995) DSM-IV and the disappearance of agoraphobia without a history of panic disorder: New data on a controversial diagnosis. *Am J Psychiatry* **152**(10): 1438–1443.

Gloger S, Grunhaus L, Birmacher B, Troudert T (1981) Treatment of spontaneous panic attacks with clomipramine. *Am J Psychiatry* **138**: 1215–1217.

Goldstein RB, Wickramaratne PJ, Horwart E, Weissman MM (1997) Familial aggregation and phenomenology of "early"-onset (at or before age 20 years) panic disorder. *Arch Gen Psychiatry* **54**(3): 271–278.

Guidano V, Liotti G (1983) *Cognitive Processes and Emotional Disorders.* New York: Guilford Press.

Hallarm RS (1978) Agoraphobia: A critical review of the concept. *Br J Psychiatry* **133**: 314–319.

Harris EL, Noyes R, Crowe RR et al. (1983) Family study of agoraphobia. *Arch Gen Psychiatry* **40**: 1061–1064.

Hoffart A (1995) Psychoanalytical personality types and agoraphobia. *J Nerv Ment Dis* **183**(3): 139–144.

Hubbard J, Realmuto GM, Northwood AK, Masten AS (1995) Comorbidity of psychiatric diagnosis with post-traumatic stress disorder in survivors of childhood trauma. *J Am Child Adolesc Psychiatry* **34**(9): 1167–1173.

Jacob RG, Furman JM, Durrant JD, Turner SM (1996) Panic, agoraphobia and vestibular dysfunction. *Am J Psychiatry* **153**(4): 503–512.

Johnson J, Weissman MM, Klerman GL (1990) Panic disorder, comorbidity and suicide attempts. *Arch Gen Psychiatry* **47**(9): 805–808.

Joyce PR, Bushnell JA, Oakley-Browne HA et al. (1989) The epidemiology of panic symptomatology and agoraphobic avoidance. *Compr Psychiatry* **30**: 303–312.

Kagan J, Reznick JS, Clarke C et al. (1984) Behavioural inhibition to the unfamiliar. *Child Dev* **55**: 2212–2225.

Kaplan DS, Masand PS, Gupta S (1996) The relationship of irritable bowel syndrome (IBS) and panic disorder. *Ann Clin Psychiatry* **8**(2): 81–88.

Katerndahl DA, Realini JP (1993) Lifetime prevalence of panic states. *Am J Psychiatry* **150**(2): 246–249.

Katerndahl DA, Realini JP (1997) Quality of life and panic-related work disability in subjects with infrequent panic and panic disorder. *J Clin Psychiatry* **58**(4): 153–158.

Kessler RC, Davis CG, Kendler KS (1997) Childhood adversity and adult psychiatric disorders in the US National Comorbidity Survey. *Psychol Med* **27**(5): 1001–1019.

Klein DF (1964) Delineation of two drug-responsive anxiety syndromes. *Psychopharmacol* **5**: 397–408.

Klein DF (1981) Anxiety reconceptualised. In Klein DF, Raskin J (eds) *Anxiety: New Research and Changing Concepts*. New York: Raven Press.

Klein DF (1987) Anxiety reconceptualised. In Klein DF (ed.) *Anxiety*. Basel: Karger.

Klein DF (1993) False suffocation alarms, spontaneous panic and related conditions: An integrative hypothesis. *Arch Gen Psychiatry* 50: 306–317.

Klein RG (1992) Adult consequences of childhood separation anxiety disorder. In Macher JQ, Crocq MA (eds) *New Prospects in Psychiatry/The Bioclinical Interface I*. Amsterdam: Elsevier Science.

Klein RG (1995) Is panic disorder associated with childhood separation anxiety disorder? *Clin Neuropharmacol* 18 Suppl: 7–14.

Klein RG, Klein DF (1988) Adult anxiety disorders and childhood separation anxiety. In Roth M, Noyes R, Burraws GD (eds) Vol. I. *Biological, Clinical and Cultural Perspectives* (pp. 213–229). Amsterdam: Elsevier Science.

Klerman GL, Weissman MM, Ouellette R et al. (1991) Panic attacks in the community. Social morbidity and health care utilization. *J Am Med Assoc* 265(6): 742–746.

Laraia MT, Stuart GV, Frye LH et al. (1994) Childhood environment of women having panic disorder with agoraphobia. *J Anxiety Disord* 8: 1–17.

Last CG, Hersen M, Kazdin A et al. (1991) A family study of childhood anxiety disorders. *Arch Gen Psychiatry* 48: 928–934.

Leckman JF, Weissman MM, Merikangas KR et al. (1983) Panic disorder and major depression: Increased risk of depression, alcoholism, panic and phobic disorders in families of depressed probands with panic disorder. *Arch Gen Psychiatry* 40(10): 1055–1060.

Lelliott P, Marks I, McNamee G, Tobena A (1989) Onset of panic disorder with agoraphobia. *Arch Gen Psychiatry* 46: 1000–1004.

Lépine JP, Chignon JM, Teherani M (1993) Suicide attempts in patients with panic disorder. *Arch Gen Psychiatry* 50: 144–149.

Lesser IM, Rubin RT, Pecknold JC et al. (1988) Secondary depression in panic disorder and agoraphobia, I: Frequency, severity, and response to treatment. *Arch Gen Psychiatry* 45: 437–443.

Lipsitz JD, Martin LY, Mannuzza S et al. (1994) Childhood separation anxiety disorder in patients with adult anxiety disorders. *Am J Psychiatry* 151: 927–929.

Maier W. Buller R (1988) The course of panic attacks and agoraphobia. *Arch Gen Psychiatry* 45: 501.

Malcolm R, Bellanger JC, Sturgis ET, Anton R (1989) Double-blind controlled trial comparing carbamazepine to oxazepam treatment of alcohol withdrawal. *Am J Psychiatry* 146: 617–621.

Marazziti D, Toni C, Pedru S et al. (1995) Headache, panic disorder and depression: Comorbidity or spectrum? *Neuropsychobiology* 31(3): 125–129.

Markowitz JS, Weissman MM, Ouellette R et al. (1989) Quality of life in panic disorder. *Arch Gen Psychiatry* 46: 984–992.

Mellman TA, Udhe TW (1989) Electroencephalographic sleep in panic disorder. *Arch Gen Psychiatry* 46: 178–184.

Merikangas KR, Angst J, Isler H (1990) Migraine and psychopathology: Results of the Zurich cohort study of young adults. *Arch Gen Psychiatry* 47(9): 849–853.

Munjack M, Moss HB (1981) Affective disorders and alcoholism in family of agoraphobics. *Arch Gen Psychiatry* 38: 869–871.

Myers JK, Weissman MM, Tischler CE et al. (1984) Sixth-month prevalence of psychiatric disorders in three communities. *Arch Gen Psychiatry* 41: 959–967.

Nagy LM, Kristal JH, Woods SW (1989) Clinical and medication outcome after short-term alprazolam in behavioral group treatment of panic disorder. *Arch J Psychiatry* 46: 993–999.

Norton GR, Harrison B, Hauch J, Rhodes L (1985) Characteristics of people with infrequent panic attacks. *J Abnorm Psychol* 94(2): 216–221.

Noyes R, Crowe RR, Harris EL et al. (1986) Relationship between panic disorder and agoraphobia: A family study. *Arch Gen Psychiatry* **43**: 227–232.

Noyes R, Reich J, Christiansen J et al. (1990) Outcome of panic disorder: Relationship to diagnostic subtypes and comorbidity. *Arch Gen Psychiatry* **47**: 809–818.

Noyes R Jr, Woodman CL, Garvey MJ et al. (1992) Generalized anxiety disorder vs panic disorder: Distinguishing characteristics and patterns of comorbidity. *J Nerv Ment Dis* **180**(6): 369–379.

Noyes R Jr, Woodman CL, Holt CS et al. (1995) Avoidant personality traits distinguish social phobic and panic disorder subjects. *J Nerv Ment Dis* **183**(3): 145–153.

Nystrom S, Lyndegard B (1975) Predisposition for mental syndromes: A study comparing predisposition for depression, neurasthenia, and anxiety state. *Acta Psychiatr Scand* **51**: 69–76.

Parker G (1979a) Parental representations of patients with anxiety neurosis. *Acta Psychiatr Scand* **63**: 33–36.

Parker G (1979b) Reported parental characteristics of agoraphobics and social phobics. *Br J Psychiatry* **135**: 555–560.

Perugi G, Deltito J, Soriani A et al. (1988) Relationship between panic disorder and separation anxiety disorder with school phobia. *Compr Psychiatry* **29**(2): 98–107.

Perugi G, Toni C, Benedetti A et al. (1998) Delineating a putative phobic–anxious temperament in 126 panic-agoraphobic patients: Toward a rapprochement of European and US views. *J Affect Disord* **47**(1–3): 11–23.

Pollak MH, Kradin R, Otto MW et al. (1996) Prevalence of panic in patients referred for pulmonary function testing as a major medical centre. *Am J Psychiatry* **153**(1): 110–113.

Pollak MH, Otto MW, Rosenbaum JF et al. (1990) Longitudinal course of panic disorder: Findings from the Massachussetts General Hospital Naturalistic Study. *J Clin Psychiatry* **51**: 12–16.

Raskin M, Peeke HVS, Dikman W et al. (1982) Panic and generalised anxiety disorders: Developmental antecedents and precipitants. *Arch Gen Psychiatry* **39**: 587–589.

Reich J, Noyes R Jr, Troughton E (1987) Dependent personality disorder associated with phobic avoidance in patients with panic disorder. *Am J Psychiatry* **144**: 323–326.

Reznick JS, Kagan J, Snidman N et al. (1986) Inhibited and uninhibited children: A follow-up study. *Child Dev* **51**: 660–680.

Rosenbaum JF, Biederman J, Bolduc-Murphy EA et al. (1993) Behavioural inhibition in childhood: A risk factor for anxiety disorders. *Harvard Rev Psychiatry* **1**: 2–16.

Rosenbaum JF, Biederman J, Gersten M et al. (1988) Behavioural inhibition in children of parents with panic disorder and agoraphobia: A controlled study. *Arch Gen Psychiatry* **45**: 463–470.

Roth M (1984) Agoraphobia, panic disorder and generalised anxiety disorder. *Psychiatr Dev* **2**: 31–52.

Roy-Byrne P, Ashleigh EA, Carr J (1988) Personality and the anxiety disorder: A review of clinical findings. In Noyes R, Roth M, Burrow GD (eds) *Handbook of Anxiety*. New York: Elsevier Science.

Roy-Byrne P, Geraci M, Uhde T (1986a) Life events and the course of illness in patients with panic disorder. *Am J Psychiatry* **143**: 1033–1035.

Roy-Byrne P, Geraci M, Uhde T (1986b) Life events and the onset of panic disorder. *Am J Psychiatry* **143**: 1424–1427.

Roy-Byrne PP, Uhde TW, Post RM et al. (1986c) The corticotropin-releasing hormone stimulation test in patients with panic disorder. *Am J Psychiatry* **143**: 896–869.

Saunders BE, Villepontaux LA, Liipovsky JA et al. (1992) Child sexual assault as a risk factor for mental disorders among women. *Interpersonal Violence* **7**: 189–204.

Scheibe G, Albus M (1992) Age at onset, precipitating events, sex distribution, and co-occurrence of anxiety disorders. *Psychopathol* **25**: 11–18.

Scupi BS, Benson BE, Brown LB, Uhde TW (1997) Rapid onset: A valid panic disorder criterion? *Depress Anxiety* **5**(3): 121–126.

Segui H, Salvador R, Canet J et al. (1995) Comorbidity of panic disorder and social phobia. *Actas Luso Esp Neurol Psiquiatr Cienc Afines* **23**(2): 43–47.

Shafar S (1970) Aspects of phobic illness: A study of 90 personal cases. *Br J Med Psychol* **49**: 211–236.

Sherbourne CD, Walls KB, Judd LL (1996) Functioning and well being of patients with panic disorder. *Am J Psychiatry* **153**(2): 213–218.

Silove D, Harris M, Morgan A et al. (1995) Is early separation anxiety a specific precursor of panic disorder-agoraphobia? A community study. *Psychol Med* **25**: 405–411.

Silove D, Manicavasagar V (1993) Adults who feared school: Is early separation anxiety specific to pathogenesis of panic disorder? *Acta Psychiatr Scand* **88**: 385–390.

Silove D, Manicavasagar Y, O'Connell D et al. (1993) Reported early separation anxiety symptoms in patients with panic and generalised anxiety disorders. *Aust N Z Psychiatry* **27**: 487–494.

Silove D, Parker G, Hadzi-Pavlovic D (1991) Parental representations of patients with panic disorder and generalised anxiety disorder. *Br J Psychiatry* **159**: 835–841.

Skodol AE, Oldham JM, Hyler SE et al. (1995) Patterns of anxiety and personality disorders comorbidity. *J Psychiatr Res* **29**(5): 361–374.

Solyom L, Silberfeld M, Soluom C (1976) Maternal overprotection in the aetiology of agoraphobia. *Can Psychiatr Assoc J* **21**: 109–113.

Starcevic V, Uhlenhuth EH, Kellner R, Pathac D (1993) Comparison of primary and secondary panic disorder: A preliminary report. *J Affect Disord* **27**: 81–86.

Stein MB, Tancer ME, Uhde TW (1990) Major depression in patients with panic disorder: Factors associated with course and reoccurrence. *J Affect Disord* **19**: 287–296.

Swanston HV, Tebbutt JS, O'Toole BJ, Oates RK (1997) Sexually abused children 5 years after presentation: A case-control study. *Pediatrics* **100**(4): 600–608.

Terhune WB (1949) The phobic syndrome. *Arch Neurol Psychiatr* **62**: 162–172.

Thyer B, Nesse R, Cameron O, Curtis G (1985a) Agoraphobia: A test of the separation anxiety hypothesis. *Behav Res Ther* **23**: 75–78.

Thyer B, Nesse R, Curtis G, Cameron O (1986) Panic disorder: A test of the separation anxiety hypothesis. *Behav Res Ther* **24**: 209–211.

Thyer BA, Parrish RT, Curtis GC et al. (1985b) Ages of onset of DSM-III anxiety disorders. *Compr Psychiatry* **26**: 113–122.

Torgersen S (1979) The nature and origin of common phobic fears. *Br J Psychiatry* **134**: 343–351.

Tucker WI (1956) Diagnosis and treatment of the phobic reaction. *Am J Psychiatry* **112**: 825–830.

Turner SM, Beidel DC, Costello A (1987) Psychopathology in the offspring of anxiety disorders patients. *J Consult Clin Psychol* **55**: 229–235.

Tweed JL, Schoenbach VJ, George LK et al. (1989) The effects of childhood parental death and divorce on six-month history of anxiety disorders. *Br J Psychiatry* **154**: 823–828.

Van der Molen G, Van den Hout M, Van Dieren A, Griez E (1989) Childhood separation anxiety and adult-onset panic disorders. *J Anxiety Disord* **3**: 97–106.

Van Valkenburg C, Akiskal HS, Puzantian V, Rosenthal T (1984) Anxious depressions: Clinical, family history and naturalistic outcome: comparison with panic and major depressive episode. *J Affect Disord* **6**: 67–82.

Vollrath M, Koch R, Angst J (1990) The Zurich Study, IX: Panic disorder and sporadic panic: symptoms, diagnosis, prevalence, and overlap with depression. *Eur Arch Psychiatry Neurol Sci* **239**: 221–230.

Wade S, Monroe S, Michelson R (1993) Chronic life stress and treatment outcome in agoraphobia with panic attacks. *Am J Psychiatry* **150**: 1491–1495.

Warshaw MG, Massion AO, Peterson LG et al. (1995) Suicidal behaviour in patients with panic disorder: A retrospective and prospective data. *J Affect Disord* **34**: 2235–2247.

Webster AS (1953) The development of phobias in married women. *Psychol Monographs* **67**: 367.

Weissman MM (1990) The hidden patient: Unrecognised panic disorder? *J Clin Psychiatry* **51** Suppl: 5–8.

Weissman MM, Bland RC, Canino JC et al. (1997) The cross-national epidemiology of panic disorder. *Arch Gen Psychiatry* **54**(4): 305–309.

Weissman MM, Klerman GL, Markowitz JS (1989) Suicidal ideation and suicide attempts in panic disorder and attacks. *N Engl J Med* **321**: 1209–1214.

Weissman MM, Leckman JF, Merikangas KR et al. (1984) Depression and anxiety disorders in parents and children: Results from the Yale Family Study. *Arch Gen Psychiatry* **41**: 845–852.

Weissman MM, Merikangas KR (1986) The epidemiology of anxiety and panic disorder: An update. *J Clin Psychiatry* **47** Suppl: 11–17.

Westphal C (1871) Die Agoraphobie eine neuropatische Erscheinung. *Archives für Psychiatrie und Nervenkrankheiten* **72**: 138–161.

Wittchen HU (1986) Epidemiology of panic attacks and panic disorders. In Hand I, Wittchen HU (eds) *Panic and Phobias: Empirical Evidences of Theoretical Models and Longterm Effects of Behavioural Treatments*. Berlin: Springer-Verlag.

Wittchen HU (1988) Natural history and spontaneous remissions of untreated anxiety disorders: Results of the Munich Follow-up Study (MFS). In Hand I, Wittchen HU (eds) *Panic and Phobias 2: Treatment and Variables Affecting Course and Outcome*. New York: Springer-Verlag.

Wittchen HV, Essam CA (1989) Comorbidity of anxiety disorders and depression: Does it affect course and outcome? *Psychiatric Psychobiol* **4**: 315–323.

Wittchen HU, Essau CA (1991) The epidemiology of panic attacks, panic disorder and agoraphobia. In Walker JR, Norton GR, Ross CA (eds) *Panic Disorder and Agoraphobia*. Monterey, CA: Brooks/Cole.

Young EA, Abelson JL, Curtis JC (1997) Childhood adversity and vulnerability to mood and anxiety disorders. *Depress Anxiety* **5**(2): 66–72.

Zitrin C, Ross D (1988) Early separation anxiety and adult agoraphobia. *J Ment Nerv Dis* **176**: 621–625.

Panic Disorder: Pathogenesis and Treatment

C. Faravelli, V. Ricca, and E. Truglia
Florence University Medical School, Florence, Italy

INTRODUCTION

The origin of panic disorder (PD) is still an open question, and a detailed overview of presently available findings and positions goes beyond the scope of this chapter. The following chapter, however, summarises the basic evidence.

PATHOGENESIS

Biological Findings

The principal research approaches when investigating possible biological mechanisms underlying PD are laboratory studies using provocative agents and pharmacological and neurochemical studies aimed at understanding the neurotransmitter systems involved in the pathogenesis of PD, and proposing neuroanatomical models.

Provocative Agents

Intravenous infusion of sodium lactate 0.5–1 M has been reported to reliably induce panic attacks in PD patients (Pitts and McClure, 1967). Twenty minutes inhalation of air containing 5% CO_2 (Gorman et al., 1984) or a single inhalation of 35% CO_2 (Griez et al., 1987) induces panic attacks in PD patients. Many hypotheses have been offered to explain the panicogenic effect of lactate and CO_2. One is that CO_2 and lactate, after being metabolised to CO_2, induce panic attacks by stimulating the respiratory centres, which are hypersensitive in PD patients (Gorman et al., 1988; Liebowitz et al., 1984). This hypothesis is consistent with the "false suffocation alarm" theory of Klein (1993). This theory supposes that PD patients have a low

Anxiety Disorders: An Introduction to Clinical Management and Research. Edited by E. J. L. Griez, C. Faravelli, D. Nutt and J. Zohar. © 2001 John Wiley & Sons, Ltd.

stimulation threshold of the "asphisiostat", a physiological mechanism of protection from potentially lethal stimuli.

Yohimbine, an alpha-2 adrenergic antagonist, increases noradrenergic firing; it induces panic attacks in PD patients (Charney et al., 1992), suggesting a noradrenergic involvement in PD.

Caffeine in high doses can be anxiogenic and even panicogenic in normal subjects. Patients with PD are more sensitive to the panicogenic effects of caffeine than normal controls (Boulenger and Uhde, 1982; Charney et al., 1985).

Also, m-chlorophenylpiperazine, a mixed 5-HT agonist-antagonist, and fenfluramine, a 5-HT releasing drug, have both been reported to provoke panic attacks in challenge paradigms (Kahan and Wetzler, 1991; Targum and Marshall, 1989), suggesting a role for 5-HT in PD pathogenesis. Cholecystokinin-tetrapeptide (CCK-4), a CCK agonist, is panicogenic in man (Bradwejn et al., 1990; Bradwejn et al., 1993; Javanmard et al., 1999).

Neurotransmitter Systems

The neurotransmitter systems more studied in PD are the noradrenergic, serotoninergic and gamma-aminobutyric acid (GABA)-ergic ones. With regard to noradrenergic system, an hyperactivity of the locus coeruleus (LC), the main central noradrenergic nucleus, has been supposed (Klein, 1964; Redmond and Huang, 1979); the increasing firing rate of the LC may be due to a dysfunction of noradrenergic receptors (Charney et al., 1992). The relationship between 5-HT and panic is complex (Bell and Nutt, 1998). There are two opposing hypotheses attempting to explain PD based on a serotoninergic dysfunction: 5-HT excess (Iversen, 1984) and 5-HT defect (Eriksson, 1993). The 5-HT excess theory suggests that patients with PD either have an increased level of 5-HT release or a supersensitivity of postsynaptic receptors. The 5-HT deficit theory proposes that, in particular brain regions, 5-HT has a restraining effect on panic behaviour and, when there is a deficit of 5-HT, this restraint is reduced and panic ensues. With regard to the GABA-ergic system, in PD patients a shift of BDZ receptor in the inverse agonist direction or relative deficiency of an hypothetical anxiolytic ligand has been proposed (Little et al., 1987; Nutt et al., 1990; Nutt and Lawson, 1993).

Furthermore, dysfunction of dopaminergic system is indicated by panic attacks induced by dopaminergic agents (Pitchot et al., 1992). Involvement of the opioid system is suggested by observation of naltrexone-induced panic attacks (Maremmani et al., 1998). Cholinergic abnormalities could also be involved; Yergani et al. (1994) suggested that altered sympatovagal balance may contribute to panicogenic effects of lactate in PD patients. Moreover, an important role for neuromodulator systems, such as CCK and CRH systems, is emerging (Bradwejn et al., 1990; Bradwejn et al., 1993; Javanmard et al., 1999; Holsboer et al., 1991; Abelson and Curtis, 1996).

Neuroanatomical Models

Gray (1988) proposed the earliest neuroanatomical model for anxiety. Such a model outlines a septohippocampal brain circuit and identifies behavioural inhibition as one of the potentially important functions for specific brain structures and their connections. Gorman et al. (1989) were the first authors to propose a neuroanatomical model specific to PD and they coherently accounted for the various clinical features of PD: panic attacks (discharge of brain stem nuclei), anticipatory anxiety (limbic activation and kindling), agoraphobia/fearful avoidance (prefrontal cortical activation).

More recently, attention has been paid to amygdala, a phylogenetically ancient structure playing a central role in conditioned fear (Le Doux et al., 1990). Dysfunction in the amygdala, due perhaps to a lack of control by more recent cerebral structures, may result in amygdaloid activation and panic attack (Grove et al., 1997; Windmann, 1998; Coplan and Lydiard, 1998).

Brain Imaging

Reiman et al., using positron emission tomography (PET), noted an exaggeration of the asymmetrical (right greater than left) parahippocampal gyrus cerebral blood flow in association with hypocapnia in lactate-sensitive PD subjects (Reiman, 1987; Reiman et al., 1989a; Reiman et al., 1989b). Nordahl et al. (1998) replicated the finding of exaggerated parahippocampal asymmetry (right greater than left) in PD patients using deoxyglucose PET. Using single positron emission tomography (SPECT), bilateral hippocampal hypoperfusion and exaggerated asymmetry (right greater than left) of inferior frontal cortical perfusion blood flow in lactate-sensitive PD subjects were noted (de Cristofaro et al., 1993). SPECT studies using the BDZ antagonist [123I]-iomazenil also showed an increased asymmetry (right greater than left) of ligand binding in the inferior and middle prefrontal cortex in PD patients (Kuikka et al., 1995). In a PET study measuring regional cerebral blood flow (r-CBF) during an unexpected panic attack, panic was associated with decreased r-CBF in the right orbitofrontal, prelimbic, anterior cingulate and anterior temporal cortices (Fischer et al., 1998). Bisaga et al. (1998) found a significant increase in glucose metabolism in the left hippocampus and parahippocampal area in PD patients at rest in comparison with that found in normal subjects. In addition, a significant decrease was found in metabolism in the right inferior parietal and right superior temporal brain regions of the PD subjects when compared with that of the normal subjects. Nordahl et al. (1998) found the same abnormally low left/right hippocampal and posterior inferior prefrontal regional cerebral glucose metabolic rates (r-CMRglc) ratios in treated PD patients and untreated PD patients. The general pattern of an exaggeration of the normally observed right to left asymmetry in panic-sensitive subjects is of interest and seems to be consistent, though it requires further investigation.

A second feature of neuroimaging in PD is the cerebral hypervasoconstriction observed during hyperventilation and panic attacks. SPECT studies of lactate infusion demonstrated generally increased cerebral blood flow (CBF), except in panic patients experiencing an attack during infusion, in which case there was a blunting or decrease in CBF. SPECT studies with yohimbine-induced anxiety also revealed vasoconstriction (Woods et al., 1988). Other groups have noted that even in healthy subjects high levels of anxiety are accompanied by decreases in CBF and brain metabolism (Gur et al., 1987). Regionally "perceived" anoxia in key areas of the brain that are activated by inadvertent hyperventilation and ensuing hypocapnea may mediate escape responses from situations that are phylogenetically selected for their occasional potential for fatal consequence (Coplan and Lydiard, 1998). More recent PET data by Reiman (1997) has posited abnormal function of internally cued alarm "systems", particularly in the anterior insular cortex and anterior temporal regions in patients with PD.

Psychological Models

Psychodynamic, behavioural and cognitive psychological models of panic disorder have been formulated.

Psychodynamic Models

Freud (1894), in his early psychoanalytic theory of anxiety, viewed anxiety as a result of failure in defence mechanisms; in a successive theory he considered anxiety as a cause and trigger of defence mechanisms (1926). More modern psychodynamic theories, as articulated by Shear et al. (1993), stress the contribution of parenting styles and early experiences to psychological vulnerability for anxiety.

Behavioural Models

Early behavioural explanation of panic focused on the role of classical or Pavlovian conditioning in PD. Generally, these models involve the pairing of physiological sensations (conditioned stimulus) such as palpitations with hyperventilation or lactation (unconditioned stimulus), which triggers panic/anxiety (Eysenk, 1968). Theories that are more recent also focused on conditioning processes (Wolpe and Rowan, 1988; Seligman, 1988; Barlow, 1988).

Cognitive Models

Among cognitive models, there are Clark's theory, Barlow's false alarm theory and anxiety sensitivity theory. According to Clark's theory, individuals who experience recurrent panic attacks have a relatively enduring tendency to interpret certain bodily sensations in a catastrophic fashion. The misinterpreted sensations are basically those involved in normal anxiety responses (e.g., palpitations, breathlessness, dizziness, paresthesias). The catastrophic misinterpretations involve perceiving these sensations as much more dangerous than they really are, and, in particular, interpreting the sensations as indicative of an *immediately* impending physical or mental disaster. Examples are perceiving a slight feeling of breathlessness as evidence of impending cessation of breathing and consequent death, perceiving palpitations as evidence of an impending heart attack, perceiving a pulsing sensation in the forehead as evidence of a brain haemorrhage, or perceiving a shaky feeling as evidence of impending loss of control and insanity (Clark, 1988, p. 149). Both external and internal stimuli can provoke panic attacks. The sequence culminating in an attack starts with the stimuli being interpreted as a sign of impending danger. This interpretation generates a state of apprehension, which is associated with a wide range of bodily sensation. If these anxiety-produced sensations are interpreted in a catastrophic fashion, a further increase in apprehension occurs, producing more bodily sensations, leading to a vicious circle that culminates in a panic attack. This theory accounts both for panic attacks preceded by raised anxiety and for panic attacks coming "out of the blue". For both types of attack, it is argued that the critical event is the misinterpretation of certain bodily sensations, caused by anxiety in one case and by a different emotional state or by an innocuous event such as exercising, in the other. When applying the cognitive theory to individual patients, it is often useful to distinguish between the first panic attack and the subsequent development of repeated panic attacks and panic disorder. Community surveys (Brown and Cash, 1990; Wilson et al., 1991) indicate about 7–28% of the normal population will experience an occasional unexpected panic attack. The cognitive theory assumes that individuals only go on to develop repeated panic attacks and panic disorder (3–5% of the general population, Wittchen and Essau, 1991) if they develop a tendency to interpret these perceived autonomic events in a catastrophic fashion. Such a tendency could either be a consequence of learning experiences that pre-date the first attack (Ehlers, 1993), or could arise as a consequence of the way the patient, physicians and significant others respond to the first attack.

Barlow describes panic as the basic emotion of fear, which is considered to be an acute reaction to perceived imminent danger when no danger is present (Barlow, 1988; Barlow, 1991). He identifies three types of alarm: true alarms (immediate danger present), false alarms (panic attacks) and learned alarms (conditioned panic attacks). Barlow's model of panic disorder includes a biological diathesis (propensity to experience arousal under stress) and a psychological vulnerability (influenced by factor such as early life events and parenting style). Psychologically vulnerable individuals fail to develop a sense of competence with respect to the world and themselves, and experience poor predictability and control over life events, such as intense emotional states. For biologically and psychologically vulnerable individuals, an initial false alarm may be followed by arousal and self-focused attention (anxious apprehension) centring on the possibility of experiencing further panic attacks and the belief that the attacks are dangerous. In addition, internal somatic or cognitive cues and sensations can become associated with the experience of false alarm (interoceptive conditioning), so that the experience of somatic symptoms triggers a panic attack. Such interoceptive-cued attacks are supposed to be learned alarms. Interoceptive sensitivity and anxious apprehension may contribute to avoidance of activities and situations associated with somatic sensations and cues. The avoidance then becomes negatively reinforced, since the individual believes that an attack has been averted owing to escape or avoidance.

According to the anxiety sensitivity theory, this is characterised by a belief that, beyond any immediate physical discomfort, anxiety and its associated symptoms may cause deleterious physical, psychological or social consequences (Taylor et al., 1992). Anxiety sensitivity differs from interoceptive conditioning in that the former does not refer to a conditioned response pattern to physical sensations, but to the individual's belief that the anxiety symptoms are harmful; thus conditioning is not necessary for anxiety sensitivity (McNally, 1994). Anxiety sensitivity is also distinguished from catastrophic misinterpretations of anxiety. Although individuals with PD may be inclined to make such misinterpretations, they may be fully aware of the causes of their sensations, and still hold an inherent belief that the sensations alone are dangerous (McNally, 1994). One of the most common measures of anxiety sensitivity is the Anxiety Sensitivity Index (Reiss et al., 1986). Anxiety sensitivity has been found to be normally distributed in the population; individuals with PD and agoraphobia have been found to score higher than individuals with other anxiety disorders, who in turn score higher than normal controls. Anxiety sensitivity is thought to put an individual at increased risk of developing anxiety disorders in general and PD with agoraphobia in particular.

In conclusion, it can be said that theoretical models of panic, from biological, psychological and, ultimately, integrative perspective, will be far more complex than the focused linear models currently undergoing evaluation. It seems likely that both biological and psychological vulnerabilities may be non-specific, and that the development of specific panic and anxiety disorders may involve a variety of experiences at different developmental stages to activate these non-specific diatheses. Future theory building should emphasise an integrated approach, considering such stages.

Areas of Controversy and Debate

Since the introduction of the DSM-III, the nosological position of PD has been controversial. Two main positions have arisen and given rise to a long-lasting debate. Most North American psychiatrists consider the panic attack to be the central feature of the disorder. Panic is seen as a pathological, primary phenomenon, central to the origin of the disorder. Its association with agoraphobia is interpreted as the avoidance behaviour being a secondary or a derived phenomenon, both aetiopathogenetically and chronologically (Klein, 1981; Klein, 1987). This position considers the panic attack as a predominantly biological event, qualitatively distinct from the others forms of anxiety. Moreover, the American view of PD is that repeated, sudden and spontaneous panic attacks are only seen in panic disorder. Panic attacks seen in other conditions are not spontaneous. Since agoraphobia is only considered a consequence of panic, this position denies its existence without panic. Several studies support this view. The fact that panic attacks could be experimentally provoked in predisposed subjects by a series of chemical challenges reinforced the hypothesis of a biological origin of PD. The possibility of provoking anxiety in normal subjects and increasing panic attacks in panic patients by the use of yohimbine or isoproterenol point to an important role for the noradrenergic system in PD (Charney et al., 1984; Charney et al., 1992; Pyke and Greenberg, 1986). Consistent with this hypothesis is the observation that drugs preventing spontaneous panic attacks appear to reduce the locus coeruleus firing rate (Svenson and Usdin, 1978), whereas the panicogenic stimuli usually increase this firing. In favour of the American view are also electroencephalographic data, which show that night panics occur outside rapid eye movement phases of sleep (Akiskal et al., 1984; Hauri et al., 1989; Mellman and Uhde, 1989). Changes in EEG (Beauclaire and Fontaine, 1986; Edlund et al., 1987; Lepola and Nousiainen, 1990) and cerebral blood flow (Reiman et al., 1984; Reiman et al., 1986; Reiman et al., 1989b), anatomical abnormalities in the mesiotemporal region on magnetic resonance imaging (Fontaine et al., 1990), hyposensitivity to benzodiazepines (Roy-Byrne et al., 1990) and neurological soft signs have all been reported in PD. As a confirmation of some biological abnormality, Nutt et al. (1990) demonstrated that flumazenil is anxiogenic in patients with PD: possible explanations of this finding are that in PD there is a relative deficiency of an anxiolytic ligand, or that the set point of the benzodiazepine receptor is shifted in the inverse agonist direction.

Not all these findings may be unequivocally interpreted as in favour of the biological view. The response to a chemical challenge, for instance, can be seen as the intrapsychic dramatisation of bodily sensations, rather than as a specific substance response. The fact that the various chemical challenges do not share any common mechanisms could be explained on this basis. In addition, the broad range of drugs effective for panic could suggest a low biological specificity. Moreover, the specificity of the response of panic anxiety to tricicylic antidepressants has not been confirmed in other trials, where other forms of anxiety, e.g., GAD, proved to respond to these drugs (Kahan et al., 1986; Klein et al., 1985).

Many European psychiatrists contend that the single panic attack is an aspecific phenomenon, which can be found in many other conditions: somatic illness, depression, alcohol abuse, borderline states, acute psychosis, etc. (Breier et al., 1984; Lesser et al., 1988; Noyes et al., 1990; George et al., 1990; Himle and Hill, 1991; Krystal et al., 1992). Isolated panic attacks are also frequent in normal subjects (Joyce et al., 1989; Klerman et al., 1991). This position therefore contends that panic *per se* is neither specific nor pathological. Panic becomes pathological when its occurrence is combined with specific premorbid vulnerability factors. Preconstitutive aspects of panic must exist either as a peculiar cognitive pattern or as a vulnerability to environmental events. The European position maintains that a phobic attitude precedes the development of panic and that specific temperamental features are necessary in order for PD to occur. There are findings that seem to support this position. All community epidemiological studies report the presence of a consistent rate of subjects affected by agoraphobia without panic attacks (Angst and Dobler-Mikola, 1985; Weissman et al., 1985; Wittchen, 1986; Faravelli et al., 1989). Patients affected by PD were reported to show prodromal symptoms before the onset of the disorder (Fava et al., 1988; Lelliott et al., 1988; Fava et al., 1992). The presence of personological-temperamental traits predisposing to agoraphobia is also supported by empirical verification. As often happens with biological data, however, all these findings may lend themselves to different interpretation. For instance, the abnormal response to life events could be due to impairment of the cerebral neuroendocrine systems that should cope with stress. Recent findings report that patients with PD show a blunted adrenocorticotropic hormone response to corticotropin-releasing hormone (CRH) in association with basal hypercortisolism (Roy-Byrne et al., 1986; Gold et al., 1988; Holsboer et al., 1991; Abelson and Curtis, 1996; Coplan et al., 1998).

The Evolutionary Perspective

The two positions briefly outlined represent two extremes, built up by following two strong ideological theories of the disorder: (1) *biological* PD is due to a brain dysfunction; (2) *psychological* PD is caused by the sequence of the previous social interactions. A third body of evidence, based on an *evolutionary* perspective is usually ignored. This theory states that:

1. Anxiety (or at least an anxiety-like phenomenon) is present in all the animal species, it is adaptive and useful both for the preparation of a fight or flight action and for the communication of danger in social animals.
2. Almost all the physical phenomena by which this process of activation are mediated by the autonomic nervous system (ANS), and namely by a sympathetic stimulation.
3. The somatic symptoms of panic are expression of an ortho-sympathetic stimulation.
4. ANS dysreactivity has been consistently reported in PD and increased values of autonomic functions are common observations in patients with PD even outside the panic attacks (Faravelli et al., 1997).
5. The cognition of danger is not necessarily acquired: a typical example is that of new-born chicks that are scared by the shadow of a hawk even though they have never experienced a predator. There is sensible support for the view that phobias could be considered to be the persistence of innate adaptive fears.
6. Agoraphobia definitely has a certain adaptive value: it contrasts the exploratory instinct and protects the offspring of any species from naturally occurring dangers. In the animal kingdom, agoraphobic-like behaviours are frequent: mice always cross a room following the walls and never cross it in a straight line or

diagonally. Many animals predispose safe ways of returning to their holes, and when such ways are interrupted, they show panic-like behaviours. Even among humans, the agoraphobic phenomenon is useful at least during the first years of life. It closely resembles innate behavioural patterns, which are present also in humans and which must be necessarily transmitted through precognitive biological pathways. On this basis, agoraphobia is more easily understandable in the evolutionary perspective rather than using purely psychological (symbolic) interpretations. Agoraphobia would represent the persistence (or the lack of suppression) of an instinct which is normal in earlier phases of development. When the transmission of agoraphobia is stronger, the disease would appear. An enhanced message would induce an increased vegetative response, provoking panic. In this perspective, the distinction between panic and agoraphobia would be more quantitative than qualitative.

The evolutionary approach could help to reduce the gap between purely biological and purely psychological positions.

TREATMENT

PD is perhaps the disorder for which the greatest number of therapeutic strategies have been tested. In spite of a very large number of treatments that have proved to be effective, PD is nevertheless one of the most difficult tasks for the therapist. In fact, while treatments are generally very useful, the compliance of the patients is perhaps the worst in the entire psychiatric panorama and the attrition rate (i.e. the number of cases that drop out during the treatment) may reach 50% (Cassano et al., 1988; Cassano et al., 1992). The main problem the therapist is facing is therefore that of vehiculating the treatment to the patient. In fact, treating PD patients is difficult for the following reasons:

1. PD patients are more responsive to some somatic side-effects of antidepressants, probably because of their vegetative dysreactivity.
2. They are more intolerant to side-effects, and often misinterpret them.
3. Their attitude towards drugs is commonly phobic, i.e., they are afraid of dependence, toxicity, etc.
4. Their need for control prevents them from completely trusting the therapist and from relaxing.

Pharmacological and cognitive-behavioural interventions are considered the most extensive treatments studied in this field.

Pharmacotherapy

Controlled clinical trials have established efficacy in the treatment of PD for two main classes of drugs: benzodiazepines (BDZs) and antidepressants (AD), including tricyclic antidepressants (TCAs), monoamine oxidase inhibitors (MAOIs), and selective serotonin re-uptake inhibitors (SSRIs) (Burrows et al., 1991; APA, 1998; Den Boer, 1998; Sheehan, 1999). Comparative studies suggest that all these classes of compounds can be efficacious. Differences are apparent with respect to speed of onset, side-effect profiles, safety and complications of long-term therapy, such as the ease of discontinuing medication. The latter consideration is particularly important, since for the majority of patients PD is a continuous, chronic disorder requiring treatment for at least 6–8 months, and longer in most cases (Ballanger, 1991).

The BDZs act rapidly (in minutes to hours), whereas the antidepressants work slower (over several weeks). Concerns about dependence and withdrawal aspects of the BDZs have led to recommendations that their use be restricted to the short-term administration, ideally less than four weeks, which will then present problems in enduring conditions such as PD. Therefore, there is a general consensus that the pharmacological treatment of PD means antidepressants. Although MAOI (mainly fenelzine) has proven to be highly effective in all the trials, in practice, the choice is limited to TCAs and SSRIs because of the difficulties and limitations of MAOIs. The general opinion is that SSRIs should be used as first-line treatment for PD as they are safer and better tolerated, having similar efficacy as TCAs. Their side-effect profile is relatively mild, especially when used in low doses at the start of treatment. Some authors, however, suggest that in some cases TCAs, especially clomipramine, should not be abandoned.

Benzodiazepines (BDZs)

Among BDZs, alprazolam and clonazepam have been reported to be efficacious in the treatment of PD. They maintain their efficacy as antipanic agents during chronic therapy. Significant tolerance to the therapeutic effects does not appear to occur, with lower doses often employed during maintenance treatment (Burrows et al., 1992). Relapse rates are high when BDZs are withdrawn, while many patients experience withdrawal syndrome even during a slow tapering off of the drug (Fyer et al., 1987; Howell et al., 1987; Du Pont and Pecknold, 1985). In BDZ-dependent patients, withdrawal reactions were observed in the majority of patients following abrupt discontinuation of the drug (Rickels et al., 1990). The effects of BDZ withdrawal are well recognised (Greenblatt and Shader, 1978; Hallstrom and Lader, 1981; Owen and Tyrer, 1983; Browne and Hauge, 1986; Tyrer and Murphy, 1987). Although a high dose and long duration of BDZ administration are most often associated with withdrawal syndromes, even normal or low doses (Hallstrom and Lader, 1981) and short-term therapy (Tyrer and Murphy, 1987) are implicated in withdrawal phenomena. Experiencing withdrawal effects of BDZs could lead to reinstitution of the drug and therefore reinforcing dependence. According to the authors, BDZ should be prescribed only for sporadic, symptomatic use.

Tricyclic Antidepressants (TCAs)

Among TCAs, imipramine and clomipramine have been extensively studied. Both drugs are efficacious in the treatment of PD, and patients' benefits concern the most important clinical aspects (panic attacks, anticipatory anxiety, and phobic avoidance behaviour). Clomipramine is suggested as being more efficacious than imipramine, indicating that drugs with predominantly serotoninergic effect may have greater antipanic effect. For this reason it is speculated that intravenous clomipramine could be a very effective agent in refractory cases because of the low desmethylation ratio (which maintains the 5-HT potency) compared with the same drug per os. The side-effects of TCAs may be a major hindrance to their wider applicability in panic patients, being very sensitive to any symptoms imitating anxiety attack. An initial exacerbation of anxiety symptoms has frequently been noticed (Munjack et al., 1988), and experts advise more gradual dose increases for panic patients than for depressed patients (Klerman et al., 1993). The delay of onset of improvement is not an argument against the use of TCAs, considering the chronicity of PD. Discontinuation symptoms have been described for antidepressants, but they have not been observed as a major problem in controlled studies, in contrast to treatment with alprazolam. The major advantages of antidepressants compared with BDZs are that physical dependence does not develop and that discontinuation can be instituted more rapidly. The optimal time to treatment discontinuation has not been determined. Patients are often initially treated for three months and responders continue treatment for 6–12 months, but some need longer maintenance treatment (Lecrubier et al., 1997).

In a comprehensive review of the course and outcome of panic patients (Roy-Byrne and Cowley, 1994) it was concluded that with modern treatment most patients will improve, but few will be cured. The presence of agoraphobia, depression and personality disorders indicates a poorer prognosis. Thus, a majority of patients may require long-term treatment. These issues were reviewed by Burrows et al. (1992) and they concluded that long-term treatment with TCAs did not lead to loss of efficacy, whereas high rates of relapse were observed after the discontinuation. A systematic double-blind comparison of maintenance therapy for up to eight months in patients treated with alprazolam, imipramine or placebo showed that the therapeutic gains obtained in short-term trial persisted in all groups. Nevertheless, fewer placebo patients remained throughout the whole study period; TCAs were well tolerated and no intolerance to their efficacy was indicated (Curtis et al., 1993). Another study of long-term treatment of PD showed that a higher percentage of patients withdrew from the placebo group than from the clomipramine and paroxetine groups. A similar distribution of percentage was obtained with patients who withdrew owing to lack of efficacy. An unexpected finding was that the early observed, large placebo response persisted (Lecrubrier et al., 1997).

Monoamine Oxidase Inhibitors (MAOIs)

In all the trials where phenelzine was used in one of the group, it came out as the most effective drug, even though not significantly so. However, there is less evidence based on controlled trials for MAOIs, both the classical irreversible and modern reversible inhibitors, than for TCAs and SSRIs. Their main mode of action may be on phobic anxiety (Roth and Argyle, 1988; Hollander et al., 1990; Van Vliet et al., 1993).

Selective Serotonin Re-uptake Inhibitors (SSRIs)

During a recent NIMH Algorithm Development Meeting, the expert panel reached the conclusion that the SSRIs had become the pharmacological treatment of choice for PD (Jobson and Potter, 1995). There is now a large body of evidence documenting that SSRIs are effective and probably deserve to be the pharmacological treatment of choice in PD for many patients (Davidson, 1998; Nutt, 1998). SSRIs have been available for a decade, and include fluvoxamine, fluoxetine, paroxetine, sertraline and citalopram. All of them have proved capable of reducing panic attacks and agoraphobia in PD patients.

A series of placebo-controlled trials have demonstrated that fluvoxamine is superior to placebo in the treatment of PD (Asnis, 1992; Hoehn-Saric et al., 1993; Hoehn-Saric et al., 1994; Woods et al., 1994; Nair et al., 1996; Holland et al., 1994). There are several studies comparing the efficacy of fluvoxamine with other agents. In a study comparing fluvoxamine with clomipramine, both drugs were effective, but the positive effects of clomipramine occurred earlier and were somewhat superior to those of fluvoxamine (Den Boer et al., 1987). In a comparison of fluvoxamine with brofaromine (a reversible MAOI), no significant differences were found (Van Vliet et al., 1996). Den Boer and Westenberg, comparing fluvoxamine with maprotiline (a specific norepinephrine re-uptake blocker), found that the patients on fluvoxamine experienced a significant decrease in panic attacks and in the other symptoms of PD. Significant improvement, however, was not seen in the maprotiline patients, but when maprotiline patients were switched to fluvoxamine, most of them responded well (Den Boer and Westenberg, 1996). According to the authors, this is one of the clearest studies suggesting that serotonin medication is more efficacious than a noradrenergic drug. On the other hand, other studies support the efficacy of noradrenergic drugs, such desipramine and nortriptyline (Munjack et al., 1988; Kalus et al., 1991; Sasson et al., 1999).

After eight weeks in an open trial with citalopram, 13 out of 17 patients had responded in terms of an antipanic effect. Sixteen of the patients continued in a 15-month long-term maintenance trial, with 11 of them completing this portion of the study. Initial gains were maintained throughout this longer period, with further improvement in some patients, including two patients who had failed to respond in the initial eight-week trial. There was no tolerance to early positive effects. The mean dose of citalopram fell from 41 mg/day after eight weeks to 38 mg/day at the end of the 15-month trial (Humble et al., 1989). Bertani et al. (1996) reported a positive response in four of the five patients on 20–40 mg/day. Longer-term follow-up studies of citalopram in PD are underway following the trial described above and preliminary results suggest maintenance of positive acute effects for over a year (Lepola, 1997).

Paroxetine was the first SSRI to obtain a licensed indication for PD (1995) and has been the most extensively studied SSRI in PD. A large trial (Oehrberg et al., 1995), carried out in 39 centres in 13 countries, provided definitive evidence of paroxetine efficacy. This trial involved 367 patients randomised to paroxetine, clomipramine and placebo. Patients from this study could choose at the end of the 12-week trial whether they wanted to enter a long-term extension of the study for nine months or be titrated off over a three-week period. Patients were abruptly discontinued from paroxetine and there was no evidence of withdrawal syndrome.

Two large, double-blind, placebo-controlled, flexible-dose trials have been completed with sertraline (Baumel et al., 1996; Wolkow et al., 1996), and will be discussed as one trial (Pollak et al., 1997; Pohl et al., 1997). In total, 342 patients from 20 US and Canadian centres were randomised to either sertraline or placebo. Dosages began at 25 mg/day for one week, and were then increased to between 50 and 200 mg/day based on clinical response and tolerability over the 10-week trial. Panic attack frequency was reduced significantly more in the sertraline group, beginning in the second week and was sustained throughout each week of the trial. Significant differences between sertraline and placebo emerged in the first week on "Panic Attack Burden" (the frequency of attacks multiplied by their severity): the percentage of patients who had no attacks was higher than the percentage on placebo, and the reduction of panic attacks was greater than for placebo as early as weeks two and four.

Although controlled trials for fluoxetine in PD are underway, these have not yet been presented or published. Results from open trials indicated efficacy of fluoxetine in PD treatment (Gorman et al., 1987; Pecknold et al., 1995; Coplan et al., 1997).

Paroxetine is the only SSRI that has a clear target dose (40 mg). For the sertraline, there is some suggestion that 100–150 mg might be the recommended dosage range. Fluoxetine in the range between 20 and 80 mg has been associated with response. Fluvoxamine has been demonstrated to be effective at 50–150 mg. The patients should begin treatment with as low a dose of the medication as can be practically arranged. Trials comparing paroxetine with clomipramine found that paroxetine's action was somewhat more rapid, there was reduction of more of the ancillary symptoms of PD in long-term maintenance on paroxetine, and paroxetine had significantly fewer side-effects (Lecrubier et al., 1997). Studies comparing fluvoxamine with clomipramine suggested that the two agents are approximately equal (Dick and Ferrer, 1983) or clomipramine was more effective than fluvoxamine in reducing anxiety and depressive symptoms (Den Boer et al., 1987). In a trial comparing citalopram and clomipramine, both drugs were effective, with little reported differences (Wade, 1995; Lepola, 1997). In the absence of adequate direct comparison, it would be difficult to compare SSRIs in terms of side-effects. They seem to share a cluster of side-effects (nausea, asthenia, etc.); whether there are lower rates of these various symptoms with one agent or another will have to wait for trials on direct comparisons. In conclusion, there is now a large body of evidence that SSRIs are effective and probably deserve to be the pharmacological treatment of first choice in PD for many patients.

Other Drugs

There have also been studies of other drug treatments (non-antidepressant and non-BDZ), with limited controlled double-blind studies of efficacy: noradrenergic receptor agonists and antagonists (Charney et al., 1992; Munjack et al., 1985), anticonvulsants (Woodman and Noyes, 1994; Tondo et al., 1989), GABA-B agonists (Breslow et al., 1989), dopaminergic agents (Pitchot et al., 1992), calcium-channel blockers (Klein and Uhde, 1988), drug active as neuropeptide receptors (Kramer et al., 1995) and strategies involving second-messenger systems (Benjamin et al., 1995). In general, despite encouraging results for many of these agents in case reports and open trials, efficacy has not been substantially established in double-blind controlled studies.

Caveat

It is commonly accepted that, in the age of the evidence-based medicine, only well-designed controlled studies should be taken into consideration to evaluate the efficacy of a treatment. However, a series of limitations prevents the simple transposition of the findings of the clinical trials into medical practice, as they are. Clinical trials in phase III are undertaken for the regulatory agencies rather than to establish a real pattern of use of drugs. The real needs of the clinicians are not entirely answered by the clinical trials: long-term treatments, concomitant medical treatments, comorbid physical and psychiatric disorders, suicidality, subjective intolerance are all examples of variants that can strongly influence the prescriptive pattern, and for which there is scant, if any, information. The newer antidepressants are surely much safer in overdose and generally better tolerated than TCAs. On the other hand, they are much more expensive and are not devoid of unwanted effects. The two main problems in the long-term treatment with traditional TCAs are not dry mouth, constipation or other side-effects, but weight gain and sexual problems. These may be also present with at least some SSRIs, such as paroxetine. Finally, there is the general bias of the commercial aspect: almost all the trials are sponsored and there is no guarantee that negative results have the same probability of being published.

Psychotherapy

Overall, psychological approaches have proved effective in the treatment of PD and PD with agoraphobia. Psychological treatment of PD has been shown to be more effective than no treatment, psychosocial "placebo" intervention and even some psychopharmacological interventions (Gould et al., 1995; Barlow and Lehman, 1996). Behavioural, cognitive and cognitive-behavioural approaches in particular have been shown to be useful in the treatment of PD. Psychodynamic interventions have not been evaluated in controlled studies, although in 1996 it was still the more frequently used form of psychotherapy (Goisman et al., 1999).

Behavioural, cognitive and cognitive-behavioural therapies are empirically validated for PD treatment. The rationale for the cognitive and cognitive-behavioural treatment of panic stems from the cognitive and behavioural theories of panic, respectively. Cognitive approaches to treatment assume that teaching patients to examine and modify their cognitive misconceptions can directly change cognition and cognitive schemata. In the cognitive therapy of PD, the therapist explains the nature of panic, anxiety and anxiety-related symptoms and identifies, or helps the patient to identify, "automatic thoughts", the central misinterpretations of panic symptoms and their consequences. The therapist then shows the patients some strategies to correct or evaluate their cognitive errors: (a) self-statement training, in which a neutral or more accurate statement is practised in place of the former negative statement; (b) probability revaluation, in which the actual probabilities of catastrophic consequences are more realistically examined; (c) decatastophising, in which the feared impact of consequences of panic are assessed more rationally; and (d) homework assignments are designed to help patients first identify and subsequently challenge the maladaptive cognition.

There are many studies evaluating the effectiveness of the cognitive treatment of PD. Two influential treatment protocols are the Panic Control Treatment, developed by Barlow (Barlow, 1988; Barlow and Cerny, 1988; Barlow and Craske, 1989), and the cognitive approach developed by Clark (Clark, 1988; Clark, 1989; Salkovskis and Clark, 1991). These protocols have been evaluated in controlled treatment studies. Recently , Bakker et al. (1999) compared paroxetine, clomipramine and cognitive therapy based on the model of Clark; in this study, the drugs induced significant improvement, whereas cognitive therapy did not differ significantly from placebo. PD is one of the most active research areas of clinical psychology, providing competing theories and new treatments. The relationship between psychological and physical treatments of PD is often a source of discussion. Drugs are easier to use, faster in the onset of attack, more available, but their effect does not seem to persist after treatment discontinuation. A combined approach seems to be the preferred choice in clinical practice. Certainly, essential elements in psychological approaches, such as explanation of clinical and pathogenetic issues and engaging the patient in a therapeutic alliance, are critical in maximising the value of drug treatment.

CONCLUSION

Panic disorder is a disabling, distressing psychiatric condition, which causes social and occupational disruption, and leads to requests for medical investigations. PD patients have a great comorbidity especially with agoraphobia and depression and show high risk for suicidal ideation and attempts.

Panic attacks and PD appear to be a privileged field of study of the interactions, which can exist in humans, between genetic, biological, psychological and behavioural factors. All of them probably contribute not only to the development of the disorder, but also to the intrafamilial, intergenerational maintenance of it.

REFERENCES

Abelson JL, Curtis GC (1996) Hypotalamic-pituitary-adrenal axis activity in panic disorder: Prediction of long-term outcome by pretreatment cortisol levels. *Am J Psychiatry* **153**: 69–73.

Akiskal HS, Lemmi H, Dickson H (1984) Chronic depression: Part 2: Sleep EEG differentiation of primary dysthymic disorders from anxious depression. *J Affect Dis* **6**: 287–295.

American Psychiatric Association (1998) Practice guideline for the treatment of patients with panic disorder. *Am J Psychiatry* **155**(5): 1–34.

Angst J, Dobler-Mikola A (1985) The Zurich Study: anxiety and phobia in young adults. *Eur Arch Psychiatr Neurol Sci* **235**: 171–178.

Asnis GM (1992) Effects of fluvoxamine on the treatment of panic disorder: A placebo-controlled trial. *Ann Psiquichiatric* (Madrid); **8** Suppl 1: 78.

Bakker A, van Dick R, Spinhoven P, van Balcom A (1999) Paroxetine, clomipramine and cognitive therapy in the treatment of panic disorder. *J Clin Psychiatry* **60**: 831–838.

Ballanger JC (1991) Long-term pharmacologic treatment of panic disorder. *J Clin Psychiatry* **52** Suppl 2: 18–23.

Barlow DH (1988) *Anxiety and its Disorders*. New York: Guilford Press.

Barlow DH (1991) Disorders of emotion. *Psychol Inquiry* **2**: 58–71.

Barlow DH, Cerny JA (1988) *Psychological Treatment of Panic*. New York: Guilford Press.

Barlow DH, Craske MG (1989) *Mastery of Your Anxiety and Panic*. Albany, NY: Graywind Publications.

Barlow DH, Lehman CL (1996) Advances in the psychosocial treatment of anxiety disorders: implications for national health care. *Arch Gen Psychiatry* **53**: 727–735.

Baumel B, Bielski R, Carman J et al. (1996) Double-blind comparison of sertraline and placebo in patients with panic disorder. Paper presented at Collegium Internationale Neuro-Psychopharmacologicum, June 1996, Melbourne, Australia.

Beauclaire L, Fontaine R (1986) Epileptiform abnormalities in panic disorders. Paper presented at the Society of Biological Psychiatry Annual Convention.

Bell CJ, Nutt DJ (1998) Serotonin and panic. *Br J Psychiatry* **172**: 465–471.

Benjamin MP, Levine J, Fux M et al. (1995) Double blind, placebo controlled, cross-over trial of inositol treatment for panic disorder. *Am J Psychiatry* **152**: 1004–1006.

Bertani A, Perna G, Politi E, Bellodi L (1996) Citalopram and panic disorder. *Depression and Anxiety* **4**: 253.

Bisaga A, Katz JL, Antonini A et al. (1998) Cerebral glucose metabolism in women with panic disorder. *Am J Psychiatry* **155**(9): 1778–1783.

Boulenger JP, Uhde TW (1982) Caffeine consumption and anxiety: Preliminary results of a survey comparing patients with anxiety disorders and normal controls. *Psychopharmacol Bull* **18**: 73–98.

Bradwejn J, Koszycki D, Bourin M (1993) CCK-4 and panic disorder. In Montgomery SA (ed.) *Psychopharmacology of Panic*. Oxford: Oxford University Press.

Bradwejn J, Koszycki D, Meterissian G (1990) Cholecystokinin-tetrapeptide induced panic attacks in patients with panic disorder. *Can J Psychiatry* **35**: 83–85.

Breier A, Charney DS, Heninger GR (1984) Major depression in patients with agoraphobia and panic disorder. *Arch Gen Psychiatry* **41**: 1129–1135.

Breslow MF, Fankhauser MP, Potter RL et al. (1989) Role of GABA in antipanic drug efficacy. *Am J Psychiatry* **146**: 353–356.

Brown TA, Cash TF (1990) The phenomenon of non-clinical panic: Parameters of panic, fear, and avoidance. *J Anxiety Disorders* **4**: 15–29.

Browne JL, Hauge KJ (1986) A review of alprazolam withdrawal. *Drug Intelligence Clin Pharmacy* **20**: 837–841.

Burrows GD, Judd FK, Norman TR (1992) Long-term drug treatment of panic disorder. *J Psychiatr Res* **27** Suppl 1: 111–125.

Burrows GD, Norman TR, Judd FK (1991) Panic disorder: A treatment update. *J Clin Psychiatry* **52** Suppl 7: 24–26.

Cassano GB, Perugi G, McNair DM (1988) Panic disorder: Review of the empirical and rational basis of pharmacological treatment. *Pharmacopsychiatry* **21**(4): 157–165.

Cassano GB, Toni C, Musetti L (1992) Treatment of panic disorder. *Adv Biochem Psychopharmacol* **47**: 449–460.

Charney DS, Heninger GR (1984) Noradrenergic dysfunction in panic anxiety: Aetiology and treatment studies. *Clin Neuropharmacol* **7** Suppl: S99.

Charney DS, Heninger GR, Breier A (1984) Noradrenergic function and panic anxiety effects of yohimbine in healthy subjects and patients with agoraphobia and panic disorder. *Arch Gen Psychiatry* **41**: 751–763.

Charney DS, Heninger GR, Jallon PI (1985) Increased anxiogenic effects of caffeine in panic disorder. *Arch Gen Psychiatry* **42**: 233–243.

Charney DS, Woods SW, Kristal JH et al. (1992) Noradrenergic neuronal dysregulation in panic disorder: The effects of intravenous yohimbine and clonidine in panic disorder patients. *Acta Psychiatr Scand* **86**: 273–282.

Clark DM (1988) A cognitive model of panic. In Rachman S, Maser J (eds) *Panic: Psychological Perspectives*. Hillsdale, NJ: Erlbaum.

Clark DM (1989) Anxiety states. In Hawton K, Salvoskis P, Kirk T, Clark DM (eds) *Cognitive Behaviour Therapy for Psychiatric Problems*. Oxford: Oxford University Press.

Coplan JD, Goetz R, Klein DF et al. (1998) Plasma cortisol concentrations preceding lactate-induced panic: Psychological, biochemical, and physiological correlates. *Arch Gen Psychiatry* **55**(2): 130–136.

Coplan JD, Lydiard RB (1998) Brain circuits in panic disorder. *Biol Psychiatry* **44**(12): 1264–1276.

Coplan JD, Papp LA, Pine D et al. (1997) Clinical improvement with fluoxetine therapy with noradrenergic function in patients with panic disorder. *Arch Gen Psychiatry* **54**: 643–648.

Curtis GC, Massana J, Udina C et al. (1993) Maintenance drug therapy of panic disorder. *J Psychiatr Res* **27** Suppl 1: 127–142.

Davidson JRC (1998) The long-term treatment of panic disorder. *J Clin Psychiatry* **59**(8): 17–21.

De Cristofaro MTR, Sessarego A, Pupi A et al. (1993) Brain perfusion abnormalities in drug-naive lactate-sensitive panic patients: A SPECT study. *Biol Psychiatry* **33**: 505–512.

Den Boer JA (1998) Pharmacotherapy of panic disorder: differential efficacy from a clinical viewpoint. *J Clin Psychiatry* **59**(8): 30–36.

Den Boer JA, Westenberg HG (1996) Effect of a serotonin and noradrenaline uptake inhibitor in panic disorder: A double-blind comparative study with fluvoxamine and maprotiline. *Int Clin Psychopharmacol* **16**: 299–306.

Den Boer JA, Westenberg HGM, Kamerbeek WDJ et al. (1987) Effect of serotonin uptake inhibitors in anxiety disorders, a double-blind comparison of clorimipramine and fluvoxamine. *Int Clin Psychopharmacol* **2**: 21–32.

Dick P, Ferrer E (1983) A double-blind comparative study of the clinical efficacy of fluvoxamine and clorimipramine. *Br J Clin Pharmacol* **15** Suppl 3: 419–425.

Du Pont RL, Pecknold JC (1985) Alprazolam withdrawal in panic disorder patients. New Research Abstracts of the 138th Annual Meeting of the American Psychiatric Association, Washington, DC.

Edlund JM, Swann AC, Clothier J (1987) Patients with panic attacks and abnormal EEG results. *Am J Psychiatry* **144**: 508–509.

Ehlers A (1993) Somatic symptoms and panic attack: A retrospective study of learning experiences. *Behav Res Ther* **31**: 269–278.

Eriksson E (1993) Brain neurotransmission in panic disorder. *Acta Psychiatr Scand* **335** Suppl: 31–37.

Eysenk HJ (1968) A theory of the incubation of anxiety/fear response. *Behav Res Ther* **6**: 319–321.

Faravelli C, Guerrini Degl'Innocenti B, Giardinelli L (1989) Epidemiology of anxiety disorders in Florence. *Acta Psychiatr Scand* **79**: 308–312.

Faravelli C, Marinoni M, Spiti R et al. (1997) Abnormal brain hemodynamic responses during passive orthostatic challenge in panic disorder. *Am J Psychiatry* **154**: 378–383.

Fava GA, Grandi S, Rafanelli C et al. (1988) Prodromal symptoms in panic disorder with agoraphobia. *Am J Psychiatry* **145**: 156.

Fava GA, Grandi S, Rafanelli C et al. (1992) Prodromal symptoms in panic disorder with agoraphobia: A reduplication study. *J Affect Disord* **26**: 85–88.

Fischer H, Andersson JL, Flumark T, Fredrikson M (1998) Brain correlates of an unexpected panic attack: A human positron emission tomographic study. *Neurosci Lett* **251**(2): 137–140.

Fontaine R, Breton G, Dery R et al. (1990) Temporal lobe abnormalities in panic disorders: A MRI study. *Arch Gen Psychiatry* **27**: 304–310.

Freud S (1894) Die Abwehr-Neuropsychosen. *Neurologisches Zentralblatt* **13**(10): 362–364 and **13**(11): 402–409.

Freud S (1926) *Hemmung, Symptom und Angst*. Internationalen Psychoanalytischer Verlag.

Freud S (1959) Inhibitions, symptoms and anxiety. In Strachey J (ed) *The Standard Edition of the Complete Psychological Works of Sigmund Freud*, Vol. 20. London: Hogarth Press.

Freud S (1962) The neuropsychosis of defense. In Strachey J (ed) *The Standard Edition of the Complete Psychological Works of Sigmund Freud*, Vol. 3. London: Hogarth Press.

Fyer AJ, Liebowitz MR, Gorman JM et al. (1987) Discontinuation of alprazolam treatment in panic patients. *Am J Psychiatry* **144**: 303–308.

George DT, Nutt DJ, Dwier BA, Linnoila M (1990) Alcoholism and panic disorder: Is the comorbidity more than a coincidence? *Acta Psychiatr Scand* **81**: 97–107.

Goisman RM, Warshaw MG, Keller MB (1999) Psychosocial treatment prescriptions for generalised anxiety disorder, panic disorder, and social phobia, 1991–1996. *Am J Psychiatry* **156**(11): 1819–1821.

Gold PW, Pigott TA, Kling MA (1988) Basic and clinical studies with corticotropin-releasing hormone: Implication for a possible role in panic disorder. *Psychiatry Clin North Am* **11**: 327–334.

Gorman JM, Askanazi J, Liebowitz JR et al. (1984) Response to hyperventilation in a group of patients with panic disorder. *Am J Psychiatry* **141**: 857–861.

Gorman JM, Fyer MR, Goetz R et al. (1988) Ventilatory physiology of patients with panic disorder. *Arch Gen Psychiatry* **46**: 145–150.

Gorman JM, Liebowitz MR, Fyer AJ et al. (1987) An open trial of fluoxetine in the treatment of panic disorder. *J Clin Psychopharmacol* **7**: 329–332.

Gorman JM, Liebowitz MR, Fyer AF et al. (1989) A neuroanatomical hypothesis for panic disorder. *Am J Psychiatry* **146**: 148–161.

Gould RA, Otto MW, Pollak MH (1995) A meta-analysis of treatment outcome for panic disorder. *Clin Psychol Rev* **15**: 819–844.

Gray JA (1988) The neuropsychological basis of anxiety. In Last GC, Hersen M (eds) *Handbook of Anxiety Disorders*. New York: Pergamon Press.

Greenblatt DJ, Shader RI (1978) Dependence, tolerance and addiction to benzodiazepines: Clinical and pharmacokinetic considerations. *Drug Metab Rev* **8**: 13–28.

Griez EJ, Lousberg H, Van Den Hout MA, Van Den Molen GM (1987) CO_2 vulnerability in panic disorder. *Am J Psychiatry* **144**: 1080–1082.

Grove G, Coplan JD, Hollander E (1997) The neuroanatomy of 5HT dysregulation and panic disorder. *J Neuropsychiatry Clin Neurosci* **9**: 198–207.

Gur RC, Gur RE, Resnick SM et al. (1987) The effect of anxiety on cortical cerebral blood flow and metabolism. *J Cereb Blood Flow Metab* **7**: 173–177.

Hallstrom C, Lader MH (1981) Benzodiazepine withdrawal phenomenon. *Int Pharmacopsychiatry* **16**: 235–244.

Hauri P, Friedman M, Ravaris CL (1989) Sleep in patients with spontaneous panic attacks. *Sleep* **12**: 323–337.

Himle JA, Hill EM (1991) Alcohol abuse and the anxiety disorders: Evidence from the Epidemiological Catchment Area Survey. *J Anxiety Disord* **5**: 237–245.

Hoehn-Saric R, Fawcett J, Munjack DJ, Roy-Byrne PP (1994) A multicentre, double-blind, placebo-controlled study of fluvoxamine in the treatment of panic disorder. In *Neuropsychopharmacology*, Part 2, Oral Communications and Poster Abstracts of the XIXth Collegium International Neuropsychopharmacologicum Congress: 27 June–1 July 1994, Washington, DC: Abst P-58-33.

Hoehn-Saric R, McLeod DR, Hispley PA (1993) Effect of fluvoxamine on panic disorder. *J Clin Psychopharmacol* **13**: 321–326.

Holland RI, Fawcett J, Hoehn-Saric R et al. (1994) Long-term treatment of panic disorder with fluvoxamine in outpatients who had completed double-blind studies. *Neuropsychopharmacology* **10** (3S, Part 2): 102S.

Hollander E, Hattarer J, Klein DF (1990) Antidepressant for the treatment of panic and agoraphobia. In Noyes R, Roth M, Burrow GD (eds) *Handbook of Anxiety*. Amsterdam: Elsevier.

Holsboer F, Staiger A, Bardeleben U et al. (1991) Role of CRH and other neuropeptides in panic disorder. Paper presented at 5th World Congress of Biological Psychiatry, Florence.

Howell SF, Laraia M, Ballenger JC, Lydiard RB (1987) Lorazepam treatment in panic disorder. In New Research Program and Abstract, 140th Annual Meeting of American Psychiatric Association, 1987: Abst NR 166, 111.

Humble M, Koczas C, Wistedt B (1989) Serotonin and anxiety: An open study of citalopram in panic disorder. In Stefanis CN, Soldatos CR, Rabavilas AD (eds) *Psychiatry Today: VIII World Congress of Psychiatry Abstracts*. New York: Elsevier.

Iversen SD (1984) 5-HT and anxiety. *Neuropsychopharmacology* **23**: 1353–1360.

Javanmard M, Shlik J, Kennedy SH et al. (1999) Neuroanatomic correlates of CCK-4 induced panic attacks in healthy humans: A comparison of two time points. *Biol Psychiatry* **45**(7): 872–882.

Jobson KO, Potter WZ (1995) International psychopharmacology algorithm project report. *Psychopharmacol Bull* **31**: 457–507.

Joyce PR, Bushnell JA, Oakley-Browne HA, Wells JE, Hornblow AR (1989) The epidemiology of panic symptomatology and agoraphobic avoidance. *Cmpr Psychiatry* **30**: 303–312.

Kahan RS, McNair DM, Lipman RS et al. (1986) Imipramine and clordiazepoxide in depressive and anxiety disorders. *Arch Gen Psychiatry* **43**: 79–85.

Kahan RS, Wetzler S (1991) m-Chlorophenylpiperazine as a probe of serotonin function. *Biol Psychiatry* **30**: 1139–1166.

Kalus O, Asnis GM, Rubinson E et al. (1991) Desipramine treatment in panic disorder. *J Affect Disord* **21**(4): 239–244.

Klein DF (1964) Delineation of two drug-responsive anxiety syndromes. *Psychopharmacol* **5**: 397–408.

Klein DF (1981) Anxiety reconceptualized. In Klein DF, Raskin J (eds) *Anxiety: New Research and*

Changing Concepts. New York: Raven Press.

Klein DF (1987) Anxiety reconceptualized. In Klein DK (ed.) *Anxiety.* Basle: Karger.

Klein DF (1993) False suffocation alarms, spontaneous panic and related conditions: An integrative hypothesis. *Arch Gen Psychiatry* **50**: 306–317.

Klein DF, Rabkin G, Gorman JM (1985) Etiological and pathophysiological inferences from the pharmacological treatment of anxiety. In Tuma AH, Maser JD (eds) *Anxiety and the Anxiety Disorders.* Hillsdale, NJ: Lawrence Erlbaum.

Klein E, Uhde T (1988) Controlled study of verapamil for treatment of panic disorder. *Am J Psychiatry* **145**: 431–144.

Klerman GL, Hirschfeld RMA, Weissman MM et al. (1993) *Panic Anxiety and its Treatments.* Washington, DC: American Psychiatric Press.

Klerman GL, Weissman MM, Onellette R et al. (1991) Panic attacks in the community. *J Am Med Assoc* **265**(6): 742–746.

Ko GN, Elsworth JD, Roth RH et al. (1983) Panic induced elevation of plasma MHPG levels in phobic-anxious patients. *Arch Gen Psychiatry* **40**: 425–430.

Kramer MS, Cutler NR, Ballanger JC et al. (1995) A placebo controlled trial of L-365,260, a CCK-B antagonist in panic disorder. *Biol Psychiatry* **37**: 462–466.

Krystal JH, Leaf PS, Bruce ML et al. (1992) Effect of age and alcoholism on the prevalence of panic disorder. *Acta Psychiatr Scand* **85**: 77–82.

Kuikka JT, Pitkanen A, Lepola U et al. (1995) Abnormal regional benzodiazepine receptor uptake in the prefrontal cortex in patients with panic disorder. *Nucl Med Commun* **16**: 273–280.

Lecrubier, Judge R, the Collaborative Paroxetine Study Investigators (1997) Long-term evaluation of paroxetine, clomipramine and placebo in the treatment of panic disorder. *Acta Psychiatr Scand* **95**: 153–160.

Le Doux JE, Cicchetti P, Xagoraris A, Ronanski LM (1990) The lateral amygdaloid nucleus: sensory interface of the amygdala in fear conditioning. *J Neurosci* **10**: 1062–1069.

Lelliott P, Marks I, McNamee C, Tobena A (1988) Onset of panic disorder with agoraphobia. *Arch Gen Psychiatry* **46**: 1000–1004.

Lepola U (1997) Long-term citalopram is effective in relieving panic disorder. Paper presented at the 17th Annual Meeting of the Anxiety Disorders Association of America, New Orleans, LA, March.

Lepola U, Nousiainen U (1990) EEG and CT findings in patients with panic disorder. *Biol Psychiatry* **28**: 721–727.

Liebowitz MR, Fyer AJ, Gorman JM et al. (1984) Lactate provocation of panic attacks. *Arch Gen Psychiatry* **41**: 764–770.

Little HJ, Nutt DJ, Taylor SC (1987) Bidirectional effects of chronic treatment with agonists and inverse agonists at the benzodiazepine receptor. *Brain Res Bull* **19**: 371–378.

Maremmani I, Marini G, Fornai F (1998) Naltrexone-induced panic attacks. *Am J Psychiatry* **155**: 3.

Marks IM (1969) *Fears and Phobias.* London: Heinemann.

McNally RJ (1994) *Panic Disorder: A Critical Analysis.* New York: Guilford Press.

Mellman TA, Uhde TW (1989) Electroencephalographic sleep in panic disorder. *Arch Gen Psychiatry* **46**: 178–184.

Munjack DJ, Rebal R, Shaner R et al. (1985) Imipramine versus propanolol for the treatment of panic attacks: A pilot study. *Compr Psychiatry* **26**: 80–89.

Munjack DJ, Usigli R, Zulueta A et al. (1988) Nortriptyline in the treatment of panic disorder and agoraphobia with panic attacks. *J Clin Psychopharmacol* **8**: 204–207.

Nair NP, Bakish D, Saxena B et al. (1996) Comparison of fluvoxamine, imipraminne and placebo in the treatment of outpatients with panic disorder. *Anxiety* **2**: 192–198.

Nordahl TE, Semple WE, Gross M et al. (1990) Cerebral glucose metabolic differences in patients with panic disorder. *Neuropsychopharmacology* **3**: 261–273.

Nordahl TE, Stein MB, Benkelfalt C et al. (1998) Regional cerebral metabolic asymmetries replicated in an independent group of patients with panic disorder. *Biol Psychiatry* **44**(10): 998–1006.

Noyes R, Reich J, Christiansen J et al. (1990) Outcome of panic disorder. *Arch Gen Psychiatry* **47**: 809–818.

Nutt DJ (1998) Antidepressants in panic disorder: Clinical and preclinical mechanisms. *J Clin Psychiatry* **59**(8): 24–28.

Nutt DJ, Glue P, Lawson C, Wilson S (1990) Flumazenil provocation of panic attacks. *Arch Gen Psychiatry* **47**: 917–925.

Nutt DJ, Lawson C (1993) Panic attacks: A neurochemical overview of models and mechanisms. *Br J Psychiatry* **160**: 165–178.

Oehrberg S, Christiansen PE, Behnek K et al. (1995) Paroxetine in the treatment of panic disorder: A randomised double blind placebo controlled study. *Br J Psychiatry* **167**: 374–379.

Owen RP, Tyrer P (1983) Benzodiazepine dependence: A review of the evidence. *Drugs* **25**: 385–398.

Pecknold JC, Luthe L, Iny I, Ramdoyal D (1995) Fluoxetine in panic disorder: A pharmacological and tritiated platelet imipramine and paroxetine binding study. *J Psychiatry Neurosci* **20**: 193–198.

Pitchot W, Ansseau M, Gonzalez MA et al. (1992) Dopaminergic function in panic disorder: Comparison with major and minor depression. *Biol Psychiatry* **32**: 1004–1011.

Pitts FM, McClure JN (1967) Lactate metabolism in anxiety neurosis. *N Engl J Med* **277**: 1329–1336.

Pohl RH, Clary C, Wolkow R (1997) Double-blind comparison of sertraline and placebo in patients with panic disorder. Paper presented at the annual meeting of the American Psychiatric Association, San Diego, May.

Pollak M, Wolkow R, Clary C (1997) Double-blind comparison of sertraline and placebo in patients with panic disorder. Paper presented at the annual meeting of the New Clinical Drug Evaluation Unit, May.

Pyke RE, Greenberg S (1986) Norepinephrine challenges in panic patients. *J Clin Psychopharmacology* **6**: 279–285.

Redmond DE, Huang YH (1979) Current concepts II: New evidence for a locus coeruleus norepinephrine connection with anxiety. *Life Sci* **25**: 2149–2162.

Reiman EM (1987) The study of panic disorder using positron emission tomography. *Psychiatr Dev* **5**(1): 63–78.

Reiman EM (1997) The application of positron emission tomography to the study of normal and pathologic emotions. *J Clin Psychiatry* **58**(16): 4–12.

Reiman EM, Raichle ME, Butler FK (1984) A focal brain abnormality in panic disorder: A severe form of anxiety. *Nature* **310**: 683–685.

Reiman EM, Raichle ME, Robins E (1986) Application of positron emission tomography to the study of panic disorder. *Am J Psychiatry* **143**: 469–477.

Reiman EM, Raichle ME, Robins E et al. (1989a) Neuroanatomic correlates of a lactate-induced anxiety attack. *Arch Gen Psychiatry* **46**: 493–500.

Reiman EM, Raichle ME, Robins E (1989b) Involvement of temporal poles in pathological and normal forms of anxiety. *J Blood Flow Metab* **9**(1): S589.

Reiss S, Peterson RA, Gurssky DM, McNally RJ (1986) Anxiety sensitivity, anxiety frequency and prediction of fearfulness. *Behav Res Ther* **24**: 1–8.

Rickels K, Schweizer E, Case WG, Greenblatt DJ (1990) Long-term therapeutic use of benzodiazepines I: Effect of abrupt discontinuation. *Arch Gen Psychiatry* **47**: 899–907.

Robins LN, Regier DA (1991) *Psychiatric Disorders in America: The Epidemiological Catchment Area Study*. New York: Free Press.

Roth M, Argyle N (1988) Anxiety, panic and phobic disorders: An overview. *J Psychiatr Res* **22** Suppl 1: 33–54.

Roy-Byrne PP, Cowley DS (1994) Course and outcome in panic disorder: A review of recent follow-up studies. *Anxiety* **1**: 151–160.

Roy-Byrne P, Cowley DS, Greenblatt DJ et al. (1990) Reduced benzodiazepine sensitivity in panic disorder. *Arch Gen Psychiatry* **47**: 534–538.

Roy-Byrne P, Uhde TW, Post RM et al. (1986) The corticotropin-releasing hormone stimulation test in patients with panic disorder. *Am J Psychiatry* **143**: 896–899.

Salkovskis PM, Clark DM (1991) Cognitive therapy for panic disorder. *J Cognitive Psychother* **5**: 15–26.

Sasson Y, Iancu I, Fux M et al. (1999) A double-blind crossover comparison of clomipramine and desipramine in the treatment of panic disorder. *Eur Neuropsychopharmacol* **9**(3): 191–196.

Seligman MEP (1988) Competing theories of panic. In Rachman S, Maser JD (eds) *Panic: Psychological Perspectives*. Hillsdale, NJ: Erlbaum.

Shear MK, Cooper AM, Klerman GL et al. (1993) A psychodynamic model for panic disorder. *Am J Psychiatry* **150**: 859–866.

Sheehan DV (1999) Current concepts in the treatment of panic disorder. *J Clin Psychiatry* **60**(18): 16–21.

Svenson TH, Usdin T (1978) Feedback inhibition of brain noradrenaline neurons by triciclic antidepressant alpha-receptor mediation. *Science* **202**: 1089–1091.

Targum SD, Marshall LE (1989) Fenfluramine provocation of anxiety in patients with panic disorder. *Psychiatry Res* **28**: 295–306.

Taylor S, Koch WJ, McNally RJ, Crockett DJ (1992) Conceptualisations of anxiety sensitivity. *Psychol Assess* **4**: 245–250.

Thyer BA, Himle J (1985) Temporal relationship between panic attack onset and phobic avoidance in agoraphobia. *Behav Res Ther* **23**(5): 607–608.

Tondo L, Burrai C, Scamonatti L et al. (1989) Carbamazepine in panic disorder. *Am J Psychiatry* **146**: 558–559.

Tyrer P, Murphy S (1987) The place of benzodiazepines in psychiatric practice. *Br J Psychiatry* **151**: 719–723.

Uhde TW, Boulenger JP, Roy-Byrne PP et al. (1985) Longitudinal course of panic disorder: Clinical and biological considerations. *Progr Neuropsychopharmacol Biol Psychiatry* **9**(1): 39–51.

Van Vliet IM, Den Boer JA, Westenberg HG et al. (1996) A double-blind comparative study of brofaromine and fluvoxamine in outpatients with panic disorder. *J Clin Psychopharmacol* **16**: 299–306.

Van Vliet IM, Westenberg HG, Den Boer JA (1993) MAO inhibitors in panic disorder: Clinical effects of treatment with brofaromine. A double blind placebo controlled study. *Psychopharmacology Berl* **112**: 483–489.

Wade AG (1995) The optimal therapeutical area for SSRIs: Panic disorder. Paper presented at the VIII Annual European College of Neuropsychopharmacology, Venice, Italy, October.

Weissman MM, Loof PJ, Holzer CE (1985) The epidemiology of anxiety disorders: A highlight of recent evidence. *Psychopharmacol Bull* **21**: 538–541.

Wilson KG, Sandler LS, Asmundson GHG et al. (1991) Effects of instructional sets on self-reports of panic attacks. *J Anxiety Disord* **5**: 43–63.

Windmann S (1998) Panic disorder from a monist perspective: Integrating neurobiological and psychological approaches. *J Anxiety Disord* **12**(5): 485–507.

Wittchen HU (1986) Epidemiology of panic attacks and panic disorders. In Hand I, Wittchen HU (eds) *Panic and Phobias: Empirical Evidences of Theoretical Models and Long-term Effects of Behavioral Treatments*. Berlin: Springer-Verlag.

Wittchen HU, Essau CA (1989) Comorbidity of anxiety disorders and depression: Does it affect course and outcome? *Psychiatric Psychobiol* **4**: 315–323.

Wittchen HU, Essau CA (1991) The epidemiology of panic attacks, panic disorder and agoraphobia. In Walker JR, Norton GR, Ross CA (eds) *Panic Disorder and Agoraphobia*. Monterey, CA: Brooks/Cole.

Wolkow R, Apter J, Clayton A et al. (1996) Double-blind comparison of sertraline and placebo in patients with panic disorder. Paper presented at Collegium Internationale Neuro-Psychopharmacologicum, June, Melbourne, Australia.

Wolpe J, Rowan VC (1988) Panic disorder: A product of classical conditioning. *Behav Res Ther* **26**: 241–250.

Woodman CL, Noyes R (1994) Panic disorder: Treatment with valoroate. *J Clin Psychiatry* **55**: 134–136.

Woods S, Black D, Brown S et al. (1994) Fluvoxamine in the treatment of panic disorder in outpatients: A double-blind, placebo-controlled study. In *Neuropsychopharmacology*, Part 2, Oral Communications and Poster Abstracts of the XIXth Collegium International Neuro-psychopharmacologicum Congress: 27 June–1 July, 1994, Washington, DC: Abst P-58-37.

Woods SW, Koster K, Kristal JK et al. (1988) Yohimbine alters regional cerebral blood flow in panic disorder. *Lancet* **ii**: 678.

World Health Organization (1992) *The ICD-10 Classification of Mental and Behavioural Disorders: Clinical and Diagnostical Guidelines*. Geneva: WHO.

Yergani VK, Spinivasan K, Pohl R et al. (1994) Sodium lactate increases sympathovagal ratios in normal control subjects: spectral analysis of heart rate, blood pressure, and respiration. *Psychiatry Res* **54**: 97–114.

6

Specific Phobias

H. Merckelbach and P. Muris

Maastricht University, Maastricht, The Netherlands

INTRODUCTION

Specific (formerly "simple" or "monosymptomatic") phobias are irrational and persistent fears of certain objects or animals. Whereas specific phobia is a relatively recent concept, descriptions of the condition to which it refers have a long tradition in medical history (Errera, 1962). For example, in his writings, Hippocrates refers to a case of a man who displayed an irrational fear of bridges. Likewise, detailed discussions of phobic symptoms can be found in the work of seventeenth- or eighteenth-century authors like Descartes, Le Camus, and Sauvages.

While descriptions of phobic behaviour have remained remarkably constant throughout history, theories to explain this behaviour have changed dramatically. In early medical texts, speculations about eye muscle dysfunction, vascular abnormalities or mysterious underground water streams were not uncommon (Errera, 1962). Over the past two decades, our understanding of the origins of specific phobias has steadily increased. This is nicely illustrated by the large number of detailed review articles that cover this domain of psychopathology (e.g., Craske, 1997; Davey, 1997; Menzies and Clarke, 1995; Merckelbach et al., 1996a; Muris and Merckelbach, 1998; Muris and Merckelbach 2000; Page, 1991; Rachman, 1998). It is now recognised that learning mechanisms and developmental processes play a crucial role in the aetiology of specific phobias. Furthermore, there are now strong indications that certain cognitive processes contribute to the maintenance of phobic symptoms. The present chapter will evaluate these elements in more detail. The first section is concerned with the symptomatology and epidemiology of specific phobias. The second section emphasises the developmental aspects of specific phobias. This is followed in the third section by a discussion of the learning mechanisms that are involved in the aetiology of specific phobias. The fourth section outlines various cognitive mechanisms that presumably intensify phobic symptoms. Next, treatment methods for specific phobias are briefly considered. The final section summarises the main points of this chapter.

Anxiety Disorders: An Introduction to Clinical Management and Research. Edited by E. J. L. Griez, C. Faravelli, D. Nutt and J. Zohar. © 2001 John Wiley & Sons, Ltd.

SYMPTOMATOLOGY, EPIDEMIOLOGY AND GENETICS

Symptomatology

The Diagnostic and Statistical Manual of Mental Disorders, fourth edition (DSM-IV: APA, 1994) lists a number of criteria for the diagnostic category of specific phobia. Briefly, DSM-IV emphasises that specific phobias are directed at a limited set of stimuli (e.g., spiders) and that confrontation with these stimuli elicits intense fear and avoidance behaviour. Furthermore, DSM-IV stresses that the fear is excessive and unreasonable to such a degree that it interferes with daily life. These characteristics deserve some comment.

To begin with, it is important to recognise that specific fears are non-randomly distributed. A number of fear survey studies (e.g., Agras et al., 1969; Costello, 1982; Arrindell et al., 1991) have shown that in the general population, some fears (e.g., fear of spiders or snakes) are far more prevalent than others (e.g., fear of electricity). In other words, most specific fears and phobias pertain to a relatively narrow class of stimuli. Seligman, Öhman, Marks and Nesse have interpreted this phenomenon in terms of evolutionary processes (Seligman, 1971; Öhman, 1996; Marks, 1987; Marks and Nesse, 1994). According to these authors, inspection of this narrow class of stimuli reveals that it consists of objects and events that were probably threatening to prehistoric man. They assume that fear of animals such as spiders and snakes promoted the survival chances of our prehistoric ancestors. As a result of natural selection, fear of these evolutionary dangers became genetically coded in the form of a primitive learning mechanism. Consequently, modern man would still possess a biological readiness or preparedness to develop specific fears of spiders, snakes and so forth. While this "evolutionary preparedness" hypothesis has attracted considerable attention, other plausible interpretations of the selectivity of fears do exist (Davey, 1995; Merckelbach and De Jong, 1997). For example, it might well be the case that the selectivity of specific fears is a consequence of the negative connotations that certain stimuli have in our culture (e.g., spiders are commonly seen as dirty; Davey, 1995). Whatever its origins, the non-random distribution of specific fears is a well-established phenomenon. In fact, the DSM-IV (APA, 1994) differentiates between four highly prevalent categories of specific phobia: animal type (e.g., spider phobia), natural environment type (e.g., phobia of heights), blood-injection-injury type (e.g., dental phobia), and situational type (e.g., claustrophobia). In addition, the DSM-IV introduces a miscellaneous category ("other type") which encompasses, for example, choking phobia. Largely, this taxonomy of specific phobias nicely fits with data that come from factor analytic studies (e.g., Fredrikson et al., 1996).

A second point that must be considered is the nature of intense fear emotions. A good framework for discussing this point is the "three-systems model" proposed by Lang (Lang, 1968; see also Hugdahl, 1981). According to this model, emotions such as fear consist of three relatively independent components: a physiological component, a subjective component, and a behavioural component. Thus, fear is reflected in autonomic symptoms (e.g., tachycardia, increased respiration, etc.), subjective feelings of apprehension, and avoidance or escape behaviour. However, the extent to which these components co-occur varies (Hugdahl, 1981; Hodgson and Rachman, 1974). Thus, it is conceivable that a mild fear of, say, spiders is accompanied by behavioural avoidance of spiders, but relatively little autonomic reactions when confronted with spiders. Although such discordance between components is not uncommon, there are reasons to believe that discordance will be less evident when fear is intense (Hodgson and Rachman, 1974). Nevertheless, the three-systems model has important implications for the study of specific phobias. To begin with, the model suggests that in diagnosis or therapy outcome evaluation, it is important to measure each component. It should be noted that good measurement instruments are available for each component. More specifically, the physiological component can be monitored using psychophysiological techniques (e.g., recording of heart rate, respiration, eye blink startle responses; Hugdahl, 1989; Lang, 1995), the subjective component can be quantified with specially constructed and validated self-report instruments (e.g., the Spider Phobia Questionnaire; Klorman et al., 1974; the Screen for Child Anxiety Related Emotional Disorders; Muris et al., 1999), while the behavioural component can be measured by standardised approach tasks (i.e., tasks which require a stepwise approach towards a phobic object; e.g., Öst et al., 1991a). The idea that one should assess all three components when studying phobic fear seems self-evident, but, as a matter of fact, studies in this area often either rely on one or two measures or make use of vague and imprecise instruments to tap the three components (Eifert and Wilson, 1991).

It is worthy of note that not all types of specific phobias display a comparable profile concerning the three components. For instance, both animal phobia and blood-injection-injury phobia are accompanied by subjective reports of distress. However, whereas in animal phobia distress usually takes the form of fear (but see Matchett and Davey, 1991), blood-injection-injury phobia is associated with strong subjective feelings of disgust and repulsion (Page, 1994). Also, confrontation with the phobic stimulus elicits sympathetic activation (e.g., tachycardia) in animal phobia, but parasympathetic activation (e.g., bradycardia) in blood-injection-injury phobia. Thus, the heightened arousal that occurs in animal phobics who are exposed to their feared stimulus stands in sharp contrast to the lowered arousal seen in blood-injection-injury phobia (Thyer et al., 1985). Referring to the peculiar characteristics of blood-injection-injury phobia (i.e., subjective feelings of disgust, bradycardia, and fainting), some authors (e.g., Rachman, 1990a) have argued that the term blood-injection-injury phobia is a misnomer. According to these authors, blood phobics do not fear blood, but the consequences of confrontation with blood (e.g., fainting). This would imply that there is an interesting connection between blood-injection-injury phobia and panic disorder inasmuch as both conditions are characterised by fear of bodily sensations.

As far as the content of subjective fear is concerned, there are also major differences between situational phobia, in particular claustrophobia, on the one hand, and animal phobia, on the other hand. Subjective fear in claustrophobia is not only focused on danger expectations (e.g., fear of suffocation), but also on anxiety expectancies (e.g., fear of going crazy) and bodily sensations. The latter components are less prominent in animal phobias (Craske et al., 1995). Thus, from a cognitive point of view, claustrophobia seems to represent a more complex fear than animal phobia. Indeed, a close look at the subjective cognitions that are involved in specific phobias makes clear that these phobias do not constitute a homogeneous class (e.g., Himle et al., 1991).

Another characteristic of specific phobias that requires some elaboration is their irrational nature. The patient suffering from, say, an intense spider phobia readily admits that her or his fear is excessive. Nevertheless, she or he is unable to inhibit fear responses when exposed to spiders. How can one account for this failure to control fear responses? According to Öhman (1996), phobic stimuli are analysed by fast and subcortical information-processing routines. These subcortical processes would provide a rough analysis of the stimulus and then initiate an immediate fear response. Consequently, even before the patient becomes fully aware of the phobic stimulus, a fear response is already on its way. This might explain why phobics experience their fears as uncontrollable. In passing, it should be noted that this view accords well with the neurobiological studies of LeDoux (1992). In his animal studies, LeDoux found evidence for a subcortical fear pathway linking the thalamus with the amygdala. This thalamo-amygdala pathway is a quick and dirty transmission route in which the thalamus carries out a crude analysis of the sensory input and then immediately activates the amygdala, which, in turn, generates an emotional response. According to LeDoux (1992, p. 276), this pathway has adaptive value in that "the thalamo-amygdala system might be especially useful as a processing channel under conditions where rapid responses are required to threatening stimuli. In such situations, it may be more important to respond quickly than to be certain that the stimulus merits a response." Thus, it is conceivable that in the case of specific phobias, learning experiences or genetic factors affect the thalamo-amygdala pathway in such a way that it becomes oversensitive to certain phobic cues (for a detailed discussion, see LeDoux, 1995). Interestingly, Fredrikson and associates (1993) found in their PET scan study of snake phobics some indications that the thalamus acts as an important relay station for phobic stimulus processing.

On the other hand, experimental studies that addressed the Öhman/LeDoux hypothesis in more depth have come up with mixed results. In order to examine fast processing routines in phobias, Öhman and Soares (1994) confronted spider fearful, snake fearful, and control subjects to subliminal presentations (i.e., 30 msec) of spiders, snakes, and neutral pictures while autonomic arousal as indexed by skin conductance responses (SCRs) were measured. The results of this study were in line with the idea that phobics immediately react to degraded phobic stimuli even when these stimuli are blocked from conscious recognition. That is, spider fearfuls were found to react with heightened SCRs to subliminal spider pictures, snake fearfuls were found to respond with heightened SCRs to subliminal snake pictures, whereas control subjects did not react with specific SCRs to any of the subliminal pictures. However, attempts to cross-validate these findings in severely phobic adults (Mayer et al., 1999a) or children (Mayer et al., 1999b) have produced disappointing results.

In conclusion, then, the Öhman/LeDoux hypothesis awaits further empirical testing.

Prevalence, Natural Course, and Genetics

Epidemiological studies indicate that lifetime prevalence rates for specific phobias may be as high as 12% (e.g., Regier et al., 1988; Kessler et al., 1994). This suggests that specific phobias belong to the most frequent mental disorders. In a community study by Costello (1982), it was found that animal fears (including fear of dogs, snakes, etc.) were the most prevalent, followed by nature (e.g., heights), and mutilation (e.g., injections) fears. In effect, animal fears occurred in nearly 43% of the women. Whether these fears represent clinical phobias remains unclear, but at the very least, Costello's results suggest that mild specific phobias are widespread. This point is further underlined by the National Comorbidity Survey conducted by Magee and associates (Magee et al., 1996). These authors not only found a high lifetime prevalence rates for specific phobias (11.3%), but also noted that specific phobias are often associated with serious role impairment (i.e., interference with daily life), even though they usually go untreated.

Another common finding in the literature is that specific phobias are diagnosed more often in women than in men. This is especially true for animal phobias (Sturgis and Scott, 1984; Öst, 1987a; see also Kirkpatrick, 1984; Fredrikson et al., 1996). There are strong indications that this sex difference cannot be fully explained by assuming that it is more socially permissible for women to report fear than for men (Cornelius and Averill, 1983). Probably, other predisposing factors (e.g., sex hormones; see below) contribute to the skewed sex distribution of fears and phobias.

With regard to the natural course of specific phobia, Wittchen (1988) summarised the results of his longitudinal community study as follows: "The natural course of simple phobias is in the majority of cases chronic and can be characterised by the persistence of mild rather than severe symptoms of anxiety over decades. Only 16% remitted completely over the follow-up period of 7 years: thus, only very few spontaneous remissions could be observed" (ibid.: 14). In passing, it should be noted that specific phobia often occur as a comorbid diagnosis in panic disorder and generalised anxiety disorder (de Ruiter et al., 1989).

Several family and twin studies have been carried out to explore to what extent genetic factors predispose to phobic fear (e.g., Kendler et al., 1992). Briefly, family studies noted that relatives of probands with specific phobias have a threefold higher risk of specific phobias than control subjects (Fyer et al., 1995; Fredrikson et al., 1997). Likewise, twin studies show that the genetic contribution to specific phobias is significant though heredity can vary considerably for the different subtypes of specific phobias, with those for animal phobias being highest (32%) and those for situational phobias being relatively low (for a review, see Smoller and Tsuang, 1998).

There is some discussion about the precise way in which genetic factors contribute to the aetiology of phobias. Some authors (Smoller and Tsuang, 1998) have suggested that their contribution is fairly specific, but there is also strong evidence for the existence of a general anxiety diathesis that may be variably expressed. This general diathesis does not refer to inheritance of a specific fear, but to inheritance of a general trait that predisposes to a broad range of anxiety complaints. In some cases these complaints amount to a specific phobia, but in others they may take the form of, for example, social phobia, agoraphobia, and so on (see also Andrews et al., 1990). In a recent article, Taylor (1998) reviewed a number of large-scale behavioural-genetic studies concerned with phobias. Although his review was not particularly focused on childhood phobias, his differentiation between general and specific genetic factors is very useful for the present discussion. According to Taylor (1998), the general (i.e., higher-order) genetic factor constitutes the biological substrate of broad temperamental traits such as negative affectivity and neuroticism and acts as a vulnerability factor for a wide range of phobic fears. In contrast, specific (i.e., lower-order) factors predispose to certain circumscribed fears. Taylor (1998, pp. 211, 212) summarised the role of both factors in phobic aetiology as follows:

> The general factor tended to make a modest contribution to agoraphobia, situational phobia, and social phobia (7–10% of variance; mean = 9%) and a greater contribution to animal phobia (35%). Conversely, specific genetic factors were more important for agoraphobia, situational phobia, and social phobia (20–29%; mean = 23%) compared to animal phobia (0%).

The importance of general genetic factors in the aetiology of specific phobias becomes obvious when one looks at comorbidity studies. These studies show that having one specific phobia also increases the likelihood of experiencing subclinical fears from other phobia subtypes (e.g., Hofmann et al., 1997). The well-established fact that phobias tend to be strongly comorbid with each other (see also Magee et al., 1996) has two important implications. First, it casts doubts on the preparedness hypothesis (see above), inasmuch as this hypothesis assumes that evolutionary pressures have resulted in the genetic transmission of specific fears and phobias rather than a general trait. Second, this finding calls for studies that address the behavioural or temperamental manifestations of general genetic factors. Obvious candidates in this respect are neuroticism, negative affectivity, but also behavioural inhibition (Zinbarg and Barlow, 1996).

DEVELOPMENTAL ASPECTS

One robust finding in clinical studies is that, in general, specific phobias are characterised by early onset ages. For example, Öst (1987a) found mean onset ages of 7 and 9 years for animal and blood-injury-injection phobias, respectively. An early onset is also found in natural environment phobias. Thus, a considerable percentage of height fearful subjects report that their fear has always been present (e.g., Menzies and Clarke, 1993). It should be noted, though, that situational fears such as claustrophobia differ from this pattern in that they have a later onset. Thus, Öst (1987a) reports a mean onset age of 20 years for his sample of claustrophobics. This late onset accords with the impression that claustrophobia is a more "sophisticated" fear, at least when one looks at the sort of cognitions that are involved. Nevertheless, generally, a substantial proportion of specific phobias begins in childhood. This finding is underlined by surveys of subclinical fears among children. In an early study by MacFarlane et al. (1954), it was found that only a small minority of a large sample of children (N = 1096) displayed no fear reactions. Lapouse and Monk (1959) reported a similar finding. In a more recent study, Muris and colleagues (2000) found that specific fears are common among four- to six-year-old children (71%), peak between ages seven to nine (87%), and then decline in 10 to 12 year olds (68%). Together, these and other studies demonstrate that mild to moderate fears are quite normal phenomena in childhood. In this connection, there are several points that deserve comment. First, studies that are evaluating specific fears in children, have consistently found that girls report more fears than boys (e.g., Ollendick and King, 1991).

Second, the mild fears seen in children often represent transient developmental phenomena. That is to say, childhood fears follow a predictable course (see for a review Marks, 1987). For example, Bauer (1976) found that fear of ghosts and fear of animals are common in children aged four to eight. In contrast, fear of injury is more often found in children aged 10 to 12. According to Bauer, these fluctuations in childhood fear are closely tied to cognitive development. Younger children would rely on global perception and animistic concepts in interpreting cause–effect relationships. This would explain why their fears are directed at ghosts and animals. Bauer's emphasis on cognitive development makes sense. For example, the visual cliff phenomenon (i.e., fear of heights) that typically occurs in young babies between four and nine months has long been interpreted as a prototype of a genetically based fear. Yet, experiments show that this phenomenon critically depends on locomotion development in infants (Bertenthal and Campos, 1984).

Third, while it is clear that the majority of childhood fears disappear spontaneously, there are also indications that in a subgroup of children, specific fears persist and tend to radicalise (e.g., Ollendick, 1979). Thus, the critical question is why, in some cases, specific fears appear to continue from childhood into adulthood. There are good reasons to believe that genetically based temperamental traits play an important role in this context. Germane to this issue are studies on behavioural inhibition (e.g., Biederman et al., 1995). Behavioural inhibition refers to the tendency of some children to interrupt ongoing behaviour and react with vocal restraint and withdrawal when confronted with unfamiliar people or settings. Behavioural inhibition is thought to be a stable and inherited trait that characterises approximately 10% to 15% of children. Cross-sectional and longitudinal data collected by Biederman and co-workers strongly suggest that this trait constitutes a risk factor for anxiety disorders. More specifically, these authors noted that compared to control children, pre-school children identified as behaviourally inhibited are more likely to have anxiety disorders (including specific phobias). This became even more prominent at a three-year follow-up. That is, in the cohort of children who were initially identified as behaviourally inhibited, the rates of specific phobias and other anxiety disorders had increased markedly. Thus, behavioural inhibition seems to be a vulnerability factor for a broad range of anxiety disorders, among which are specific phobias. It is not surprising, therefore, that this trait has been linked to other higher-order constructs such as neuroticism, trait anxiety (Craske, 1997), and negative affectivity (Clark et al., 1994). Recent studies have sought to elucidate the neurobiological underpinnings of these higher-order traits. According to some authors (e.g., Rosen and Schulkin, 1998), hyperexcitability in the amygdala is associated with behavioural inhibition. This hyperexcitability would promote a development from normal, adaptive fear states into pathological anxiety. Other authors have found that response styles such as behavioural inhibition are subserved by hyperactivity in the right frontal areas (e.g., Calkins et al., 1996), a finding that accords well with the hypothesis that the anterior cortex is involved in avoidance behaviour (see below). The precise biological parameters of behavioural inhibition await further clarification. Meanwhile, it should be stressed that about 70% of the children classified as behaviourally inhibited remain free of any anxiety disorder. Apparently, then, learning experiences determine whether genetically transmitted vulnerabilities culminate in specific phobias.

LEARNING EXPERIENCES

As previously explained, early medical literature provides a number of speculative ideas to account for specific phobia. However, the first real breakthrough in the study of phobias occurred when Watson and Rayner (1920) proposed that phobias are the product of conditioning processes. This proposal had several important and testable implications. For example, if phobias are learned, they should be reversible. In the decades that followed, implications of this sort were subjected to empirical research. This contributed to a further extension and refinement of the conditioning interpretation of phobias. However, gradually it became clear that conditioning is only one pathway to phobias and that other, more subtle pathways (i.e., negative information and modelling) may also contribute to the acquisition of fears.

Classical Conditioning

Watson and Rayner's "little Albert study" (Watson and Rayner, 1920; see also Harris, 1979) was quite simple: little Albert was an infant who initially showed no fear of live animals. However, he did react with fear whenever noise was produced by hitting a steel bar with a hammer. Watson and Rayner then exposed Albert to a white rat and produced a loud noise with the hammer and steel. Albert was given six trials of white rat and noise. Eventually, little Albert reacted with crying and avoidance as soon as he was confronted with the white rat. Watson and Rayner, as well as many researchers after them, argued that the little Albert case illustrates that phobias can be understood as the outcome of aversive Pavlovian or classical conditioning. In technical terms: the phobic object (e.g., a rat) is a "conditioned stimulus" (CS) that initially elicits no fear. An aversive event (e.g., a loud startling noise) is an "unconditioned stimulus" (UCS) that by virtue of its biological features reliably induces a fear response. This fear response is therefore termed the "unconditioned response" (UCR). If the CS is paired with the UCS, a fear response occurs and becomes associated with the CS. Thereafter, the CS is able to elicit a full-blown fear response, even in the absence of the UCS. The fear response has then become a conditioned response (CR) to the CS and, consequently, the CS has turned into a phobic object.

The basic finding of Watson and Rayner, (i.e., fear can be conditioned by pairing a neutral CS with an aversive or traumatic UCS), has been replicated time and again. For example, in a study by Campbell et al. (1964), subjects listened to a 75 dB tone (CS) that was followed by an injection of scoline. This injection produced a temporary respiratory paralysis (UCS) and, consequently, intense fear (UCR). Even weeks after this single conditioning trial, subjects reacted with strong sympathetic responses (CR) to isolated presentations of the tone (i.e., the tone was not followed by paralysis). While laboratory findings such as these illustrate that conditioning processes can, in principle, produce phobia-like fears, they do not prove that in everyday life, classical conditioning is the primary antecedent of phobias. However, a compelling case can be made that even outside the laboratory, classical conditioning processes may heavily contribute to the acquisition of phobias. For example, Kuch et al. (1994) reported that of 55 survivors of road vehicle accidents (UCS), 21 (38%) developed a phobia of driving (CS). Likewise, choking phobia, which the DSM-IV classifies as a specific phobia "other type", is nearly always the result of a traumatic incident in which the patient chokes on, for example, a fishbone (Greenberg et al., 1988).

The classical conditioning model of specific phobias explains why persons react with subjective fear and physiological arousal when they are exposed to the phobic CS. It does not, however, account for the persistent avoidance behaviour that phobics display. The influential two-stage theory of Mowrer (1960) attempts to incorporate this point. Briefly, Mowrer's theory assumes that the development of phobias involves two stages. During the first stage, a pairing of a neutral CS and an aversive UCS results in a conditioned fear response to the CS. During the second stage, the person learns that fear responses to the CS can be reduced by avoiding the CS. A reduction in fear levels that follows avoidance is experienced as a positive state. Consequently, avoidance behaviour is reinforced, and in time becomes an integral part of the phobic fear. Again, research shows that the scenario depicted by the two-stage theory works in the laboratory. Thus, when subjects are confronted with pairings of light (CS) and shock (UCS) and then are given the opportunity to react with an escape response every time the CS appears, persistent avoidance responding occurs (Malloy and Levis, 1988).

The two-stage theory of phobic fear has straightforward treatment implications. According to this theory, avoidance behaviour maintains phobic fear because it prevents prolonged exposure to the phobic object. Consequently, phobic subjects have no opportunity to experience that an aversive UCS no longer accompanies the phobic CS. The treatment lesson to be learned from this is that one should confront phobic subjects with their phobic CS while ensuring that they do not react with avoidance to this CS. This strategy, known as exposure therapy, has proven to be very successful in the treatment of specific phobias (Marks, 1987; Öst, 1989; Öst, 1997). It should be added, though, that more recent work has made it clear that the connection between avoidance behaviour and the maintenance of phobias is considerably more complex than previously thought. Thus, under some conditions, exposure plus escape behaviour might be as effective in reducing fear levels as exposure alone, a finding that is difficult to reconcile with the traditional Mowrerian idea that avoidance/escape necessarily maintains phobic fear (Rachman et al., 1986). Probably, other factors such as overprediction of fear and the presence of safety signals determine whether avoidance/escape maintains phobic fear (for a detailed discussion, see Rachman, 1998).

Shortcomings of the Traditional Conditioning Account

In the 1970s, several authors drew attention to the fact that the classical conditioning model of phobias and its extension, Mowrer's two-stage theory, suffer from a number of serious shortcomings (e.g., Rachman, 1977; Eysenck, 1979). First, the conditioning approach fails to explain why specific fears are non-randomly distributed. Indeed, from a conditioning point of view, one would expect that each object could become a phobic stimulus (CS), if it is followed by an aversive event (UCS). As explained before, this is obviously not the case. After all, fear of snakes occurs more often than fear of electricity, although there is no obvious reason to suspect that snakes are more frequently associated with UCSs than electricity (Agras et al., 1969).

Second, in clinical literature, excellent illustrations can be found of aversive situations (UCSs; e.g., air raids, sieges, accidents) in which, contrary to all predictions that can be derived from the classical conditioning model, people did not acquire phobic fears (e.g., Saigh, 1984). In the above cited study by Kuch et al. (1994), not all accident survivors developed a fear of driving. Similarly, there is abundant evidence to show that aversive experiences (UCSs) with spiders, dentists or dogs *per se* do not give rise to spider phobia, dental phobia or dog phobia, respectively (Merckelbach et al., 1992; Lautch, 1971; diNardo et al., 1988). Obviously, then, trauma (UCS) without subsequent phobia occurs.

Third, over the years, it has become clear that not all specific phobias can be traced back to a confrontation with a traumatic or aversive event (UCS). In other words, some people develop a fear response to a CS, although this CS has never been directly paired with an UCS (Wolpe et al., 1985). In other words, phobia without preceding trauma (UCS) occurs.

These and other shortcomings of the traditional conditioning approach to phobias, paved the way for two types of revision. The first type of revision stressed that conditioning concepts should be connected with biological notions in order to understand the aetiology of phobias. The above-mentioned preparedness hypothesis

(Seligman, 1971) is a good example of such a biologically orientated revision. Recall that this hypothesis assumes that conditioning interacts with evolutionary processes to produce phobic fear. Thus, aversive events (UCSs) in the context of a evolutionary recent objects (e.g., electricity) would not produce a phobic fear, whereas such events in the context of evolutionary relevant items (e.g., snakes) would easily give rise to a phobic fear. Several experiments have tested this idea in the laboratory. Mainly, the results of these experiments are disappointing in that they found no evidence for a connection between ease of conditioning and evolutionary relevance of the CS (Hugdahl and Johnsen, 1989). Furthermore, the preparedness hypothesis raises some difficult theoretical points. For example, this hypothesis assumes that evolutionary pressure acted on fear of certain objects. But why should evolution have favoured fear behaviour rather than, for instance, aggressive behaviour? In conclusion, the preparedness hypothesis does not seem to provide a successful revision of the conditioning model of phobias (see reviews by Davey, 1995; McNally, 1987; Merckelbach and de Jong, 1997).

Another attempt to revise the conditioning model along biological lines proposes that the phobogenic effects of CS-UCS pairings interact with the neurohormonal state of the organism. In Kelley's (1987, p. 403) words: "neuroses equals conditioning times neurohormones". More specifically, Kelley argued that high levels of adrenocorticotrope hormone (ACTH) and vasopressin enhance the effects of CS-UCS pairings whereas high levels of endogenous opioids (i.e., endorphins) attenuate these effects. Accordingly, individual differences in neurohormonal levels could explain why, for example, an automobile accident produces a driving phobia in some people, but not in others. That is, some subjects are more vulnerable to CS-UCS pairings because they habitually have heightened levels of ACTH and vasopressin and/or lowered endorphin levels. Although it is evident that phobic fear is accompanied by elevated or reduced levels of certain (neuro)hormones (for review, see Cameron and Nesse, 1988), Kelley's proposal has not been put to a direct test. All that can be concluded from the evidence at hand is that lowering the endorphin levels by applying naltrexone, an opioid antagonist, intensifies fear in subjects who are already phobic (Merluzzi et al., 1991; Arntz et al., 1993). However, there are no indications that neurohormones such as endorphins are directly involved in the aetiology of specific phobias. In fact, laboratory experiments have failed to find that endorphins enhance the effects of conditioning in non-phobic subjects (Merckelbach et al., 1993a). Obviously, it remains to be seen whether ACTH and vasopressin are involved in the aetiology of specific phobias.

A related line of research has stressed the involvement of sex hormones in the acquisition of phobic fear. For example, in their review, Cameron and Nesse (1988, p. 291) conclude that: "sex hormone fluctuations in women during the menstrual cycle may be related to changes in anxiety levels, although fluctuations have not always been observed". Interestingly, Van der Molen et al. (1988) found that pre-menstrual women show an increased susceptibility to fear conditioning. Thus, sex hormone fluctuations may explain why specific phobias are more often found in women than in men.

Other studies have focused on the role of stress hormones like cortisol, adrenaline, and noradrenaline in potentiating the effects of classical conditioning. In general, animal studies have documented that post-conditioning peripheral administration of these neurohormones (or their precursors) enhances conditioned fear responses (for a review, see Rosen and Schulkin, 1998). It remains to be seen to what extent these findings can be generalised to human classical conditioning. More specifically, this domain of research would benefit from studies looking at stable individual differences in baseline levels of stress hormones, and whether such differences may explain vulnerability to the phobogenic effects of aversive classical conditioning. Note that there are some indications that individual differences in, for example, cortisol are intimately linked to higher-order traits like neuroticism and behavioural inhibition (cf. supra; see also Schmidt et al., 1997). Furthermore, it is obvious that individuals who possess such traits acquire fear responses with relative ease compared with control individuals (e.g., Gershuny and Sher, 1998). Thus, we await studies that delineate the precise connections between higher-order traits, hormones, and the phobogenic potential of classical conditioning.

The Neoconditioning Approach

The second type of revision of the classical conditioning model is more cognitively orientated. Advocates of this approach point out that conditioning is not the blind, reflexive process that it is often assumed to be (e.g., Davey, 1992). Take the example of little Albert. Did conditioning result in a reflexive connection between the white rat stimulus (CS) and the fear response (CR)? Or did little Albert learn that the white rat stimulus (CS) predicts the onset of the noise stimulus (UCS) and was it this knowledge that elicited a CR? The first scenario is called S-R learning, while the second is known as S-S learning. There are reasons to believe that in humans, S-S learning is the most common classical conditioning scenario. That is to say, conditioning is usually a cognitive process during which one learns that the CS predicts the UCS (Rescorla, 1988). This is not the place to summarise the evidence for this conclusion. However, it is important to note that a S-S approach (i.e., the neoconditioning model) has a number of interesting ramifications and is able to avoid some of the inadequacies of the traditional conditioning model (Rachman, 1991; Davey, 2000). To illustrate this, we will briefly discuss the phenomena of latent inhibition and UCS inflation.

Suppose a subject has extensive experience with a CS (e.g., light) that is not followed by an aversive UCS. What happens when later this subject is exposed to a new situation in which a painful UCS (e.g., electric shock) suddenly accompanies the CS? Will the CS now elicit a conditioned fear response? The answer is no. Laboratory experiments show that it is difficult to condition fear responses to a familiar CS that was formerly never associated with an aversive UCS (e.g., Booth et al., 1989). Recall that during conditioning subjects learn that a CS is predictor of an UCS. If the subject has experienced a number of times that the CS predicts nothing, an incidental co-occurrence of the CS with an aversive UCS is not powerful enough to make the subject believe that the CS has changed into a predictor of the UCS. In other words, prior experiences with the CS inhibit fear conditioning. A study by Doogan and Thomas (1992) nicely illustrates that the mechanism of latent inhibition is relevant when one tries to understand how trauma (UCS) without subsequent phobia can occur. These researchers found that both subjects with fear of dogs and subjects without fear of dogs report traumatic encounters with dogs. However, the latter group reported previous non-aversive contact with dogs. In other words, the non-fearful subjects had experienced many occasions on which dogs (CS) did not attack. This suggests that in the non-fearful group, latent inhibition helped to minimise the effects of fear conditioning (see also Davey, 1989a). Likewise, de Jongh et al. (1995) noted that painful dental treatments (UCSs) do not produce dental phobia when subjects have extensive non-aversive experiences with dental treatment prior to their first painful dental treatment.

A second phenomenon emphasised by neoconditioning theorists is termed UCS inflation (Davey, 1989b). This phenomenon refers to a situation in which subjects are exposed to pairings of a CS and a mild UCS. Because of this, subjects acquire an S-S association. However, given the low intensity of the UCS, this S-S association leads to a weak conditioned fear response (CR). Now the following may happen: if subjects during a next phase learn that the UCS is nevertheless dangerous, this post-conditioning information will lead to an inflation of the UCS value. Consequently, the conditioned fear response will grow in strength. A clinical example taken from White and Davey (1989, p. 165) illustrates how this scenario may account for cases in which conditioned fear emerges without pertinent trauma:

> [A]n individual may witness an unknown person die of a heart attack on a bus or a train. On future occasions, riding on public transport may evoke memories of this incident but no anxiety . . .. Subsequently, however, that individual may be present when a close friend or relative dies of a heart attack, thus inflating the aversive properties of heart attacks. This may then give rise to acute anxiety when riding on public transport. In this particular scenario, public transport has never been directly associated with anxiety-eliciting trauma, but the public transport phobia results from a prior learned association between public transport and heart attacks, and subsequent independent inflation of heart attacks as aversive events.

Several case histories of phobia can be interpreted in terms of UCS inflation (Davey et al., 1993a). However, laboratory experiments indicate that in human subjects, it is not easy to produce robust fear conditioning through UCS inflation (De Jong et al., 1994). Thus, it seems that UCS inflation does occur, but only under specific conditions that are not entirely understood.

To recapitulate, neoconditioning concepts such as latent inhibition and UCS inflation can deal with some inadequacies of the traditional conditioning approach. More specifically, latent inhibition can explain why UCS trauma does not always lead to phobia, while UCS inflation can explain why phobia without pertinent UCS trauma is possible. Apart from that, these concepts have implications for the treatment of phobias (Davey, 1992). For example, one may use the principle of latent inhibition as a immunisation strategy against the effects of subsequent CS-UCS trials. Giving dental patients a series of painless "sham" treatments will probably reduce the likelihood that a subsequent painful treatment results in a dental phobia. As another example, the principle of UCS inflation suggests that during treatment, it might be worthwhile to systematically "devaluate" the UCS. In the case of dental phobia, this could mean that one stresses that aversive dental treatment may promote healthy teeth.

Indirect Pathways to Phobia: Modelling and Information

The classical conditioning pathway to fear assumes that the subject has direct experience with the CS and the UCS. This is true for straightforward conditioning in which a CS is paired with a traumatic UCS as well as for subtle conditioning scenarios such as latent inhibition and UCS inflation. However, there are cases in which subjects develop a specific phobia although they have no history of direct experience with the CS (i.e., phobic object) and/or UCS (Rachman, 1977; Rachman, 1990b; Rachman, 1991). In these cases, indirect pathways of fear acquisition may play a pivotal role. Rachman (Rachman, 1977; Rachman, 1990b; Rachman, 1991) provides a detailed description of two indirect pathways that are important in this context: modelling (i.e., vicarious transmission of fear) and negative information.

The modelling pathway assumes that phobic fears can be acquired by watching parents or peers reacting fearfully to a stimulus (e.g., a spider). Animal and human laboratory studies support this assumption. For example, Cook and Mineka (1989) found that rhesus monkeys can acquire a fear of snakes through watching video tapes of two model monkeys reacting fearfully to toy snakes. Likewise, Hygge and Öhman (1978) demonstrated that subjects respond with sympathetic activation to pictures of e.g., snakes when they have previously watched others reacting fearfully to these pictures. The reverse is also true. The pioneers of behaviour therapy already knew that one can eliminate specific fears by presenting non-fearful models and enhancing social learning through modelling (Kornfeld, 1989). In turning now to negative information, it seems obvious that verbal information about certain stimuli provided by books, television or significant others may give rise to fear of these stimuli. If this was not the case, prevention programmes concerned with smoking or AIDS would make no sense. While there is a scarcity of experimental studies on the fear-evoking characteristics of negative information, social psychological studies show that subjects assign more value to negative than to positive information. There might be good evolutionary reasons for this asymmetry (Pratto and John, 1991).

Historical literature offers some perfect illustrations of the role of negative information in the development of fear. A case in point is Riley (1986) who provides us with a lively description of how scientists' discoveries of pathogens on insects around the turn of the century were communicated to health authorities and lay people. Riley writes that this development "provoked a sudden change in attitudes toward certain insects, especially the common fly. Whereas people had previously shown an attitude of friendly tolerance to insects, specialists suddenly advised them as dangerous pests" (p. 844; see also Arrindell, 2000). Note that Riley's description of how negative information about insects led to aversion and disgust of these stimuli is, again, difficult to reconcile with a preparedness view. By this view, one would not have anticipated an attitude of "friendly tolerance" to stimuli that evidently may threaten biological fitness. Riley's example can better be explained in terms of disgust-relevance and disgust sensitivity. There is now abundant evidence that phobias of snakes, spiders, slugs, snails, and rats have to do with the disgust-evoking status of these animals (e.g., Davey et al., 1993b). That is, contemporary culture associates disease, illness, and contamination with these animals. Accordingly, people who are high on disgust sensitivity will react with fear and avoidance to these animals. As can be expected, subjects with small animal phobias have heightened scores on instruments measuring disgust sensitivity (Merckelbach et al., 1993b; Tolin et al., 1997). Disgust sensitivity is a stable trait and there are some indications of its familial transmission. For example, parents' disgust sensitivity has been found to be a powerful predictor of children's animal phobias (Davey et al., 1993b; De Jong et al., 1997). Perhaps, then, disgust sensitivity qualifies as the behavioural expression of what Taylor (1998) termed a lower-order (i.e., specific) genetic factor that interacts with culturally determined disgust connotations to produce small animal phobias.

Retrospective Clinical Studies

A number of studies have examined to what extent the three pathways to fear play a role in the aetiology of specific phobia (e.g., Öst, 1987a; Merckelbach et al., 1992; Kleinknecht, 1994). Most of these studies relied on the Phobic Origin Questionnaire (POQ; Öst and Hugdahl, 1981), a retrospective self-report instrument that asks phobic patients to indicate to what degree their phobia developed along a direct (i.e., conditioning) and/or an indirect (i.e., modelling; negative information) pathway.

Several interesting findings have emerged from the POQ studies. First, while each of the three pathways is represented in the various types of specific phobia, there appear to be significant differences between the types. For example, animal phobics and blood-injection-injury phobics more often ascribe their fears to modelling and negative information than claustrophobics. Interestingly, Öst (1987a) found evidence to suggest that modelling and negative information are associated with an early onset age. In contrast, the conditioning pathway is more pronounced in claustrophobia than in animal, blood-injection-injury illness or height phobia (e.g., Öst, 1987a; Menzies and Clarke, 1993). It is worthwhile speculating a bit about the type of conditioning that might occur in situational phobias (e.g., claustrophobia). The neoconditioning approach (cf. supra) has made it clear that UCSs are not necessarily restricted to external and painful events. Internal experiences such as isolated panic attacks may also function as powerful UCSs. Himle et al. (1991) noted that almost half of their sample of situational phobics ascribed the onset of their complaints to a panic-like experience in specific situations that subsequently became the object of their fear. A similar finding has been reported for people with driving phobia (Ehlers et al., 1994). Thus, it may well be the case that situational phobias are the joint product of panic-like conditioning experiences and an exaggerated fear of suffocation. An exaggerated fear of suffocation is thought to reflect a biological and possibly heritable trait (see also Verburg et al., 1994).

Second, several studies (e.g., Merckelbach et al., 1991; Ollendick and King, 1991) have found that fearful individuals often report more than one pathway. There are even indications that individuals with "mixed" pathways (e.g., conditioning and modelling) have higher levels of fear. Third, the three pathways to fear are also found in fearful children aged 9 to 14 years (Ollendick and King, 1991; see also Doogan and Thomas, 1992).

An interesting speculation about the interrelationship between the three pathways to fear, the three symptoms systems of fear, and treatment interventions was put forward by Rachman (e.g., 1977; De Silva and Rachman, 1981). Rachman proposed that there might be a systematic connection between aetiology of phobia, symptom profiles of phobia, and treatment of phobia. More specifically, he argued that phobias based on a direct conditioning pathway would be dominated by behavioural and physiological symptoms, whereas indirectly acquired phobias would be characterised by cognitive symptoms. Consequently, the first class of phobias would profit more from exposure-based interventions while the second class of phobias would benefit from cognitive interventions (see also Wolpe, 1981). So far, attempts to evaluate the empirical merits of Rachman's suggestions have largely produced disappointing results (Eifert and Wilson, 1991; but see Öst, 1987b). As said before, phobic patients often attribute their complaints to two or three pathways. Moreover, several studies have failed to find a significant association between pathways to fear and loadings on the three symptoms systems (e.g., Öst, 1991). However, Eifert and Wilson (1991) rightly remarked that these studies were based on rather imprecise methods for measuring symptom profiles. Obviously, Rachman's suggestion warrants further investigation.

A potential problem with the POQ studies is, of course, that phobics are invited to provide a retrospective judgement as to the cause of their complaints. With such retrospective research strategy, all kinds of biases (e.g., memory distortions) may occur. For example, the large-scale prospective study by Henry and co-workers (1994) shows that adolescents are not very good at reporting their own behavioural problems (e.g., phobias, depression) at ages 9 to 11. In that study, correlation between retrospective and concurrent reports were often well below 0.20. To circumvent the potential biases of retrospective accounts, researchers have begun to conduct studies in which phobic adults' or children's reports about onset events are compared with those of knowledgeable informants. Kheriaty et al. (1999) reported that a majority of their dog and blood-injection fearful participants reported conditioning and, to a lesser extent, modelling onset events and a significant number of these events were confirmed by their parents. Similar results were reported by Merckelbach et al. (1996b) and Merckelbach and Muris (1997) in their studies on children with severe spider phobia children. Taken together, these findings suggest that Rachman's three-pathway model is a valuable framework for conceptualising the role of learning experiences in the development of childhood fears and phobias.

COGNITIVE BIASES

Specific phobias are the end products of a complex interplay between genetically linked traits (behavioural inhibition, disgust sensitivity, fear of suffocation) and direct or indirect learning experiences. How are phobic fears maintained, once they are acquired? Mowrer's two-stage model mentioned earlier suggests that avoidance behaviour is responsible for the conservation of phobic fear. That is, avoidance would minimise direct and prolonged contact with the phobic object and, hence, phobics would not have the opportunity to learn that the CS is a neutral object. However, apart from avoidance behaviour, there seem to be other mechanisms playing a role in the conservation of fear. These mechanisms are cognitive in nature and have been the object of extensive research in the past two decades (for a review, see Williams et al., 1997). There is agreement among most researchers in this field that pathological anxiety (e.g., specific phobia) is not accompanied by a general cognitive dysfunction. In other words, it is not the case that pathological anxiety is associated with overall deficits in memory, attention, motor function, and so on. Instead, cognitive dysfunctions in specific phobias take on a highly restricted form. Briefly, phobic subjects show evidence of dysfunctions in attentional and judgmental processes rather than memory. As well, the attentional and judgmental biases that characterise phobias are content dependent. That is to say, these biases become apparent if and only if phobics are confronted with fear-relevant stimuli (e.g., the word "spider" in case of a spider phobic subject).

Attentional Bias

Attentional bias refers to hyperattention to threatening material. This hyperattention occurs even with verbal material that is not relevant to the primary task in which the subject is involved. One frequently employed technique for demonstrating attentional bias is the modified Stroop colour task. During this task, subjects are confronted with rows of words that are printed in different colours (e.g., red, green, yellow, and blue). Subjects are required to name the colour of a word while ignoring the meaning of that word. A consistent finding in Stroop studies with anxious patients is that their colour naming of threatening words is slower than that of neutral words (e.g., see for a review Williams et al., 1996). For example, spider phobics display retarded colour-naming times when they are confronted with spider-related words (e.g., "spider", "creepy"), but not when they have to colour name neutral words (e.g., "car"). This is due to the fact that spider phobics automatically direct their attention to the content of the threatening words and this interferes with their main task (i.e., colour naming).

As to the clinical consequence of attentional bias, it seems likely that an increased focus on danger and threat stimuli may serve to maintain phobic fear. That is, attentional bias implicates an increased encoding of threatening material and this, in turn, will elevate fear levels. Interestingly, clinical improvement of specific phobias due to exposure therapy is accompanied by a disappearance or reduction of attentional bias on the Stroop task (Lavy et al., 1993). The relevance of findings such as these is twofold. To begin with, they suggest that the modified Stroop colour task and related cognitive tasks are potentially useful clinical assessment tools for measuring symptom severity and treatment prognosis. Note that performance on these cognitive tasks is quite different from completing a self-report questionnaire. That is, unlike questionnaires, these tasks do not require introspection or conscious monitoring. Rather, they directly tap cognitive processes that are involuntary and automatic (for a review, see McNally, 1995). Germane to this issue are studies that succeeded in documenting attentional bias phenomena for subliminally presented threat words. In these studies, normal subjects high or low on trait anxiety saw ultra short (e.g., 30 msec) presentations of neutral and threat words that were immediately followed by supraliminal coloured masks. Subjects were asked to identify the colour of the masks. Although subjects were not able consciously to identify the neutral or threat words, high-trait anxious, but not low-trait anxious participants displayed retarded colour naming (i.e., attentional bias) after threatening, but not after neutral target words (Van den Hout et al., 1995). With this procedure, MacLeod and Hagan (1992) were able to show that attentional bias towards threat-related material is a better predictor of vulnerability to emotional distress elicited by stressful life events than are scores on self-report questionnaires.

A second point is that experimental tools such as the modified Stroop task offer good opportunities for studying the way in which fundamental traits interact with stressful events to maintain psychopathology. Attentional bias phenomena have been found to occur in a number of anxiety disorders (e.g., specific phobia, panic disorder, generalised anxiety disorder), but, as was pointed out above, also in high-trait anxious individuals. Trait anxiety is closely related to higher-order traits like neuroticism and behavioural inhibition (e.g., Eysenck, 1992). Thus, it appears that these traits point in the direction of a hypervigilant cognitive style that gives high processing priorities to threat-related stimuli, thereby promoting escalation of fear. In the words of MacLeod (1991, p. 289): "high trait anxious individuals are those people who, at an automatic non-conscious level of processing, respond to elevations in state anxiety or arousal by increasing the degree to which generally threatening information selectively is encoded from the environment".

Judgmental Bias

There are two types of judgmental bias that probably play a role in the maintenance of specific phobia. The first type is the co-variation bias, which refers to the tendency to overestimate the association between phobic stimuli and aversive outcomes

(Tomarken et al., 1989). The experimental demonstration of co-variation bias in phobias is straightforward. Phobic and normal subjects are shown a series of slides consisting of fear-relevant pictures (e.g., spiders) and fear-irrelevant pictures (e.g., flowers). Slide offset is followed by one of three outcomes: an aversive shock, a tone or nothing. Fear-relevant and fear-irrelevant pictures are equally often followed by each of the outcomes. After the series of slides, subjects are asked to estimate the contingencies between slides and outcomes ("if a spider picture appeared, how great was the chance that this picture was followed by a shock?"). Under these experimental conditions, phobic subjects systematically overestimate the contingency between phobic stimuli and aversive outcomes. Again, in successfully treated spider phobics, the co-variation bias disappears (De Jong et al., 1992). Furthermore, De Jong et al. (1995a) noted that there is a strong and positive correlation ($r = 0.61$) between residual co-variation bias in treated spider phobics and relapse. That is, the stronger the (post-treatment) overestimation of the contingency between spider picture and aversive shock, the higher the spider fear at two-year follow up. In sum, then, phobics have a tendency to attribute aversive experiences to the phobic object and this, in turn, will sustain their fear.

A second judgmental bias that may occur in specific phobias is a style of reasoning known as *ex consequentia* inference. Like other people, phobics believe that dangerous situations elicit anxiety. However, unlike many non-phobic subjects, spider phobics seem to believe that anxiety symptoms imply the presence of danger (e.g., a dangerous spider; Arntz et al., 1995). The *ex consequentia* inference probably serves to legitimate the phobic fear and, thus, may maintain the phobia. However, more studies are needed firmly to establish the role of this reasoning style in the maintenance of fear.

The Origins of Cognitive Biases

It is interesting to speculate about the origins of cognitive biases. For example, is it possible to link these biases to neurobiological processes (McNally, 1998)? One hypothesis that deserves consideration is that cognitive biases emerge from a right hemisphere mode of information processing (Merckelbach et al., 1990). Most researchers agree that the left and right hemisphere have different cognitive characteristics. Whereas the left hemisphere would mediate analytic and serial operations, the right hemisphere would sustain holistic and imaginal operations. Tucker and Newman (1981) have argued that the left hemisphere-processing mode is very effective in controlling emotional reactions. In contrast, the right hemisphere mode would lead to an intensification of affect. This suggestion makes sense because one may expect that the global and imprecise approach of the right hemisphere enhances hyperattention to threat and overestimation of aversive outcome. Interestingly, studies by Davidson (1998) indicate that there are stable individual differences in frontal EEG asymmetry. More specifically, Davidson's work shows that habitual right frontal overactivation (as indexed by EEG background activity) is, indeed, related to an affective style that is characterised by lowered thresholds for avoidance behaviour and negative affect. Thus, it may well be the case that a chronic right hemisphere overactivity is involved in cognitive biases and the maintenance of fear. Although there is some experimental work that supports this causal relationship (De Jong et al., 1995b), further research is needed to examine whether habitual right hemisphere overactivation is the source of the cognitive biases that occur in anxiety disorders. Studies that are more recent, reviewed by Heller and Nitschke (1998), suggest that theoretical progress in this research domain depends on a more fine-grained analysis of the behavioural functions of frontal and parieto-temporal regions. According to these authors, one needs to distinguish between anxious apprehension, which seems to be a function of left frontal regions, and anxious arousal which seems to be driven by right parieto-temporal areas.

TREATMENT OF SPECIFIC PHOBIAS

Surveys (e.g., Magee et al., 1996) have shown time and time again that only a small minority of people with specific phobias ever seek professional help. Meanwhile, the prospects for treating this condition are extremely good. Exposure *in vivo* is the treatment of choice for specific phobias (Marks, 1987; Rachman, 1990b). Exposure treatment involves graded and prolonged confrontation with the phobic object. Meanwhile the therapist encourages the patient to approach the phobic object and to refrain from avoidance behaviour. Exposure is often combined with other techniques such as modelling by the therapist in the case of animal phobias (Öst, 1989), applied tension to prevent fainting in the case of blood-injection-injury phobias (Öst et al., 1991b), and cognitive interventions to correct catastrophic misinterpretations of bodily symptoms in the case of claustrophobia (Craske et al., 1995). Exposure treatments yield good results in that success percentages of 90% are not exceptional. Furthermore, controlled studies show that the efficacy of exposure is maintained at long-term follow-up (Öst et al., 1991a). Recently, Öst (1997) summarised the results of some 25 randomised clinical trials involving rapid (i.e., one-session) exposure treatment for different subtypes of specific phobias. This author concluded that "across the different specific phobias the rapid treatment methods yield 74–94% clinically improved patients after 2–3 hours of treatment" (ibid., p. 244).

The precise mechanism underlying the beneficial effects of exposure is a matter of some debate. Some authors have favoured an "extinction" or "habituation" interpretation of exposure effects (e.g., Marks, 1987; Watts, 1979). According to these authors, exposure is the extinction or habituation of a fear CR to a CS that is no longer followed by an UCS. Others have argued that exposure effects are linked to cognitive changes rather than response habituation (e.g., Foa and Kozak, 1986). These authors emphasise that during exposure, the patient learns that the phobic object is not associated with catastrophic events. This will eventually lead to a correction of the phobic fear. Note, in passing, that this formulation is compatible with the S-S view of phobic fear (Eysenck, 1987), but also with cognitive theories about phobic fear (Last, 1987). There is preliminary evidence that interpretations of exposure that emphasise cognitive change are closer to the truth than extinction/ habituation accounts. For example, Shafran et al. (1993) recently showed that treatment of claustrophobia is successful to the degree that it corrects certain essential cognitions (e.g., "I will suffocate"). Similarly, in their study of one-session exposure treatment of spider phobia, Öst and colleagues (1991a, p. 421) remark that

> [T]he clinical impression from treating these patients is that the most important factor in the one-session treatment is making explicit the patients' catastrophic thoughts concerning the phobic situation and devising the exposure situation in such a way that these can be tested out.

Despite the superiority of *in vivo* exposure treatment for specific phobias, some clinicians have promoted alternative therapies for this condition. One of them is eye movement desensitisation and reprocessing (EMDR). EMDR is a relatively new technique that was originally proposed as a treatment method for post-traumatic stress disorder (PTSD; Shapiro, 1989). During EMDR, patients imaginably expose themselves to a traumatic or aversive memory, while simultaneously engaging in lateral eye movements that are induced by the therapist. The idea is that through eye movements, negative memories are emotionally processed and assimilated. The therapist-induced eye movements would simulate the inhibitory function of Rapid Eye Movement (REM) sleep. Some authors have claimed that EMDR treatment is not only effective in PTSD, but also in specific phobias (e.g., Marquis, 1991; De Jongh et al., 1999). However, this claim rests largely on miraculous case studies. Controlled outcome studies designed to compare the effectivity of EMDR and exposure *in vivo* in the treatment of specific phobias clearly indicate that exposure yields superior results (Acierno et al., 1994; Muris and Merckelbach, 1999). It is not stretching the point too far to say that EMDR is effective insofar as it contains an element of exposure (Acierno et al., 1994). So far, laboratory studies have found no evidence for the claim that the lateral eye movements during an EMDR procedure possess the potential to inhibit negative emotions (Tallis and Smith, 1994; Merckelbach et al., 1994). With these findings in mind, it is disturbing to see that in the past five years or so, EMDR has gained great popularity among psychotherapists. Its rapid proliferation follows the dissemination pattern of what some have called "Power Therapies" (Rosen et al., 1998), that is therapies that promise rapid cures for an ever widening array of disorders in the total absence of empirical justifications. Needless to say that "well established cognitive and behavioural principles are more likely to serve patients' needs" (Rosen et al., 1998, p. 98).

There is abundant evidence showing that benzodiazepines have anxiolytic effects (e.g., Rickels, 1978). Furthermore, animal research indicates that benzodiazepines inhibit conditioned fear responses. Consequently, one would predict that benzodiazepines could be useful in the treatment of specific phobias. However, studies designed to evaluate the effect of benzodiazepines on phobic avoidance have generally yielded disappointing results (e.g., Bernadt et al., 1980; Sartory et al., 1990).

Although benzodiazepines might inhibit subjective fear during phobic confrontation, they do not increase approach behaviour (Sartory et al., 1990). Gray (1987) has gone one step further and suggested that benzodiazepines might even be harmful in that they create state dependency effects. That is, phobics learn to approach the phobic stimulus when drugged, but this learning is not transferred to a non-drugged state.

CONCLUSION

Specific phobias have been well researched in the past decades. As a result, we now have a rather complete picture of the important elements that constitute this diagnostic category. To summarise the most important points, specific phobias form a heterogeneous class of disorders (Himle et al., 1991). The most radical difference is that between small animal phobias and situational phobias (e.g., claustrophobia). Compared with animal phobias, situational phobias are characterised by a more elaborated set of cognitions, a later age of onset, a more pronounced role of conditioning experiences in their aetiology (e.g., Öst, 1987a), and a higher comorbidity with panic attacks and panic disorder (Himle et al., 1991). Accordingly, in situational phobias, but not in animal phobias, effects of exposure treatment are enhanced when the treatment is combined with cognitive interventions (Craske et al., 1995).

As we have explained in more detail elsewhere (Muris and Merckelbach, 2000), the aetiologically diversity of specific phobias can best be handled by a multifactorial model that comprises, at least, the following four elements.

1. Generally, on one hand, there is continuity between normal developmental fears that occur in the large majority of children and adolescents, and on the other hand, there is severe specific phobia that affect a sizeable minority of adults. This continuity has to do with the fact that in a subgroup of children and adolescents, normal fears tend to escalate.
2. This escalation occurs against the general background of higher-order genetic vulnerabilities that manifest themselves in behavioural patterns (e.g., behavioural inhibition) and temperamental traits (e.g., neuroticism, negative affectivity, trait anxiety).
3. The precise content of specific phobias is a product of an interaction between lower-order genetic vulnerabilities (e.g., disgust sensitivity, hypersensitive suffocation detectors) and certain learning experiences dictated by conditioning, modelling, and/or negative information.
4. Once a specific phobia exists, it is maintained by avoidance behaviour, but also by cognitive biases such as attentional bias and co-variation bias. Consequently, in most cases, the natural course of specific phobias is chronic. However, exposure-based treatments are very effective in reducing specific phobias.

Several questions remain. Most importantly, the precise dynamics between the four factors specified above are far from clear. For example, do aversive learning experiences contribute to a radicalisation of developmental fears only during a critical period? Or is it the case that learning experiences together with behavioural inhibition and other genetically linked traits may reinstate developmental fears that disappeared during a previous phase? The only way to resolve these issues is to gather longitudinal general population data. Of course, such studies are not easy to conduct, but further progress will depend critically on them. In the meantime, this research domain could profit from a more concentrated research focus on normal childhood fears and how they relate to higher- and lower-order traits.

The skewed sex distribution of specific phobias is another issue that is not well understood. It might well be the case that sex hormones interact with conditioning processes. While there is some tentative laboratory evidence showing that conditioning of autonomic responses varies with the menstrual cycle (Van der Molen et al., 1988), more research is needed to evaluate this hypothesis. In more general terms, it might be worthwhile to subject Kelley's hypothesis "neurosis equals conditioning times neurohormones" to rigorous empirical testing.

Another point that is still elusive, is the non-random distribution of specific fears. Why is it that phobic fears are more often directed at, say, snakes than at, for example, electricity? It is clear that the "evolutionary preparedness" interpretation of this phenomenon is not very satisfactory. A more plausible interpretation of the non-random distribution of fears points to the role of culturally transmitted ideas and values about certain phobogenic stimuli (Kirkpatrick, 1984). That is, children might learn from their parents that stimuli such as snakes, spiders, etc. are associated with disease, contamination or dirt. As was discussed above, there is good evidence for the role of disgust in, at least, small animal phobias (Matchett and Davey, 1991) and there are also indications that parents' disgust predicts animal fear in their offspring (Davey et al., 1993b). These findings are consistent with a cultural interpretation of the non-random distribution of fears, but they also fit with the idea that disgust sensitivity is genetically transmitted. Clearly, large-scale cross-cultural studies are needed to determine how genetic and cultural factors shape the non-random distribution of fear. Research along these lines has only just begun. For example, Davey et al. (1998) noted in their study on animal fears in seven different western and Asian countries that the category of disgust-evoking animals (e.g., spiders, frogs, cockroaches) seems to be rather universal. Yet, these authors also found considerable cross-cultural differences in subjects' fear ratings of these animals. Parametric studies examining the links between specific fears, disgust, and disgust sensitivity in parents and children from different cultures may prove to be one fruitful avenue for future research.

A final point concerns the role of exposure in fear reduction. Empirical research leaves no doubt that exposure-based interventions are very effective in reducing and eliminating specific fears and phobias (see also Eysenck, 1994). However, it remains to be seen whether *in vivo* exposure is a necessary prerequisite for the reduction of phobic fear. Some authors have argued that it is not (De Silva and Rachman, 1981; Rachman, 1990b). These authors emphasise that fear can be acquired along indirect learning pathways (modelling and/or negative information). Consequently, it should be possible to reduce fear by providing corrective information. Indeed, preliminary results suggest that a pure cognitive intervention without exposure does reduce claustrophobic fear (Booth and Rachman, 1992). However, it may well be the case that this positive finding is closely connected to the peculiar nature of claustrophobic fears (e.g., later onset, strong involvement of certain "fear of fear" cognitions) and cannot be generalised to other specific phobias. Other researchers tend to regard exposure as a necessary but not sufficient therapeutic component for fear reduction (e.g., Marks, 1987). So far, no critical experiment has been performed that allows us to choose among these different positions.

More than two decades ago, the Dutch psychologist Barendregt (1976, p. 137) remarked with regard to phobic disorders that "one fool can think of more hypotheses than ten wise men can test". Plainly, since Barendregt, our understanding of specific phobias has advanced up to a point where the number of problems and sensible hypotheses is limited. Further theoretical progress will critically dependent on increasingly complex research designs. Yet, it should be noted that this undertaking is not only important in its own right, but may also have heuristic value for our understanding of other anxiety disorders.

REFERENCES

Acierno R, Hersen M, Hasselt VB, Tremont G, Hueser KT (1994) Review of the validation and dissemination of eye movement desensitisation and reprocessing: A scientific and ethical dilemma. *Clinical Psychology Review* **14**: 287–299.

Agras S, Sylvester D, Oliveau D (1969) The epidemiology of common fears and phobias. *Comprehensive Psychiatry* **10**: 151–156.

American Psychiatric Association (1994) *Diagnostic and Statistical Manual of Mental Disorders* (4th edition). Washington, DC: American Psychiatric Association.

Andrews G, Stewart G, Morris-Yates A, Holt P, Henderson S (1990) Evidence for a general neurotic syndrome. *Br J Psychiatry* **157**: 6–12.

Arntz A, Merckelbach H, De Jong PJ (1993) Opioid antagonist affects behavioural effects of exposure in vivo. *J Consulting and Clin Psychology* **61**: 865–870.

Arntz A, Rauner M, Van den Hout MA (1995) "If I feel anxious, there must be danger": Ex-consequentia reasoning in inferring danger in anxiety disorders. *Behav Res Ther* **33**: 917–925.

Arrindell WA (2000) Phobic dimensions: IV. The structure of animal fears. *Behav Res Ther*, in press.

Arrindell WA, Pickersgill MJ, Merckelbach H, Ardon AM, Cornet FC (1991) Phobic dimensions: III. Factor analytic approaches to the study of common phobic fears: An updated review of findings with adult subjects. *Advances in Behav Res Ther* **13**: 73–130.

Barendregt JT (1976) Phobias and phobics. In HM van Praag (ed) *Research in Neurosis*. Utrecht: Bohn, Scheltema & Holkema.

Bauer DH (1976) An exploratory study of developmental changes in children's fears. *J Child Psychology and Psychiatry* **17**: 69–74.

Bernadt MW, Silverstone T, Singleton W (1980) Behavioural and subjective effects of beta-adrenergic blockade in phobic subjects. *B J Psychiatry* **137**: 452–457.

Bertenthal BL, Campos JJ (1984) A re-examination of fear and its determinants on the visual cliff. *Psychophysiology* **21**: 413–417.

Biederman J, Rosenbaum JF, Charloff J, Kagan J (1995) Behavioural inhibition as a risk factor for anxiety disorders. In JS March (ed) *Anxiety Disorders in Children and Adolescents*. New York: Guilford.

Booth ML, Siddle DAT, Bond NW (1989) Effects of conditioned fear-relevance and pre-exposure on expectancy and electrodermal measures of human Pavlovian conditioning. *Psychophysiology* **26**: 281–291.

Booth R, Rachman S (1992) The reduction of claustrophobia. *Behav Res Ther* **30**: 207–222.

Calkins SD, Fox NA, Marshall TR (1996) Behavioural and physiological antecedents of inhibited and uninhibited behaviour. *Child Development* **67**: 523–540.

Cameron OG, Nesse RM (1988) Systemic hormonal and physiological abnormalities in anxiety disorders. *Psychoneuroendocrinology* **13**: 287–307.

Campbell D, Sanderson RE, Laverty SG (1964) Characteristics of a conditioned response in human subjects during extinction trials following a single traumatic conditioning trial. *J Abnorm Social Psychol* **68**: 627–639.

Clark LA, Watson D, Mineka S (1994) Temperament, personality, and the mood and anxiety disorders. *J Abnorm Psychol* **103**: 103–116.

Cook M, Mineka S (1989) Observational conditioning of fear to fear-relevant versus fear-irrelevant stimuli in rhesus monkeys. *J Abnorm Psychol* **98**: 448–459.

Cornelius RR, Averill JR (1983) Sex differences in fear of spiders. *J Personality and Social Psychology* **45**: 377–383.

Costello CG (1982) Fears and phobias in women: A community study. *J Abnorm Psychol* **91**: 280–286.

Craske MG (1997) Fear and anxiety in children and adolescents. *Bull Menninger Clinic* **61**: 4–36.

Craske MG, Mohlman J, Yi J, Glover D, Valeri S (1995) Treatment of claustrophobia and snake/spider phobias: Fear of arousal and fear of context. *Behav Res Ther* **33**: 197–203.

Davey GCL (1989a) Dental phobics and anxieties: Evidence for conditioning processes in the acquisition and modulation of a learned fear. *Behav Res Ther* **27**: 52–58.

Davey GCL (1989b) UCS revaluation and conditioning models of acquired fears. *Behav Res Ther* **27**: 521–528.

Davey GCL (1992) Classical conditioning and the acquisition of human fears and phobias: A review and synthesis of the literature. *Advances in Behav Res Ther* **14**: 29–66.

Davey GCL (1995) Preparedness and phobias: Specific evolved associations or a generalised expectancy bias? *Behavioural and Brain Sciences* **18**: 289–325.

Davey GCL (1997) *Phobias: A Handbook of Theory, Research, and Treatment*. Chichester: Wiley.

Davey GCL (2000) Multiple pathways to specific phobias: Divergent aetiologies within a common conceptual framework. Manuscript submitted for publication.

Davey GCL, de Jong PJ, Tallis F (1993a) UCS inflation in the aetiology of a variety of anxiety disorders: Some case histories. *Behav Res Ther* **31**: 495–498.

Davey GCL, Forster L, Mayhew G (1993b) Familial resemblances in disgust sensitivity and animal phobias. *Behav Res Ther* **31**: 41–50.

Davey GCL, McDonald AS, Hirisave U, Prabhu GG, Iwawaki S, Im Jim C, Merckelbach H, De Jong PJ, Leung PWL, Reimann BC (1998) A cross-cultural study of animal fears. *Behav Res Ther* **36**: 735–750.

Davidson RJ (1998) Affective style and affective disorders: Perspectives from affective neuroscience. *Cognition and Emotion* **12**: 307–330.

De Jong PJ, Andrea H, Muris P (1997) Spider phobia in children: Disgust and fear before and after treatment. *Behav Res Ther* **35**: 559–562.

De Jong PJ, Merckelbach H, Arntz A, Nijman H (1992) Co-variation detection in treated and untreated spider phobics. *J Abnorm Psychol* **101**: 724–727.

De Jong PJ, Merckelbach H, Koertshuis G, Muris P (1994) UCS inflation and acquired fear responses in human conditioning. *Advances in Behav Res Ther* **16**: 131–165.

De Jong PJ, Merckelbach H, Nijman H (1995b) Hemisphere preference, anxiety, and co-variation bias. *Personality and Individual Differences* **18**: 363–371.

De Jongh A, Muris P, Ter Horst G, Duyx M (1995) Acquisition and maintenance of dental anxiety: The role of conditioning experiences and cognitions. *Behav Res Ther* **33**: 205–210.

De Jongh A, Ten Broeke E, Renssen MR (1999) Treatment of specific phobias with eye movement desensitisation and reprocessing (EMDR): Protocol, empirical status, and conceptual issues. *J Anx Dis* **13**: 69–85.

De Jong PJ, Van den Hout MA, Merckelbach H (1995a) Co-variation bias and the return of fear. *Behav Res Ther* **33**: 211–213.

De Ruiter C, Rijken H, Garssen B, Van Schaik A, Kraaimaat F (1989) Comorbidity among the anxiety disorders. *J Anx Dis* **3**: 57–68.

De Silva P, Rachman S (1981) Is exposure a necessary condition for fear reduction? *Behav Res Ther* **19**: 227–232.

DiNardo PA, Guzy LT, Bak RM (1988) Anxiety response patterns and etiologic factors in dog-fearful and non-fearful subjects. *Behav Res Ther* **26**: 245–252.

Doogan S, Thomas GV (1992) Origins of fear of dogs in adults and children: The role of conditioning processes and prior familiarity with dogs. *Behav Res Ther* **30**: 387–394.

Ehlers A, Hofmann SG, Herda CA, Roth WT (1994) Clinical characteristics of driving phobia. *J Anx Dis* **8**: 323–339.

Eifert GH, Wilson PH (1991) The triple response approach to assessment: A conceptual and methodological reappraisal. *Behav Res Ther* **29**: 283–292.

Errera P (1962) Some historical aspects of the concept phobia. *Psychiatric Quarterly* **36**: 325–336.

Eysenck HJ (1979) The conditioning model of neurosis. *Behav Brain Sciences* **2**: 155–199.

Eysenck HJ (1987) Behaviour therapy. In Eysenck HJ, Martin I (eds) *Theoretical Foundations of Behaviour Therapy*. New York: Plenum Press.

Eysenck MW (1992) *Anxiety: The Cognitive Perspective*. Hove: Erlbaum.

Eysenck HJ (1994) The outcome problem in psychotherapy: What have we learned? *Behav Res Ther* **32**: 477–495.

Foa EB, Kozak MJ (1986) Emotional processing of fear: Exposure to corrective information. *Psychological Bulletin* **99**: 20–35.

Fredrikson M, Annas P, Fischer H, Wik G (1996) Gender and age differences in the prevalence of specific fears and phobias. *Behav Res Ther* **34**: 33–39.

Fredrikson M, Annas P, Wik G (1997) Parental history, aversive exposure, and the development of snake and spider phobia in women. *Behav Res Ther* **35**: 23–28.

Fredrikson M, Wik G, Greitz T, Eriksson L, Stone-Elander S, Ericson K, Sedvall G (1993) Regional cerebral blood flow during experimental phobic fear. *Psychophysiology* **30**: 126–130.

Fyer AJ, Manuzza S, Chapman TF, Martin LY, Klein DF (1995) Specificity in familial aggregation of phobic disorders. *Arch General Psychiatry* **52**: 564–573.

Gershuny BS, Sher KJ (1998) The relation between personality and anxiety: Findings from a 3-year prospective study. *J Abnorm Psychol* **107**: 252–262.

Gray JA (1987) Interactions between drugs and behaviour therapy. In Eysenck HJ, Martin I (eds) *Theoretical Foundations of Behaviour Therapy*. New York: Plenum Press.

Greenberg DB, Stern TA, Weilburg JB (1988) The fear of choking: Three successfully treated cases. *Psychosomatics* **29**: 126–129.

Harris B (1979) Whatever happened to little Albert? *Am Psychologist* **34**: 151–160.

Hekmat H (1987) Origins and development of human fear reactions. *J Anx Dis* **1**: 197–218.

Heller W, Nitschke JB (1998) The puzzle of regional brain activity in depression and anxiety: The importance of subtypes and comorbidity. *Cognition and Emotion* **12**: 421–447.

Henry B, Moffitt TE, Caspi A, Langley J, Silva PA (1994) On the remembrance of things past: A longitudinal evaluation of the retrospective method. *Psychological Assessment* **6**: 92–101.

Himle JA, Crystal D, Curtis GC, Fluent TE (1991) Mode of onset of simple phobia subtypes: Further evidence of heterogeneity. *Psychiatry Research* **36**: 37–43.

Hodgson R, Rachman S (1974) Desynchrony in measures of fear. *Behav Res Ther* **12**: 319–326.

Hofmann SG, Lehman CL, Barlow DH (1997) How specific are specific phobias? *J Behav Ther Experimental Psychiatry* **28**: 233–240.

Hugdahl K (1981) The three-systems-model of fear and emotion: A critical examination. *Behav Res Ther* **19**: 75–85.

Hugdahl K (1989) Simple phobias. In Turpin G (ed) *Handbook of Clinical Psychophysiology*. Chichester: Wiley.

Hugdahl K, Johnsen B (1989) Preparedness and electrodermal fear conditioning: ontogenetic vs phylogenetic explanations. *Behav Res Ther* **27**: 269–278.

Hygge S, Öhman A (1978) Modelling processes in the acquisition of fears: Vicarious electrodermal conditioning to fear-relevant stimuli. *J Personality and Individual Differences* **36**: 271–279.

Kelley MJ (1987) Hormones and clinical anxiety: An imbalanced neuromodulation of attention. In Eysenck HJ, Martin I (eds) *Theoretical Foundations of Behavior Therapy*. New York: Plenum Press.

Kendler KS, Neale MC, Kessler RC, Heath AC, Eaves LJ (1992) The genetic epidemiology of phobias in women: The interrelationship of agoraphobia, situational phobia, and simple phobia. *Arch General Psychiatry* **49**: 273–281.

Kessler RC, McGonagle K, Zhao S, Nelson C, Hughes M, Eschelemann S, Wittchen HU, Kendler KS (1994) Lifetime and 12-months prevalence of DSM-III-R psychiatric disorders in the United States: Results from the National Comorbidity Survey. *Arch General Psychiatry* **51**: 8–19.

Kheriaty E, Kleinknecht RA, Hyman IE (1999) Recall and validation of phobia origins as a function of structured interview versus the phobia origins questionnaire. *Behav Modification* **23**: 61–78.

Kirkpatrick DR (1984) Age, gender and patterns of common intense fears among adults. *Behav Res Ther* **22**: 141–150.

Kleinknecht RA (1994) Acquisition of blood, injury, and needle fears and phobias. *Behav Res Ther* **32**: 817–823.

Klorman R, Weerts TC, Hastings JE, Melamed BG, Lang PJ (1974) Psychometric description of some specific fear questionnaires. *Behav Ther* **5**: 401–409.

Kornfeld AD (1989) Mary Cover Jones and the Peter case: Social learning versus conditioning. *J Anx Dis* **3**: 187–195.

Kuch K, Cox BJ, Evans RE, Shulman I (1994) Phobias, panic, and pain in 55 survivors of road vehicle accidents. *J Anx Dis* **8**: 181–187.

Lang PJ (1968) Fear reduction and fear behaviour: Problems in treating a construct. In Schlien JM (ed) *Research in Psychotherapy* Vol. III. Washington, DC: APA.

Lang PJ (1995) The emotion probe: Studies of emotion and attention. *Am Psychologist* **50**: 372–385.

Lapouse R, Monk MA (1959) Fears and worries in a representative sample of children. *American Journal of Orthopsychiatry* **29**: 803–813.

Last C (1987) Simple phobias. In Michelson L, Ascher M (eds) *Anxiety and Stress Disorders*. New York: Guilford Press.

Lautch H (1971) Dental phobia. *B J Psychiatry* **119**: 151–158.

Lavy EH, Van den Hout M, Arntz A (1993) Attentional bias and spider phobia: Conceptual and clinical issues. *Behav Res Ther* **31**: 17–24.

LeDoux J (1992) Emotion as memory: Anatomical systems underlying indelible neural traces. In Christianson SA (ed) *The Handbook of Emotion and Memory: Research and Theory*. Hillsdale, NJ: Erlbaum.

LeDoux J (1995) Emotion: Clues from the brain. *Annual Review of Psychology* **46**: 209–235.

MacFarlane JW, Allen L, Honzik MP (1954) *A Developmental Study of the Behavior Problems of Normal Children between 21 Months and 14 Years*. Berkeley, CA: University of California Press.

MacLeod C (1991) Clinical anxiety and the selective encoding of threatening information.

International Review of Psychiatry **3**: 279–292.

MacLeod C, Hagan R (1992) Individual differences in the selective processing of threatening information and emotional responses to a stressful life event. *Behav Res Ther* **30**: 151–161.

Magee WM, Eaton WW, Wittchen HU, McGoanagle KA, Kessler RC (1996) Agoraphobia, simple phobia, and social phobia in the National Comorbidity Survey. *Arch General Psychiatry* **53**: 159–168.

Malloy P, Levis DJ (1988) A laboratory demonstration of persistent human avoidance. *Behav Ther* **19**: 229–241.

Marks I (1987) *Fears, Phobias, and Rituals*. Oxford: Oxford University Press.

Marks I, Nesse RM (1994) Fear and fitness: An evolutionary analysis of anxiety disorders. *Ethology and Sociobiology* **15**: 247–261.

Marquis JN (1991) A report of seventy-eight cases treated by eye movement desensitisation. *J Behav Ther Experimental Psychiatry* **22**: 187–192.

Matchett G, Davey GCL (1991) A test of a disease avoidance model of animal phobias. *Behav Res Ther* **29**: 91–94.

Mayer B, Merckelbach H, De Jong PJ, Leeuw I (1999a) Skin conductance responses of spider phobics to backwardly masked phobic cues. *J Psychophysiology* **13**: 152–159.

Mayer B, Merckelbach H, Muris P (1999b) Spider phobic children do not react with differential skin conductance responses to masked phobic stimuli. *J Psychopathology and Behavioral Assessment* **21**: 237–248.

McNally RJ (1987) Preparedness and phobias: A review. *Psychological Bulletin* **101**: 283–303.

McNally RJ (1995) Automaticity and the anxiety disorders. *Behav Res Ther* **33**: 747–754.

McNally RJ (1998) Information processing abnormalities in anxiety disorders: Implications for cognitive neuroscience. *Cognition and Emotion* **12**: 479–495.

Menzies RG, Clarke JC (1993) The aetiology of fear of heights and its relationship to severity and individual response patterns. *Behav Res Ther* **31**: 355–366.

Menzies RG, Clarke JC (1995) The aetiology of phobias: A non-associative account. *Clinical Psychology Review* **15**: 23–48.

Merckelbach H, Arntz A, De Jong PJ (1991) Conditioning experiences in spider phobics. *Behav Res Ther* **29**: 333–335.

Merckelbach H, Arntz A, De Jong PJ, Schouten E (1993a) Effects of endorphin blocking on conditioned SCR in humans. *Behav Res Ther* **31**: 775–779.

Merckelbach H, Arrindell WA, Arntz A, De Jong PJ (1992) Pathways to spider phobia. *Behav Res Ther* **30**: 543–546.

Merckelbach H, De Jong PJ (1997) Evolutionary models of phobias. In Davey GCL (ed.) *Phobias: A Handbook of Theory, Research, and Treatment*. Chichester: Wiley.

Merckelbach H, De Jong PJ, Arntz A, Schouten E (1993b) The role of evaluative learning and disgust sensitivity in the aetiology and treatment of spider phobia. *Advances in Behaviour Research and Therapy* **15**: 243–255.

Merckelbach H, De Jong PJ, Muris P, Van den Hout MA (1996a) The aetiology of specific phobias: A review. *Clinical Psychology Review* **16**: 337–361.

Merckelbach H, Hogervorst E, Kampman M, De Jongh A (1994) Effects of eye movement desensitisation on emotional processing in normal subjects. *Behavioural and Cognitive Psychotherapy* **22**: 331–335.

Merckelbach H, Muris P (1997) The etiology of childhood spider phobia. *Behav Res Ther* **35**: 1031–1034.

Merckelbach H, Muris P, De Jong PJ (1990) Hemisphere preference, phobia, and depression. *International Journal of Neuroscience* **55**: 119–123.

Merckelbach H, Muris P, Schouten E (1996b) Pathways to fear in spider phobic children. *Behav Res Ther* **34**: 935–938.

Merluzzi TV, Taylor CB, Boltwood M, Götestam KG (1991) Opioid antagonist impedes exposure. *Journal of Consulting and Clinical Psychology* **59**: 425–430.

Mowrer O (1960) *Learning Theory and Behaviour.* New York: Wiley.

Muris P, Merckelbach H (1998) Specific phobias. In Bellack AS, Hersen M (eds) *Comprehensive Clinical Psychology.* Vol. 6. *Adults: Clinical Formulation and Treatment.* Oxford: Pergamon Press.

Muris P, Merckelbach H (1999) Traumatic memories, eye movements, phobia, and panic: A critical note on the proliferation of EMDR. *J Anx Dis* **13**: 209–233.

Muris P, Merckelbach H (2000) The aetiology of childhood specific phobias: A multifactorial model. In Vasey MW, Dadds MR (eds) *The Developmental Psychopathology of Anxiety.* New York: Oxford Univerity Press.

Muris P, Merckelbach H, Gadet B, Moulaert V (2000) Fears, worries, and scary dreams in 4- to 12-year old children: Their content, developmental pattern, and origins. *Journal of Clinical Child Psychology* **29**: 43–52.

Muris P, Merckelbach H, Schmidt H, Mayer B (1999) The revised Screen for Child Anxiety Related Emotional Disorders (SCARED-R): Factor structure in normal children. *Personality and Individual Differences* **26**: 99–112.

Öhman A, Soares JJF (1994) Unconscious anxiety: Phobic responses to masked stimuli. *J Abnorm Psychol* **103**: 231–240.

Öhman A (1996) Preferential pre-attentive processing of threat in anxiety: Preparedness and attentional biases. In Rapee R (ed) *Current Controversies in the Anxiety Disorders.* New York: Guildford.

Ollendick TH (1979) Fear reduction techniques with children. In Miller P, Eisler R (eds) *Progress in Behavior Modification,* Vol. 8. New York: Academic Press.

Ollendick TH, King NJ (1991) Origins of childhood fears: An evaluation of Rachman's theory of fear acquisition. *Behav Res Ther* **29**: 117–123.

Öst LG (1987a) Age of onset in different phobias. *J Abnorm Psychol* **96**: 223–229.

Öst LG (1987b) Individual response patterns and the effect of different behavioural methods in the treatment of phobias. In Magnusson D, Öhman A (eds) *Psychopathology: An Interactional Perspective.* New York: Academic Press.

Öst LG (1989) One-session treatment for specific phobias. *Behav Res Ther* **27**: 1–8.

Öst LG (1991) Acquisition of blood and injection phobia and anxiety response patterns in clinical patients. *Behav Res Ther* **29**: 323–332.

Öst LG (1997) Rapid treatment of specific phobias. In Davey GCL (ed.) *Phobias: A Handbook of Theory, Research, and Treatment.* Chichester: Wiley.

Öst LG, Fellenius J, Sterner U (1991b) Applied tension, exposure in vivo, and tension-only in the treatment of blood phobia. *Behav Res Ther* **29**: 561–575.

Öst LG, Hugdahl K (1981) Acquisition of phobias and anxiety response patterns in clinical patients. *Behav Res Ther* **19**: 439–447.

Öst LG, Salkovskis PM, Hellström K (1991a) One-session therapist-directed exposure vs self-exposure in the treatment of spider phobia. *Behav Ther* **22**: 407–422.

Page AC (1991) Simple phobia. *International Review of Psychiatry* **3**: 175–187.

Page AC (1994) Blood-injury phobia. *Clinical Psychology Review* **14**: 443–461.

Pratto F, John OP (1991) Automatic vigilance: The attention grabbing power of negative social information. *Journal of Personality and Social Psychology* **61**: 380–391.

Rachman S (1977) The conditioning theory of fear acquisition: A critical examination. *Behav Res Ther* **15**: 375–387.

Rachman S (1990a) *Fear and Courage.* New York: Freeman.

Rachman S (1990b) The determinants and treatment of simple phobias. *Advances in Behaviour Research and Therapy* **12**: 1–30.

Rachman S (1991) Neoconditioning and the classical theory of fear acquisition. *Clinical Psychology Review* **11**: 155–173.

Rachman S (1998) *Anxiety.* Hove: Psychology Press.

Rachman S, Craske M, Tallman K, Solyom C (1986) Does escape behaviour strengthen agoraphobic avoidance?: A replication. *Behav Ther* **17**: 366–384.

Regier DA, Boyd DH, Burke JD, Rae DS, Myers JK, Kramer M, Robins LN, George LK, Karno M, Locke BZ (1988) One-month prevalence of mental disorders in the United States. *Archives of General Psychiatry* **45**: 977–986.

Rescorla RA (1988) Pavlovian conditioning: It is not what you think it is. *American Psychologist* **43**: 151–160.

Rickels K (1978) Use of anti-anxiety agents in anxious outpatients. *Psychopharmacology* **58**: 1–17.

Riley JC (1986) Insects and the European mortality decline. *American Historical Review* **91**: 833–858.

Rosen GM, Lohr GM, McNally RJ, Herbert JD (1998) Power therapies, miraculous claims, and the cures that fail. *Behavioural and Cognitive Psychotherapy* **26**: 97–99.

Rosen JB, Schulkin J (1998) From normal fear to pathological anxiety. *Psychological Review* **105**: 325–350.

Saigh PA (1984) Pre- and post-invasion anxiety in the Lebanon. *Behav Ther* **15**: 185–190.

Sartory G, MacDonald R, Gray JA (1990) Effects of diazepam on approach, self-reported fear and psychophysiological responses in snake phobics. *Behav Res Ther* **28**: 273–282.

Schmidt LA, Fox NA, Rubin KH, Sternberg EM, Gold PW, Smith CC, Schulkin J (1997) Behavioural and neuroendocrine responses in shy children. *Developmental Psychobiology* **30**: 127–140.

Seligman MEP (1971) Phobias and preparedness. *Behav Ther* **2**: 307–320.

Shafran R, Booth R, Rachman S (1993) The reduction of claustrophobia: Cognitive analyses. *Behav Res Ther* **31**: 75–85.

Shapiro F (1989) Efficacy of the eye movement desensitisation procedure in the treatment of traumatic memories. *Journal of Traumatic Stress* **2**: 199–223.

Smoller JW, Tsuang MT (1998) Panic and phobic anxiety: Defining phenotypes for genetic studies. *Am J Psychiatry* **155**: 1152–1162.

Sturgis ET, Scott R (1984) Simple phobia. In Turner SM (ed) *Behavioral Theories and Treatment of Anxiety*. New York: Plenum Press.

Tallis F, Smith E (1994) Does rapid eye movement desensitisation facilitate emotional processing? *Behav Res Ther* **32**: 459–461.

Taylor S (1998) The hierarchic structure of fears. *Behav Res Ther* **36**: 205–214.

Thyer BA, Himle J, Curtis GC (1985) Blood-injury-illness phobia: A review. *Journal of Clinical Psychology* **41**: 451–459.

Tolin DF, Lohr JM, Sawchuck CN, Lee TC (1997) Disgust and disgust sensitivity in blood-injection-injury and spider phobia. *Behav Res Ther* **35**: 949–953.

Tomarken AJ, Mineka S, Cook M (1989) Fear relevant selective associations and co-variation bias. *J Abnorm Psychol* **98**: 381–394.

Tucker DM, Newman JP (1981) Verbal versus imaginal cognitive strategies in the inhibition of emotional arousal. *Cognitive Therapy and Research* **5**: 197–202.

Van den Hout MA, Tenney N, Huygens K, Merckelbach H, Kindt M (1995) Responding to subliminal threat cues is related to trait anxiety and emotional vulnerability: A successful replication of MacLeod and Hagan (1992). *Behav Res Ther* **33**: 451–454.

Van der Molen GM, Merckelbach H, Van den Hout MA (1988) The possible relation of the menstrual cycle to susceptibility to fear acquisition. *J Behaviour Therapy and Experimental Psychiatry* **19**: 127–133.

Verburg K, Griez E, Meijer J (1994) A 35% carbon dioxide challenge in simple phobias. *Acta Psychiatr Scand* **90**: 420–423.

Watson J, Rayner R (1920) Conditioned emotional reactions. *J Experimental Psychology* **3**: 1–22.

Watts FN (1979) Habituation model of systematic desensitisation. *Psychological Review* **86**: 627–637.

White K, Davey GCL (1989) Sensory preconditioning and UCS inflation in human fear conditioning. *Behav Res Ther* **27**: 161–166.

Williams JMG, Mathews A, MacLeod C (1996) The emotional Stroop task and psychopathology. *Psychological Bull* **120**: 3–24.

Williams JMG, Watts FN, MacLeod C, Mathews A (1997) *Cognitive Psychology and Emotional Disorders* (2nd edition). Chichester: Wiley.

Wittchen H (1988) Natural course and spontaneous remissions of untreated anxiety disorders. In Hand I, Wittchen H (eds) *Panic and Phobias: Treatment and Variables Affecting Course and Outcome*. Berlin: Springer Verlag.

Wolpe J (1981) The dichotomy between classical conditioned and cognitively learned anxiety. *Journal of Behaviour Therapy and Experimental Psychiatry* **12**: 35–42.

Wolpe J, Lande SD, McNally RJ, Schotte D (1985) Differentiation between classically conditioned and cognitively based neurotic fears: Two pilot studies. *Journal of Behavior Therapy and Experimental Psychiatry* **16**: 287–293.

Zinbarg RE, Barlow DH (1996) Structure of anxiety and the anxiety disorders: A hierarchical model. *J Abnorm Psychol* **105**: 181–193.

7

Social Phobia

C. Faravelli, T. Zucchi, A. Perone, R. Salmoria and B. Viviani

Florence University Medical School, Florence, Italy

INTRODUCTION

Social phobia (SP) is a condition characterised by an intense, irrational, persistent fear of being scrutinised or evaluated by others, with the patient anticipating humiliation or ridicule. The fear may involve most social interactions/situations where it is possible to be judged or be confronted with specific public performance. Anticipation of these situations is also experienced with uneasiness, distress or fear. The course of SP is that of a chronic, unremitting lifelong disease and secondary complications as depression, substance abuse (alcohol or tranquillisers) and suicide attempts may be associated with it, thus making the disorder severely disabling. SP is increasingly recognised as one of the more common anxiety disorders. Only with recent large-scale epidemiological studies of psychiatric disorders has the true prevalence of SP been recognised. Lifetime prevalence has been reported to vary between 2% and 4% in most epidemiological studies (Faravelli et al., 1989; Wittchen et al., 1992; Davidson et al., 1993, Lindal and Stefansson, 1993; Degonda and Angst, 1993; Lépine and Lellouch, 1995) with other epidemiological surveys (Wacker et al., 1992; Kessler et al., 1994; Magee et al., 1996) reporting rates even three times as higher.

SP is a relatively recent diagnosis as it was first described by Marks and Gelder as "fears of eating, drinking, shaking, speaking, writing, and so on in presence of other people", the central feature being the fear of seeming ridiculous to others (Marks and Gelder, 1966). SP has been found to differ from panic disorder (PD) with or without agoraphobia and from other phobias as regards age of onset, sex occurrence, response to provocation challenges, course and response to treatment (Marks, 1970; Amies et al., 1983; Liebowitz et al., 1985a; Munjack et al., 1987; Goldstein 1987; Stein et al., 1989). Marks and Gelder's definition included patients with specific social fears and those with more generalised forms of social anxiety (i.e. fears of initiating conversations, meeting new people, members of opposite sex, people in authority). Social phobia did not became an officially recognised diagnosis until DSM-III was

Anxiety Disorders: An Introduction to Clinical Management and Research. Edited by E. J. L. Griez, C. Faravelli, D. Nutt and J. Zohar. © 2001 John Wiley & Sons, Ltd.

published (APA, 1980). As Liebowitz et al. (1985b) emphasised, this common disorder was among the most neglected of the major anxiety disorders. DSM-III described SP as a circumscribed phobia, involving anxiety about a situation in which the individual is exposed to possible scrutiny by others, implying that patients with multiple fears or more generalised SP are rare or should be included in other diagnostic categories; the diagnosis of SP had to be excluded if the criteria for avoidant personality disorder were fulfilled. Because of the lack of empirical bases, the rule of exclusion of SP in the presence of the axis II disorder was omitted in DSM III-R (APA, 1987) and a generalised type of SP was included. The DSM III-R criteria for SP and avoidant personality disorder have a high degree of similarity and overlap. DSM-IV (APA, 1994), that have not changed markedly from those found in DSM III-R, did not clarify much this distinction. In general, APD should be characterised by the absence of intense fears reactions with a much milder, less pervasive pattern of discomfort in social situations in which the patients feel they are exposed to evaluation or scrutiny (Judd, 1994). As a rule, however, SP and APD coexist in the majority of cases complaining of social anxiety.

CLINICAL FEATURES

As mentioned above, the central feature of social phobia is a marked and persistent fear of one or more social or performance situations in which the person is exposed to unfamiliar people or feels to be under scrutiny. The psychopathological foundations of SP are rather specific and typically phobic: exaggeration of autonomic responses, anticipation, repeated presentation of the fear and the awareness that the fear is unreasonable and excessive, accompanied by the feeling of being unable to control these emotions. Therefore, anxiety emerges when the patient is exposed to the phobic stimulus or contemplates future contact with the feared situations. This anxiety reaction may be experienced sometimes as a full-blown panic attack with the characteristic fears of losing control, dying or going mad, accompanied by autonomic responses.

For SP patients the most commonly trigger situations are interactions as speaking or eating in public, writing in front of others, attending a party, meeting new people, contacting members of opposite sex, interacting with people in authority, using public bathrooms. The types of social situations feared by children and adults with SP are similar; one exception are the fears of meetings, a situation not generally encountered during childhood (Beidel, 1998). The range of feared situations is an important element to subclassify the disorder. The subtypes uniformly accepted are "nongeneralised" and "generalised" social phobia. The first one is usually confined to a fear of one or two social or performance situations, of which the most common is speaking in public; the second form of SP is pervasive and more extensive, and regards most interactions and social situations. Generalised social phobia has been observed to be highly familiar, more severe and disabling, more persistent, with higher rates of comorbidity, higher incidence of help-seeking behaviour and often requires more intensive medical intervention. The boundary between this latter form of social phobia and avoidant personality disorder is blurred.

It is important to distinguish the "normal" anxiety experienced by most individuals in social and performance situations and the exceptional anxiety experienced by the individual with social phobia. The first one usually reaches a peak at the beginning with adaptive advantage (greater efficacy) and it attenuates over the course of any given performance or social encounter, while the intense social phobics' anxiety increases during the course of the social event or performance and this can result in impediment of functional ability.

The clinical symptoms of SP can present at physical, cognitive and behavioural level and play a role in vicious circles that may contribute maintaining the disorder. Blushing is the principal physical symptom and with tachycardia, sweating and trembling suggests heightened autonomic arousal. Muscle tension, dry throat and gastrointestinal distress, such as nausea or diarrhoea are other common symptoms. SP patients have an exaggerated awareness of minimal somatic symptoms associated with a tendency to overreact with great anxiety to them and with an exaggerated fear that others may notice that they are anxious, distressed or unfit. Then, these physical indicators of anxiety may become part of a vicious circle: as social phobics anticipate or face feared social encounters, they experience an increase of somatic discomfort, which alerts them that they have become more anxious. This event leads to distraction, feelings of embarrassment or humiliation, these latter lead to further symptoms and then to more distraction, perception of impaired performance, and so on. The resulting negative experience fuels further anticipatory anxiety when faced with future social situations. Compared with agoraphobics, social phobics have significantly more cardiovascular symptoms, sweating and tremor and fewer respiratory symptoms during their situational panics (Liebowitz et al., 1985b; Rapaport et al., 1995). This may have a role in determining SP since blushing, sweating and trembling may be more easily noticed by the others. Children and adults have a similar somatic presentation, the only difference being that children frequently report "butterflies in their stomach", an expression that may reflects children's limited ability to say what they feel (Beidel, 1998).

Cognitive symptoms include maladaptive thoughts about social situations. Sufferers may have rigid concepts of appropriate social behaviour, they exaggerate the impact of social blunders and ruminate about them afterwards. These beliefs are important in adults whereas are absent in children. Other features of SP are: an unrealistic tendency to experience others as critical or disapproving, associated with hypersensitivity to rejection or criticism, low assertiveness al least in phobic situations and low self-esteem.

The behavioural symptoms include a freezing response, in which the sufferer may perform badly in social situations, and phobic avoidance. Avoidance of feared situation relieves anxiety, thus reinforcing further avoidance behaviour. The latter prevents the sufferer from being able to have positive experiences of social situations, and therefore negative expectations during interactions with others are perpetuated. A broad avoidance pattern frequently exacerbates problems with education, occupational, social functioning and increases the individual's distress. SP may therefore become a disabling disorder leading to an egodystonic social isolation, unstable employment record, poor achievement and often financial dependence for the patients (Schneier et al., 1992; Davidson et al., 1994; Montgomery, 1995; Weiller et al., 1996; Wittchen and Beloch, 1996). However, social disability and the discomfort determinated by SP are not fully explained by the severity of the disorder. It is the resultant of a combination of personal skills (of which SP is an important factor), actual needs for social performances and social pressures.

It is noteworthy that individuals with SP are reticent to seek help in view of the nature of the symptoms since pathological anxiety is often mistaken for shyness without the awareness that treatment is possible. Sometimes SP sufferers use alcohol in an attempt to self-medicate their distressing anxiety symptoms. Anxiety, depressive and substance abuse problems may then follow (Schneier et al., 1992; Lecrubier, 1998; Lépine and Pelissolo, 1998). When the disorder does not present these complications, sleep discomfort, appetite and sexual distress are usually absent.

AGE OF ONSET

The onset of social phobia generally occurs early in childhood or in adolescence, between five and 20 years. In an epidemiological sample (Schneier et al., 1992), the mean age at onset for social phobia is reported as being between 11 and 15 years, and onset after the age of 25 years is rare. Nevertheless, even if the data from epidemiological studies and from retrospective reports of adults with social phobia indicate that the mean age at onset is in mid-adolescence (Thyer et al., 1985; Schneier et al., 1992; Turner et al., 1992), social phobia can be detected in children as young as eight years of age (Beidel and Turner, 1998). In effect it has been seen that sufferers from social phobia frequently recalled the onset of the disorder as being "since early childhood", or "ever since I can remember" (Stein et al., 1990).

Since SP usually has had an early onset, it may interfere with development of social and educational skills, leaving the individual at a social and occupational disadvantage. It was suggested that part of the disability induced by SP might be a consequence of this very early burden (Lecrubier, 1998). Subtypes of social phobia may have different mean ages at onset. It is reported (Mannuzza et al., 1995) that the generalised subtype appears earlier, with patients having a mean age at onset of 11 years in contrast to a mean age at onset of 17 years for patients with the specific subtype. Recovery is less likely if the condition started in early childhood (Davidson et al., 1993). In addition, it was found that there is a difference in the level of comorbidity linked to the age at onset of SP. In patients with early onset (< 15 years of age) there is a higher risk of developing further depressive comordibity compared with that in those with a late onset (> 15 years of age) of the disorder (Lecrubier, 1998). The onset of SP usually predates the onset of depressive symptoms, suggesting that SP may have a role in the development of other psychiatric disorders.

COMORBIDITY

The SP seldom occurs in its "pure" form and it has been estimated in most of epidemiological studies that a large part of patients with SP (from 70–80% to 92% in various general population samples) have at least one other psychiatric disorder during their life. The commonest comorbid disorders with SP, considering lifetime diagnosis, are panic disorder with agoraphobia (PDA), generalised anxiety disorder (GAD), major depressive episode (MDE), obsessive-compulsive disorder (OCD), AGO, simple phobia, eating disorders, alcohol and substance abuse/dependence. Moreover, SP often coexists with axis II disorders, especially avoidant personality disorder and obsessive-compulsive personality disorder (Turner et al., 1991). Comorbidity increases severity of social anxiety, causes greater disability and increases suicidality. The overall burden of the comorbid disease is greater both for the patient (greater disability) and for the health care services (greater use of medical services). However, comorbidity in SP may result in at least one positive thing: increased recognition and treatment, because in absence of comorbidity the level of recognition of the disorder is very low.

The presence of comorbidity increases the number of suicide attempts: Davidson et al. (1993) showed that the proportion of patients with suicidal thoughts rose from approximately 40% in those with SP and one comorbid disorder to about 60% in those with two or more comorbid disorders. Similarly, lifetime suicide attempts increased from 2% to 21%. Overall, the level of suicidality in SP is comparable with that for panic disorder.

Recent findings (the NCS) have reported that the prevalence of comorbid conditions is higher in patients with complex (generalised) SP than in patients with speaking-only SP. This is especially true for mood disorders and other anxiety disorders whereas substance abuse showed little difference. Using DSM-IV criteria for detecting comorbidity, some association may be artificially increased, as different categories may have overlapping criteria, but it is clear that some relationship between SP and other disorder does exist. They may be interpreted in three ways:

1. SP is a common precursor (or risk factor) for other anxiety and depressive disorder.
2. SP is a consequence or a complication of other disorders.
3. There is a common ground.

When the temporal relationship between SP and comorbid psychiatric disorder has been investigated, SP precedes the comorbid disorder in the majority of patients. SP seems to be rarely a secondary complication of other disorders or to have an onset in the same year or in the same episode as another disorder. This consideration suggests that SP may be a risk factor for additional psychiatric disorders, but it is unclear whether SP is an aetiologic factor in the development of other disorders or whether SP and comorbid disorders result from common predisposing factors. It may also be that the occurrence of another disorder worsens social anxiety, thus rendering SP clinically evident. Major depression is one of the commonest conditions associated with SP. SP may have an aetiologic role for it; alternatively, major depression may be a consequence of the chronic disability associated with SP.

For the SP sufferers, the extreme anxiety associated with social or performance situations often results in the abuse of, and ultimately dependence on, alcohol and BDZ. However, excessive alcohol consumption may actually precipitate anxiety symptoms, and thus a vicious circle between anxiety and alcoholism is established: in fact, although the subjects showed decreased anxiety shortly after drinking, they reported an increase in anxiety and dysphoria as they continued to drink. The physical consequences of prolonged and heavy drinking such as gastrointestinal disturbances and sleep disturbances may overlap with anxiety symptoms.

Generalised anxiety disorder is also highly prevalent in all the anxiety disorders and its presence in social phobic patients indicates that a large number of them suffer from a pervasive pattern of maladaptive anxiety in addition to their more circumscribed social fears.

The coexistence of SP with axis II diagnosis, as avoidant personality disorder and obsessive-compulsive disorder, may suggest that the fear of criticism and rejection, along with the tendency to be obsessional, are important features in the personality make-up of social phobics.

COURSE AND CONSEQUENCES

The clinical course of SP is chronic, unremitting, and life-long. Patients often enter treatment later in life, frequently reporting suffering from severe symptoms for many years before seeking treatment. As already mentioned, the presence of a comorbid disorder in SP has important implications in term of prognosis. The combination of a very early onset together with a chronic lifetime course indicates that SP is responsible for many years of disability and life distortion for patients. Compared with sufferers of other mood and anxiety disorders, SP sufferers experienced a worse quality of life in the domains of work, friendship, and partnership (Bech and Angst, 1996). The consequences of this impairment include academic underachievement, inability to work, underperformance at work, and thus financial dependency; moreover, there is evidence that more than half of all SP are single, divorced, or separated. Utilisation of treatment (morbidity) is increased in SP patients: SP overall is associated with significantly elevated rates of seeking any outpatient treatment for emotional problems and of psychiatric outpatient treatment. In the Florence Psychiatric Survey (Faravelli et al., 1989), 78.4% of SP patients sought help from their general practitioner, 21% were referred to a public psychiatrist, 14.9% underwent psychotherapy and 13.5% used other outpatient facilities.

However, a consistent portion of the long-term consequences and burden of SP seems to be due to the association with other disorders. The ECA study reports that only 5.4% of patients with uncomplicated SP sought help from a mental health specialist.

The socio-economic impact of SP is no less significant. By disrupting schooling in adolescence, the disorder limits educational attainment and career progression. Throughout the working lives of sufferers, continuing functional impairment has an economic impact, reflected in the loss of working days to illness and reduced work performance. The NCS study also found that patients with complex (generalised) SP, compared with patients with speaking-only SP, were more likely to report that their phobia interfered with their lives, more likely to have received treatment for phobia, more likely to have seen a mental health specialist, and more likely to have taken medication for their phobia (Kessler et al., 1998). Although many sufferers may organise their working and social lives to accommodate the condition, and thus may not perceive an actual deterioration in quality of life, they are clearly not realising their full potential (Montgomery, 1996). Thus, as well as the considerable personal burden of SP, the condition also places a burden on society as a whole.

AETIOLOGY

It is unclear whether there is a continuum between normal and pathological social anxiety or whether they are categorically distinct. A certain degree of social or performance anxiety is ubiquitous and may have some evolutionary adaptive advantage by motivating preparation and rehearsal of important interpersonal events. It is also likely that social anxiety has a role in determining hierarchical ranks in animal groups. In contrast with anxiety in normal subjects, social anxiety does not seem to attenuate during the course of a single social event or performance. Social phobics seem to lack the ability to habituate in social or performance situations.

Current theories consider the development of SP to be due to a combination of genetic and environmental factors (Rosenbaum et al., 1994). A family study (Fyer et al., 1993) reported significant increased risk for SP in the first-degree relatives of social phobics. In this study, 16% of the relatives of the "pure" social phobics had SP themselves, compared with 5% in the never mentally ill control group. Data from twin studies have identified specific genetic factors and influences as well. Torgersen (1979) compared social fears in a small subject sample of monozygotic and dizygotic twin pairs: the MZ twins were significantly more concordant for such social phobic features as discomfort when eating with strangers or when being watched working, writing, or trembling, suggesting a genetic contribution to social anxiety. In a large study of female twins, Kendler et al. (1992) reported significantly higher concordance rates for most phobias in MZ twins when compared with DZ twins. Their conclusion was that there are definite genetics factors in SP, agoraphobia, and animal phobias, but not in situational phobias. A range of early childhood environmental factors may also contribute to the development of the disorder. Social phobics were often noted to report that their parents were more rejecting, overprotective, and lacking in emotional warmth. However, the same parental traits and attitudes have also been identified in a variety of other mental disorders, especially in the overall phobic group (Parker, 1979; Arrindell et al., 1983). It is possible that behavioural inhibition in early childhood, defined as having excessive fears of unfamiliar settings, people, and objects, are a general aspecific risk factor for the development of anxiety and phobia. The investigation of SP at the neurobiological level is still at an early stage. The majority of studies in normal volunteers suggest that β-adrenergic blockers are helpful in reducing performance anxiety, which supports the peripheral catecholamine mediation of SP symptoms, and this differently from panic attacks. Tancer (1993) published a placebo-controlled challenge study where probes for the dopaminergic, noradrenergic and serotonergic systems were used: using the cortisol response to fenfluramine as a measure for the serotonergic function, patients with SP showed a significantly greater response compared with controls. These findings could suggest that patients with SP might have a dysregulation in the serotonergic function, namely post-synaptic receptor supersensitivity. In contrast, SP responded to clonidine challenges with blunted growth hormone responses. Significant additional research will be necessary before a clear picture can be constructed of the underlying pathophysiological brain mechanisms of SP.

Finally, Nichols (1974) has catalogued a variety of psychological and somatic traits, observed in a SP sample. Examples of these traits are a low self-evaluation, an unrealistic tendency to experience others as critical or disapproving, a negative fantasy-producing anticipatory anxiety, an increased awareness and fear of scrutiny by others, an exaggerated awareness of minimal somatic symptoms of anxiety, and so on. Nevertheless, it is unclear which among these factors are causal, which are consequences of, and which are not even specifically related to SP.

DIAGNOSIS

Difficulties in the Diagnosis of Social Phobia

In 1970, Marks was the first to discuss SP as a clinical syndrome distinct from other anxiety disorders. As explained before, SP was not officially recognised as a diagnostic entity until the publication of the third edition of the *Diagnostic and Statistical Manual of Mental Disorder*. The original DSM-III description of SP emphasised the difficulty for the clinician in identifying SP from other psychiatric disorders. SP was defined "a persistent, irrational fear of, and compelling desire to avoid a situation, in which the individual is exposed to possible scrutiny by others and fears that he or she may act in a way that will be humiliating or embarrassing" (APA, 1980). Anticipatory anxiety and avoidance occur when the individual is under scrutiny while speaking or performing publicly, eating with others, writing in public, or using public bathrooms. In the revised DSM-III, the pervasiveness of impairment across situations was explicitly recognised by the creation of a generalised subtype (GSP), in which distress is found in all or most social situation (APA, 1987). DSM-IV does not change much and the difficulty in diagnosing SP is implicitly expressed by the fact that there are two exclusion criteria where the sentence "not better accounted for by" is reported. Apart from inclusion of physical symptoms (as blushing, tremor, nausea) and the specification that the fear of scrutiny is associated with situations involving comparatively small groups of people, ICD-10 is no more precise or helpful to the diagnosis than DSM-IV in defining the criteria for SP.

Basically, the problems in the diagnosis of SP are the following:

1. The difficulty of distinguishing between shyness and SP, since quantitative rather than qualitative criteria are often used; moreover the level at which shyness is considered acceptable, or even culturally desirable, varies in different cultures and countries. In most languages, the word "shameless" represent an insult.

2. In the epidemiological studies uneasiness, distress and avoidance of social situations were considered important diagnostic elements; however, these may be due to lack of interest and motivation (as may be the case with several disorders, e.g. schizoid disorder, depression, schizophrenia) or difficulty in dealing with the situation. The latter, in turn, may be due to factors related to psychopathological conditions other than the fear of being under scrutiny (e.g. psychotic suspiciousness, depression, body dysmorphic disorder, eating disorders). In other cases the uneasiness and the avoidance may be due to the fact that the situation is actually too demanding for the capacities of the individual. Finally, the explication of inability in social situations is solely possible when the subject requires to deal with such situations. The phobia of speaking in public, for instance, may be a serious problem for a teacher, but may not be felt as such in a nun.

3. The boundaries between generalised SP (GSP) and APD (avoidant personality disorder) are uncertain and it is unclear if they represent qualitatively distinct nosological entities or whether they reflect quantitative variants of essentially the same spectrum of psychopatology. DSM-IV recognised APD as "a pervasive pattern of social inhibition, feelings of inadequacy, and hypersensitivity to negative evaluation" that begins at least by early adulthood.

Differential Diagnosis

Avoidant personality disorder appears to imply more severe social dysfunction and therefore it could be a severe variant of GSP. Nevertheless, these disorders are defined differently: SP in terms of phobic anxiety and APD in terms of social dysfunction. Further research is needed to distinguish them.

From a clinical point of view, there is considerable overlap in the symptomatology of SP and panic disorder with or without agoraphobia, since the anxiety reaction in social phobics may be experienced sometimes as a full-blown panic attack. However, the nature of the fear, feared situations, prevalent somatic symptoms, social-demographic data, biological and treatment studies are useful to distinguish between these disorders. The essential feature of agoraphobia is anxiety about being in places or situations from which escape might be difficult (or embarrassing) or in which help may not be available in the event of having a panic attack or panic-like symptoms (DSM-IV). Even if most agoraphobics also express fears of losing control, going insane, embarrassing themselves and others, in SP the fear of negative evaluation is central and associated with concerns about embarrassment and humiliation in front of others. Consequently, whereas patients with panic disorder and agoraphobia have panic attacks in a variety of non-social situations (tunnels, supermarkets, subways, bridges) and are comforted by the presence of a familiar figure when experiencing anxiety, in social phobics panic attacks are bound or predisposed to occur in only the social situations feared by the patients, and the subjects feel more comfortable if they can be alone and eschew contact with others. In SP patients, differently from agoraphobic patients, the avoided situations stand out quickly and avoidance does not extend, but remain constant. In addition, panic attacks in patients with panic disorder with or without agoraphobia can occur at any time in any setting, even awakening the patient from sleep and are accompanied by severe, acute, bodily symptoms: circulatory, respiratory, neurological-like, sweating, nausea or abdominal distress, chill or hot flushes. Patients with agoraphobia and SP also differ with respect to the type of somatic symptoms. Individuals with agoraphobia are more likely to report problems with limb weakness, feeling faint or dizzy, breathing problems, fear of passing out, and tinnitus, whereas individuals with SP are more likely to complain of blushing and muscle twitches. The kind of phobic stimuli may therefore be associated with a different somatic symptom pattern: shortness of breath is a common symptom in panic attacks associated with agoraphobia, whereas blushing is common in panics related to social or performance anxiety. On an epidemiological point of view, compared with agoraphobia, SP is less prevalent (in the community as well as the clinic), is about equally represented among males and females who seek treatment for the disturbance (in comparison to a preponderance of females among agoraphobics), and has an earlier age of onset. Results of biological challenge and treatment studies suggest that SP and panic disorder/agoraphobia may also be characterised by different pathophysiological mechanisms.

Social phobics appear distinct from schizoid patients. Although both may avoid social interaction, by definition, the social phobics desire social contact, but are blocked by anxiety, while schizoid patients lack interest in social interaction.

Clinical observations suggest that patients with Body Dysmorphic Disorder (BDD) resemble those with SP in their tendency to feel ashamed, defective, and socially anxious, as well as in their fear of being embarrassed, ridiculed, and isolated. Patients with body dysmorphic disorder are substantially more concerned about their body's appearance and perceived ugliness than about problems of performance in a social setting.

Atypical depression, with its marked anxiety and rejection-sensitivity, overlaps with SP. However, the presence of reversed vegetative symptoms of hypersomnia and hyperphagia and an unusual heaviness sometimes described as "leaden paralysis" goes well beyond the symptoms of typical SP and these symptoms are properly classified as a depressive disorder.

The distinction between SP and shyness raises the question of whether these concepts represent different aspects of one united domain of interpersonal difficulties. In 1910 Hartemberg described several forms of social anxiety under the generic term of shyness (timidity, performance anxiety, personality disorders). The features used to define shyness, such as impairment in social performances, inhibition of adequate behaviour, avoidance of interpersonal situations and autonomic symptoms are the same as SP. People suffering from dispositional shyness and those with a diagnosis of SP seem to make similar somatic responses to social situations and to have similar fears of negative evaluations. Social phobics, however, seem to avoid social settings and to suffer from more impaired day-to-day functioning than those who are shy. Besides, the prevalence of SP is estimated as between 3 and 13%, while the prevalence of shyness is around 40%. Shyness, being a stable early onset characteristic, is often considered a personality or temperamental feature. Its considerable similarity with SP and APD (avoidant personality disorder) suggests a certain overlap, and it is possible that those terms describe different degrees of severity of the same condition. However, in clinical experience, some patients with SP do not report feeling uneasy in interpersonal relationships other than the specific feared situation.

Developmental Aspects

Kagan et al. (1966) reported that behavioural inhibition in childhood might be a risk factor for the later development of anxiety and mood disorders. Social anxiety, behavioural inhibition, and interpersonal sensitivity seem to constitute often morbid antecedents of various mental disorders; SP and APD are in fact frequently in comorbidity with various anxiety and mood disorders and tend to precede their onset. From a pathogenic perspective, this may be considered either a predisposing factor, or as early expression of the disorder that will evolve, in less severe forms also. This finding implies that diagnostic categories, utilised for classification of pathological phenomena related to social anxiety, are still widely discussed. Insecurity in interpersonal and social situations, and perception of inadequacy in front of others are important variables for a correct clinical lecture of various psychopathological syndromes.

TREATMENT

In recent years, there have been major advances in the therapy of social phobia; the importance of recognising and properly treating SP is emphasised by its surprisingly high prevalence and the accompanying marked disability. Treatments with demonstrated efficacy for SP include pharmacotherapy, cognitive-behaviour therapy and psychopharmacotherapy, a combination of pharmacotherapy and psychological interventions.

Pharmacotherapy

There are three main goals of drug treatment. The first step in pharmacotherapy of SP is that of reducing and controlling pathological anxiety and related phobic avoidance of feared situations in the short term. Second, assuring adequate treatment of depression or other comorbid conditions is also an important issue. Third, as SP is a chronic condition, the choice of treatment which can be well tolerated over long periods will enhance compliance (Lydiard, 1998). Severe, generalised SP is a serious disorder that in many cases merits aggressive treatment (including pharmacological therapy) to prevent or reverse the significant disability which accompanies untreated SP. An increasing number of drugs from different pharmacological classes are being evaluated in SP. The consensus panel considered the quality of clinical evidence for the effectiveness of current therapeutic options in social anxiety disorder: SSRIs, monoamine oxidase inhibitors (MAOIs) and benzodiazepines (Ballenger et al., 1998). They show important differences in terms of tolerability, safety and side-effect profile.

Selective Serotonin Re-uptake Inhibitors (SSRIs)

A growing number of studies have evaluated members of the SSRI class of antidepressant. Two open clinical trials of *paroxetine* have suggested efficacy both in symptom distress and disabilities (Mancini and Van Ameringen, 1996; Stein et al., 1996a). A large-scale, 12-week, double-blind, placebo-controlled trial involving 187 patients has demonstrated the efficacy of paroxetine in reducing work and social life disabilities as well as fear and anticipatory anxiety (Gergel et al., 1997). Paroxetine has also been found to be effective in placebo-controlled studies in treating a number of anxiety disorders such as panic disorder (Oehrberg et al., 1995) and obsessive-compulsive disorder (Zohar and Judge, 1996) that often coexist with SP; for this reason this drug can be considered one of the main options for first-line treatment of choice in SP patients with comorbidity (Montgomery, 1998). The appropriate dosage has been defined for paroxetine: an initial dose of 20 mg/day for two to four weeks, then increased as necessary to obtain a response. An adequate trial of treatment is generally six to eight weeks, but treatment may have to be continued for several months to consolidate response and achieve a full remission (Ballenger et al., 1998).

For the other members of the SSRI drug class, only limited clinical data are available. *Fluvoxamine* was the first SSRI shown to be superior to placebo in the treatment of SP, in a parallel, double-blind, 12-week study involving 30 patients. In this study, approximately three-quarters of the sample had the generalised subtype of SP (Van Vliet et al., 1994). Further studies will have to investigate whether specific subtypes do better or worse in specific treatments.

Sertraline has also been reported to be potentially useful as treatment for SP (Van Ameringen et al., 1994; Katzelnick et al., 1995), but further controlled data are needed to confirm these early encouraging results.

An open study with *fluoxetine* in 16 patients reported that 10 of the subjects were considered to be responders at the end of treatment (Van Ameringen et al., 1993) while a case series regarding patients with social phobia treated with *citalopram* has suggested the efficacy of this drug in this disorder (Lepola et al., 1994).

Overall, it seems reasonable to affirm that all the SSRIs, though with varying levels of evidence due to the different depth in which they have been studied, are effective in SP. Efficacy and tolerability of this class of drugs permit application as a true first-line drug therapy, especially considering the long-lasting treatment of SP. Limitations of SSRIs are their cost, and some side-effects that, though fewer than with antidepressants, should be taken into account for a chronic treatment, e.g. sexual problems.

Monoamine Oxidase Inhibitors (MAOIs)

The earliest placebo-controlled evidence for the efficacy of this therapeutic class was obtained with *phenelzine*, and its efficacy is well established (Gelertner et al., 1991; Versiani et al., 1992) Concerns about its tolerability and safety, however, make it a difficult choice of first-line therapy.

There are some concerns about the efficacy of *moclobemide*, a reversible inhibitor of monoamine oxidase-A, in the treatment of SP. Earlier trials by Versiani et al. (1992) and The International Multicenter Clinical Trial Group (1997) had reported that moclobemide had greater efficacy than placebo, and a European study reported that moclobemide 600 mg/day was effective in controlling the symptoms of SP (Burrows et al., 1997). However, other studies did not confirm this result (Noyes et al., 1997; Schneier et al., 1998). *Brofaromine* has also been used in social phobia with a significantly better response than placebo (Van Vliet et al., 1992), but this drug is not commercially available.

Benzodiazepines (BDZs)

Both *alprazolam* and *clonazepam* have demonstrated their efficacy in a number of open studies (Reich et al., 1989; Munjack et al., 1990; Ontiveros and Fontaine, 1990; Reiter et al., 1991). Nevertheless, it is known that benzodiazepines (BDZs) are contra-indicated in patients who abuse alcohol (a condition that often co-occurs with SP), and that the chronic use of these drugs can cause physical dependence. Thus, they are not considered a good choice for monotherapy for long-term use in anxiety disorders such as SP. BDZs can only be useful either in association with other drugs, such as antidepressants or as purely symptomatic remedies for sporadic use.

Beta-blockers

Beta-blockers are used when cardiovascular symptoms and tremor are prominent, appear to be of use in specific SP, such as public speaking or other performance phobias (Liden and Gottfried, 1974; Gottschalk et al., 1974), whereas they have a limited efficacy in the generalised form of SP (Liebowitz et al., 1992). Their use is not generally indicated since they may have deleterious effects, especially in patients with asthma.

Psychotherapy

There is good evidence for the effectiveness of exposure-based strategies of cognitive-behavioural therapy in social anxiety disorders. The three principal forms of treatment that have been found useful in SP patients are desensitisation (*in vivo* or by imaginable exposure), social skills training, and cognitive restructuring (Heimberg et al., 1985; Mattick et al., 1989; Mersch, 1995). Behavioural strategies are designed to directly address avoidance behaviour and eliminate emotional or anxious arousal, whereas cognitive-behavioural strategies seek to change the way patients perceive and respond to threatening or fear-producing stimuli or thoughts. From a cognitive perspective, "catastrophic cognition" is believed to be an important element of SP, independently of the anxious emotional arousal.

It has been hypothesised that exposure plus cognitive restructuring would be a particularly effective combination, and several methodologically sound studies have examined this combination (Heimberg and Juster, 1994). Recently two programmes of cognitive-behavioural therapy have developed: *cognitive-behavioural group therapy* (Heimberg and Juster, 1994) and *social effectiveness therapy* (Turner et al., 1994). These treatments both involve exposure, which is the key element that influences therapy outcome. The difference is that the cognitive-behavioural group therapy (CBGT) focuses on cognitive restructuring whereas social effectiveness training (SET) is based on exposure plus social skills training (Shear and Beidel, 1998).

Overall, the clinical observation suggests that an initially effective treatment for SP, regardless of the form, may trigger a positive process of improvement in most patients: the reduction of the fears and of the anticipation of failure usually renders the subjects more willing to face situations that were formerly avoided. This, in turn, brings a sort of automatic self-exposure, which has further positive therapeutic value.

REFERENCES

American Psychiatric Association (1980) *Diagnostic and Statistical Manual of Mental Disorder*, 3rd edition. Washington, DC: American Psychiatric Association.
American Psychiatric Association (1987) *Diagnostic and Statistical Manual of Mental Disorder*, 3rd edition revised. Washington, DC: American Psychiatric Association.
American Psychiatric Association (1994) *Diagnostic and Statistical Manual of Mental Disorder*, 4th edition. Washington, DC: American Psychiatric Association.
Amies PL, Gelder MG, Shaw PM (1983) Social phobia: A comparative clinical study. *Br J Psychiatry* 142: 174–179.
Arrindell WA, Emmelkamp PMG, Monsma A et al. (1983) The role of perceived parental

rearing practices in the aetiology of phobic disorders: A controlled study. *Br J Psychiatry* **143**: 183–187.

Ballenger JC, Davidson JRT, Lecrubier Y, Nutt DJ, Bobes J, Beidel DC, Ono Y, Westenberg HGM (1998) Consensus statement on social anxiety disorder from the international consensus group on depression and anxiety. *J Clin Psychiatry* **59** Suppl 17: 54–60.

Barlow DH (1985) The dimensions of anxiety disorders. In Tuma AH, Maser JD (eds) *Anxiety and the Anxiety Disorders*. Hillsdale, NJ: Lawrence Erlbaum, 479–500.

Bech P, Angst J (1996) Quality of life in anxiety and social phobia. *Int Clin Psychopharmacol* **11** Suppl 3: 97–100.

Beidel DC (1998) Social anxiety disorder: Aetiology and early clinical presentation. *J Clin Psychiatry* **59** Suppl 17: 27–31.

Beidel DC, Turner SM (1998) *Shy Children, Phobic Adults: The Nature and Treatment of Social Phobia*. Washington, DC: American Psychological Association.

Brooks RB, Baltazar PL, Munjack DJ (1989) Co-occurrence of personality disorders with panic disorder, social phobia and generalized anxiety disorder: A review of the literature. *J Anx Dis* **3**: 259–285.

Burrows G, Evans L, Baumhackl U, Hebenstreit H, Katschnig H, Schony W (1997) Moclobemide in social phobia: A double-blind, placebo-controlled clinical study. *Eur Arch Psychiatry Clin Neurosci* **247**: 71–80.

Davidson JRT, Hughes DL, George LK, Blazer DG (1993) The epidemiology of social phobia: Findings from the Duke Epidemiological Catchment Area Study. *Psychol Med* **23**: 709–718.

Davidson JRT, Hughes DC, George LK, Blazer DG (1994) The boundary of social phobia. *Arch Gen Psychiatry* **51**: 975–983.

Degonda M, Angst J (1993) The Zurich Study XX: Social phobia and agoraphobia. *Eur Arch Psychiatry Clin Neurosci* **243**: 95–102.

Di Nardo PA, Barlow DH, Cerny JA, Vermilyea BB, Vermilyea JA, Himaldi WG, Waddell MT (1986) Anxiety Disorders Interview Schedule-Revised (ADIS-R). Unpublished manuscript, State University of New York, Albany.

Faravelli C, Guerrini DEG, Innocenti B, Giardinelli L (1989) Epidemiology of anxiety disorders in Florence. *Acta Psychiatr Scan* **79**: 308–312.

Fyer AJ, Mannuzza S, Chapman TF et al. (1993) A direct interview family study of social phobia. *Arch Gen Psychiatry* **50**: 286–293.

Gelertner CS, Uhde TW, Cimbolic P et al. (1991) Cognitive-behavioural and pharmacological treatments of social phobia: A controlled study. *Arch Gen Psychiatry* **48**: 938–945.

Gergel I, Pitts C, Oakes R, Kumar R (1997) Significant improvement in symptoms of social phobia after paroxetine treatment. *Biol Psychiatry* **42** (26S), Abs. 14-12.

Goldstein S (1987) Three cases of overlap between panic disorder, social phobia and agoraphobia. *J Clin Psychiatry* **48**: 452–453.

Gottschalk LA, Stone WN, Gleser CG (1974) Peripheral vs central mechanisms accounting for antianxiety effects of propanolol. *Psychosom Med* **36**: 47–56.

Heimberg RG, Juster HR (1994) Treatment of social phobia in cognitive behavioural groups. *J Clin Psychiatry* **55** Suppl 6: 38–46.

Heimberg RJ, Becker RE, Vermilyea JA (1985) Treatment of social phobia by exposure, cognitive restructuring and homework assignments. *J Nerv Ment Dis* **173**: 236–245.

Herbert JD, Hope DA, Bellack AS (1992) Validity of the distinction between generalized social phobia and avoidant personality disorder. *J Abnorm Psychol* **101**: 332–339.

Judd LL (1994) Social phobia: a clinical overview. *J Clin Psychiatry* **55** Suppl 6: 5–9.

Kagan J (1989) Temperamental contributions to social phobia behavior. *Am Psychol* **44**: 668–674.

Kagan J, Pearson L, Welch L (1966) Modifiability of an impulsive tempo. *J Educat Psychology* **57**(6): 359–365.

Kasper S (1998) Social phobia: The nature of the disorder. *J Affect Disord* **50**: S3–S9.

Katzelnick DJ, Kobak KA, Greist JH, Jefferson JW, Mantle JM, Serlin RC (1995) Sertraline for social phobia: A double-blind, placebo-controlled crossover study. *Am J Psychiatry* **152**: 1368–1371.

Kendler KS, Neale MC, Kessler RC et al. (1992) A population-based twin study of major depression in women: The impact of varying definition of illness. *Arch Gen Psychiatry* **49**: 257–266.

Kessler RC, McGonagle KA, Zhao S, Nelson CB, Hughes M, Eshelman S, Wittchen HU, Kendler KS (1994) Lifetime and 12-month prevalence of DSM-III-R psychiatric disorders in the United States: Results from National Comorbidity Survey. *Arch Gen Psychiatry* **51**: 8–19.

Kessler RC, Stein MB, Berglund P (1998) Social phobia subtypes in the National Comorbidity Survey. *Am J Psychiatry* **155**: 613–619.

Klein DF (1964) Delineation of two drug responsive anxiety syndromes. *Psychopharmacol* **5**: 397–408.

Kushner MG, Sher KJ, Beitman BD (1990) The relation between alcohol problems and the anxiety disorders. *Am J Psychiatry* **147**: 685–695.

Lecrubier Y (1998) Comorbidity in social anxiety disorder: Impact on disease burden and management. *J Clin Psychiatry* **59** Suppl 17: 33–37.

Lecrubier Y, Weiller E (1997) Comorbidities in social phobia. *Int Clin Psychopharmacol* **12** Suppl 6: 17–21.

Lépine JP, Lellouch J (1995) Diagnosis and epidemiology of agoraphobia and social phobia. *Clin Neuropharmacol* **18** Suppl 2: S15–S26.

Lépine JP, Pelissolo A (1998) Social phobia and alcoholism: A complex relationship. *J Affect Disord* **50**: S23–S28.

Lepola U, Koponen H, Leinonen E (1994) Citalopram in the treatment of social phobia: A report of three cases. *Pharmacopsychiatry* **27**: 186–188.

Liden S, Gottfried CG (1974) Beta-blocking agents in the treatment of catecholamine-induced symptoms in musicians. *Lancet* **ii**: 529–535.

Liebowitz MR, Fyer AJ, Gorman JM, Dillon D, Davies S, Stein JM, Cohen BS, Klein DF (1985a) Specificity of lactate infusion in social phobia versus panic disorder. *Am J Psychiatry* **142**: 947–950.

Liebowitz MR, Gorman JM, Fyer AJ, Klein DF (1985b) Social phobia: Review of a neglected anxiety disorder. *Arch Gen Psychiatry* **42**: 729–736.

Liebowitz MR, Schneier F, Campeas R, Hollander E, Hatterer J, Fyer AJ, Gorman J, Papp L, Davies S, Gully R, Klein DF (1992) Phenelzine vs Atenolol in social phobia: A placebo-controlled comparison. *Arch Gen Psychiatry* **49**: 290–300.

Lindal E, Stefansson JG (1993) The lifetime prevalence of anxiety disorders in Iceland as estimated by the US National Institute of Mental Health Diagnostic Interview Schedule. *Acta Psychiatr Scand* **88**: 29–34.

Lydiard RB (1998) The role of drug therapy in social phobia. *J Affect Disord* **50**: S35–S39.

Magee WJ, Eaton WW, Wittchen HU, McGonable KA, Kessler RC (1996) Agoraphobia, simple phobia and social phobia in the National Comorbidity Survey. *Arch Gen Psychiatry* **53**: 159–168.

Mancini C, Van Ameringen MV (1996) Paroxetine in social phobia. *J Clin Psychiatry* **57**: 519–522.

Mannuzza S, Fyer AJ, Liebowitz MR, Klein DF (1990) Delineating the boundaries of social phobia: Its relationship to panic disorders and agoraphobia. *J Anxiety Disorders* **4**: 41–59.

Mannuzza S, Schneier FR, Chapman TF, Liebowitz MR, Klein DF, Fyer AJ (1995) Generalized social phobia: Reliability and validity. *Arch Gen Psychiatry* **52**: 230–237.

Marks IM (1970) The classification of phobic disorders. *Br J Psychiatry* **116**: 377–386.

Marks IM, Gelder MG (1966) Different age of onset in varieties of phobia. *Am J Psychiatry* **123**: 218–221.

Mattick RP, Peters L, Clarke JD (1989) Exposure and cognitive restructuring for social phobia: A controlled study. *Behav Ther* **20**: 3–23.

Merikangas KR, Angst J (1995) Comorbidity and social phobia: Evidence from clinical, epidemiological, and genetic studies. *Eur Arch Psychiatry Clin Neurosci* **244**: 297–303.

Mersch PPA (1995) The treatment of social phobia: The differential effectiveness of exposure in vivo and an integration of exposure in vivo, rational emotive therapy and social skills training. *Behav Res Ther* **33**: 259–269.

Montgomery SA (1995) *Social Phobia*. London: Science Press.

Montgomery SA (1996) Need for treatment and measurement of outcome: Workshop Report 2. *Int Clin Psychiatry* **11** Suppl 3: 103–108.

Montgomery SA (1998) Implications of severity of social phobia. *J Affect Disord* **50**: S17–S22.

Munjack DJ, Baltazar PL, Bohn PB, Cabe DD, Appleton AA (1990) Clonazepam in the treatment of social phobias: A pilot study. *J Clin Psychiatry* **51** Suppl 5: 35–40.

Munjack DJ, Brown RA, McDowell DE (1987) Comparison of social anxiety in patients with social phobia and panic disorder. *J Nerv Ment Dis* **175**: 49–51.

Nichols KA (1974) Severe social anxiety. *Br J Med Psychol* **47**: 301–306.

Noyes Jr R, Moroz G, Davidson JRT et al. (1997) Moclobemide in social phobia: A controlled dose-response trial. *J Clin Psychopharmacol* **17**: 247–254.

Oehrberg S, Christiansen PE, Behnke K, Borup AL, Severn B, Soegaard J, Calberg H, Judge R, Ohrstrom JK, Manniche PM (1995) Paroxetine in the treatment of panic disorder a randomised, double-blind, placebo-controlled study. *Br J Psychiatry* **167**: 374–379.

Offord DR, Boyle MH, Campbell D, Goering P, Lin E, Wong M, Racine YA (1996) One year prevalence of psychiatric disorder in Ontarians 15 to 64 years of age. *Can J Psychiatry* **41**: 559–563.

Ontiveros A, Fontaine R (1990) Social phobia and clonazepam. *Can J Psychiatry* **35**: 439–441.

Parker G (1979) Reported parental characteristics of agoraphobics and social phobics. *Br J Psychiatry* **135**: 555–560.

Phillips KA, Gunderson CG, Mallya G, McElroy SL, Carter WA (1998) Comparison study of body dysmorphic disorder and obsessive-compulsive disorder. *J Clin Psychiatry* **59**: 568–575.

Potts NLS, Davidson JRT (1992) Social phobia: Biological aspects and pharmacotherapy. *Prog. Neuropsychopharmacol. Biol. Psychiatry* **16**: 635–646.

Rapaport MH, Paniccia G, Judd LL (1995) Advances in the epidemiology and therapy of social phobia: Directions for the nineties. *Psychopharmacol Bull* **31**(1): 125–129.

Reich J, Noyes Jr R, Yates W (1989) Alprazolam treatment in avoidant personality traits in social phobic patients. *J Clin Psychiatry* **50**: 91–95.

Reich JH, Perry VC, Shera D, Dyck I, Vasile R, Goisman RM, Rodriguez-Villa F, Massion AO, Keller M (1994) Comparison of personality disorders in different anxiety disorders diagnosis: Panic, Agoraphobia, Generalized Anxiety and Social Phobia. *Ann Clin Psychiatry* **6**: 125–134.

Reiter SR, Otto MW, Pollack MH, Rosenbaum JF (1991) Major depression in panic disorder patients with comorbid social phobia. *J Affect Dis* **3**: 171–177.

Rosenbaum JF, Biederman J, Pollock RA, Hirshfeld DR (1994) The etiology of social phobia. *J Clin Psychiatry* **55** Suppl 6: 10–16.

Schneier FR, Goetz D, Campeas R et al. (1998) Placebo-controlled trial of moclobemide in social phobia. *Br J Psychiatry* **172**: 70–77.

Schneier FR, Johnson J, Horning CD, Liebowitz MR, Weissman MM (1992) Social phobia: Comorbidity and morbidity in a epidemiologic sample. *Arch Gen Psychiatry* **49**: 282–288.

Schneier FR, Spitzer RL, Gibbon M, Fyer AJ, Liebowitz MR (1991) The relationship of social phobia subtype and avoidant personality disorder. *Compr Psychiatry* **32**: 496–502.

Schuckit MA, Hesselbrock V (1994) Alcohol dependence and anxiety disorders: What is the relationship? *Am J Psychiatry* **151**: 1723–1734.

Shear MK, Beidel DC (1998) Psychotherapy in the overall management strategy for social anxiety disorder. *J Clin Psychiatry* **59** Suppl 17: 39–44.

Stein MB, Chartier MJ, Hazen AL (1996a) Paroxetine in the treatment of generalized social phobia: Open-label treatment and double-blind placebo-controlled discontinuation. *J Clin Psychopharmacol* **16**: 218–222.

Stein MB, Chavira DA (1998) Subtypes of social phobia and comorbidity with depression and other anxiety disorders. *J Affect Disord* **50**: S11–S16.

Stein MB, Shea CA, Uhde TW (1989) Social phobic symptoms in patients with panic disorder: Practical and theoretical implications. *Am J Psychiatry* **146**: 235–238.

Stein MB, Tancer ME, Gelernter CS, Vittone BJ, Uhde TW (1990) Major depression in patients with social phobia. *Am J Psychiatry* **147**: 637–639.

Stein MB, Walker JR, Forde DR (1996b) Public speaking fears in a community sample: Prevalence, impact on functioning, and diagnostic classification. *Arch Gen Psychiatry* **53**: 169–174.

Stockwell T, Hodgson R, Rankin H (1982) Tension reduction and the effects of prolonged alcohol consumption. *Br J Psychiatry* **77**: 65–73.

Tancer ME (1993) Neurobiology of social phobia. *J Clin Psychiatry* **54** Suppl 12: 26–30.

The International Multicentre Clinical Trial Group on Moclobemide in Social Phobia (1997) Moclobemide in social phobia: A double-blind, placebo-controlled clinical study. *Eur Arch Psychiatry Clin Neurosci* **247**: 71–80.

Thyer BA, Parrish RT, Curtis GC, Nesse RM, Cameron OG (1985) Ages of onset of DSM III anxiety disorders. *Compr Psychiatry* **26**: 113–121.

Torgersen S (1979) The nature and origin of common phobic fears. *Br J Psychiatry* **134**: 343–351.

Turner SM, Beidel DC, Borden JW, Stanley MA, Jacob RG (1991) Social phobia: Axis I and II correlates. *J Abnorm Psychol* **100**: 102–106.

Turner SM, Beidel DC, Cooley MR, et al. (1994) A multicomponent behavioural treatment for social phobia: social effectiveness therapy. *Behav Res Ther* **32**: 381–390.

Turner SM, Beidel DC, Townsley RM (1992) Social phobia: A comparison of specific and generalized subtypes and avoidant personality disorder. *J Abnorm Psychol* **101**: 326–331.

Van Ameringen M, Mancini C, Streiner DL (1993) Fluoxetine efficacy in social phobia. *J Clin Psichiatry* **54**: 27–32.

Van Ameringen M, Mancini C, Streiner DL (1994) Sertraline in social phobia. *J Affect Disord* **31**: 141–145.

Van Ameringen M, Mancini C, Styan G, Donison D (1991) Relationship of social phobia with other psychiatric illness. *J Affect Disord* **21**: 93–99.

Van Vliet IM, Den Boer JA, Westenberg HG (1992) Psychopharmacological treatment of social phobia: Clinical and biochemical effects of brofaromine, a selective MAO-A inhibitor. *Eur Neuropsychopharmacol* **2**: 21–29.

Van Vliet IM, Den Boer JA, Westenberg HG (1994) Psychopharmacological treatment of social phobia: A double-blind, placebo-controlled study with fluvoxamine. *Psychopharmacol* **115**: 128–134.

Versiani M, Nardi AE, Mundim FD, Alves AB, Liebowitz MR, Amrein R (1992) Pharmacotherapy of social phobia: a controlled study with moclobemide and phenelzine. *Br J Psychiatry* **161**: 353–360.

Wacker HR, Mulleians R, Klein KH, Battegay R (1992) Identification of cases of anxiety disorders and affective disorders in the community according to ICD/10 and DSM III-R by using the composite international diagnostic interview (CIDI). *Int J Methods Psychiatr Res* **2**: 91–100.

Weiller E, Bisserbe JC, Boyer P, Lépine JP, Lecrubier Y (1996) Social phobia in general health care: An unrecognised undertreated disabling disorder. *Br J Psychiatry* **168**: 169–174.

Widiger TA (1992) Generalized social phobia versus avoidant personality disorder: A commentary on three studies. *J Abnorm Psychol* **101**: 340–343.

Wittchen HU, Beloch E (1996) The impact of social phobia on quality of life. *Int Clin Psychopharmacol* **11** Suppl 3: 15–23.

Wittchen HU, Essau CA, Zerssen D, Von Krieg D, Zaudig M (1992) Lifetime and six-month prevalence of mental disorders in the Munich follow-up study. *Eur Arch Psychiatry Clin Neurosci* **241**: 247–258.

Zohar J, Judge R (1996) Paroxetine versus clomipramine in the treatment of obsessive-compulsive disorder. *Br J Psychiatry* **169**: 468–474.

8

Obsessive-compulsive Disorder: Diagnostic Considerations and an Epidemiological Update

Y. Sasson, M. Chopra, R. Amiaz, I. Iancu and J. Zohar

Sheba Medical Center, Tel Hashomer and Sackler School of Medicine, Tel Aviv University, Tel Aviv, Israel

INTRODUCTION

Obsessive-compulsive disorder (OCD) is a common, chronic, and disabling disorder characterized by obsessions and/or compulsions. These symptoms are ego-dystonic and cause significant distress to patients and their families. Up until the early 1980s, OCD was considered a rare, treatment-refractory, chronic condition, of psychological origin. Since then, however, several researchers have reported that the prevalence of OCD is around 2% in the general population (Robins et al., 1984; Weissmann et al., 1994) and it is almost equally distributed between males and females.

HISTORY

An overview of the development of the OCD entity during the last 100 years is useful for understanding the history of psychiatry in general and of OCD in particular.

The famous case history of the Rat Man, an early twentieth-century description of a case of "obsessional neurosis", constitutes one of the earliest detailed descriptions of what is today termed OCD. This young man was treated by Freud due to distressing obsessive thoughts: he developed fears that his loved ones would suffer various punishments or mishaps because of his actions. Due to his repetitive thoughts, he had the urge to commit certain acts (compulsions) in order to prevent harm to his relatives and friends (such as moving a rock from the road in order to prevent a carriage from stepping over it). Freud proposed a relationship between the present obsession and a very early sexual experience of the patient that was coupled with fear of punishment from his father (and also with anger towards the father). Sadistic feelings were the basis of the symptoms, together with fears of punishment, and the present disorder

Anxiety Disorders: An Introduction to Clinical Management and Research. Edited by E. J. L. Griez, C. Faravelli, D. Nutt and J. Zohar. © 2001 John Wiley & Sons, Ltd.

was a repetition of past experiences. Once the basis of the Rat Man's neurosis was understood, the analysis moved on smoothly and the neurosis cleared completely. Unfortunately, the patient was killed in combat during the First World War.

Since this description, psychiatry has significantly progressed with regard to therapy, research methodology and the etiology of mental disorders. Notwithstanding Freud's critical contributions, modern psychiatry is now far more evidence-based and it seems that the pendulum has swung from "psychological" psychiatry to "biological" psychiatry. This is reflected in the use of large double-blind placebo-controlled studies and sophisticated modern techniques which include specific pharmacological and behavioral challenges, intracellular transduction, candidate genes and functional brain imaging, replacing open studies and single case reports.

CLINICAL FEATURES

The diagnosis of OCD according to DSM-IV is based on the presence of either obsessions or compulsions. Obsessions are recurrent, intrusive and distressing thoughts, images or impulses, while compulsions are repetitive, seemingly purposeful behaviors that a person feels driven to perform. Obsessions are usually unpleasant and increase a person's anxiety, whereas carrying out compulsions reduces a person's anxiety. Resisting carrying out a compulsion however, results in increased anxiety. The patient usually realizes that the obsessions are irrational and experiences both the obsession and the compulsion as egodystonic.

The obsessions and compulsions should cause marked distress, be time-consuming (more than one hour per day) and interfere significantly with the person's normal routine and social and occupational activities. At some point during the course of the disorder, but not necessarily during the current episode, the diagnosis requires for the person to have recognized that the obsessions or compulsions are excessive or unreasonable. However, if during most of the current episode the patient does not have this recognition, the diagnosis of OCD with poor insight might be most appropriate.

If another Axis I disorder is present, it is mandatory that the content of the obsessions or compulsions not be restricted to it (e.g. preoccupation with food or weight in eating disorders or guilt ruminations in the presence of Major Depressive Episode—MDD). The disturbance should not be due to the direct effects of a substance (e.g. a drug of abuse or a medication) or a general medical condition.

The DSM-IV diagnostic criteria for OCD are presented below. Patients with both obsessions and compulsions constitute a large proportion of affected patients. Most patients present with multiple obsessions and compulsions. The symptoms may shift and a patient who had washing rituals during childhood may present with checking rituals as an adult.

OCD can be expressed through many different symptoms. The classical presentations include washing and checking. A very common pattern is for an obsession of contamination by dirt or germs, to be followed by washing or avoidance of presumably contaminated objects (doorknobs, electrical switches, newspapers, people's

A. Either obsessions or compulsions

Obsessions as defined by (1), (2), (3), and (4)
(1) recurrent and persistent thoughts, impulses, or images
(2) the thoughts, impulses, or images are not simply excessive worries about real life problems
(3) the person attempts to ignore or suppress such thoughts, impulses, or images, or to neutralize them
(4) the person recognizes that the obsessional thoughts, impulses, or images are a product of his or her own mind (not imposed from without as in thought insertion)

Compulsions are defined by (1) and (2):
(1) repetitive behaviors (e.g., hand washing, ordering, checking) or mental acts (e.g., praying, counting, repeating words silently) that the person feels driven to perform
(2) the behaviors or mental acts are aimed at preventing or reducing distress or preventing some dreaded event or situation

B. At some point during the course of the disorder, the person has recognized that the obsessions or compulsions are excessive or unreasonable. Note: This does not apply to children.

C. The obsessions or compulsions cause marked distress, are time-consuming (take more than 1 hour a day), or significantly interfere with the person's normal routine.

D. If another Axis 1 disorder is present, the content of the obsessions or compulsions is not restricted to it (e.g., preoccupation with food in the presence of an Eating Disorder; ruminations in the presence of Major Depressive Disorder).

E. The disturbance is not due to the direct physiological effects of a substance (e.g. a drug of abuse, a medication) or a general medical condition.

Specify if:
With Poor Insight: if, for most of the time during the current episode, the person does not recognize that the obsessions and compulsions are excessive or unreasonable.

hands, phones). Patients wash their hands excessively and sometimes avoid leaving home due to a fear of germs. However, the feared object is difficult to avoid (for example, feces, urine, dust, or germs).

A second common pattern is for an obsession of doubt, to be followed by a compulsion of checking. Patients check whether they have turned off the stove or locked the door, either remaining at home for hours of repeated checking, or making multiple trips back home to check the stove, for example. Since instead of resolving uncertainty, the checking will often contribute to even greater doubt, this leads to further checking. Often these patients will enlist the help of family and friends to ensure they have checked enough or correctly. Ultimately, by some inscrutable means the patient resolves a particular doubt, only to have it replaced by a new obsessional doubt. Resistance, which in this case is the attempt to refrain from checking, leads to difficulty in concentrating and to exhaustion from the endless intrusion of nagging uncertainties.

Another pattern is one with merely intrusive obsessional thoughts, without a compulsion. The pure obsessional patient experiences repetitive, intrusive thoughts which are usually somatic, aggressive, or sexual, and are always reprehensible. In the absence of what appears to be discrete compulsion, these obsessions may be associated with impulses (which have been called "horrific temptations") or fearful images. When the obsession is an aggressive impulse, it is most often directed at the one person most valuable to the patient. The obsession may also be a fear of acting on other impulses (e.g. to kill somebody, to rob a bank, to steal) or a fear of being held responsible for something terrible (e.g. fire, plague). Often, there may be subtle rituals around these obsessive thoughts. For example, a mother who was afraid she would stab her daughter struggled with this impulse by avoiding sharp objects, then by avoiding touching her daughter and ultimately by leaving the house altogether. Although such avoidant behavior may not appear as an actual repetitive behavior or compulsion, it does share other properties of compulsion in that it is an intentional attempt to neutralize an obsession. Patients may seek treatment claiming they have a phobia, when actually their avoidance is motivated by obsessions. Often, close examination of patient history will reveal the presence of other obsessions or compulsions as well.

Sexual obsessions include forbidden or perverse sexual thoughts, images, or impulses that may involve children, animals, incest, homosexuality, etc. Obsessional thoughts may also be of a religious nature, rather than sexual or violent. Such thoughts may be experienced as blasphemous, leading to repetitive silent prayer, or confession or resulting in more obvious rituals such as repeated bowing or trips to church. Such behavior presents a particular problem to both clinicians and clergy as they attempt to draw the line between disorder and devotion.

Another pattern is the need for symmetry or precision, which leads to a compulsion of slowness. Patients can take hours to shave, in an attempt to do things "just right". Obsessional slowness involves the obsession to have objects or events in a certain order or position, to do and undo certain motor actions in an exact form, or to have things exactly symmetrical. Such patients require an inordinate amount of time to complete even the simplest of tasks; thus getting dressed alone may take a couple of hours. Unlike most obsessive-compulsive patients, these patients usually do not resist their symptoms. Instead, they seem to be consumed with the obsession of how to complete their routine precisely. Although this subtype of OCD is quite rare, aspects of slowness often appear along with other obsessions and compulsions and may be the major source of interference in daily functioning. Hoarding behavior is another subtype. Patients may refuse to throw out junk mail, old newspapers or used tissues, for example, because of doubt of throwing away something important in the process.

Many, if not most, OCD patients have a combination of symptoms, although one symptom type, be it washing, checking, pure obsessions or obsessional slowness, may predominate. In addition to the lack of pure subtypes is the phenomenon of symptom shifting. At different points in the course of their illness, patients report that different OCD symptoms are predominant. Thus, a patient who in childhood may have had predominantly washing rituals may have checking rituals in adulthood. The most important point in noting this symptom shift is not in terms of treatment but in terms of diagnosis, in increasing the level of confidence in making the OCD diagnosis.

Recent dimensional approaches have been utilized in order to analyze these characteristic subtypes, and present the different symptoms in an innovative way. Leckman et al. (1997) have examined the symptom dimensions of OCD in two groups of OCD patients (N = 300) using factor analysis. Four factors emerged: obsessions and checking, symmetry and ordering, cleanliness and washing, and hoarding, in total, accounting for more than 60% of the variance.

Although OCD is an anxiety disorder in the DSM-IV classification, according to the ICD-10 it belongs to the "Neurotic, Stress-related and Somatoform Disorders" group as a stand-alone disorder (and not to the "Anxiety Disorders" group). According to this classification, the obsessions or compulsions (or both) should be present for a period of at least two weeks. Otherwise, the diagnostic criteria and clinical features are similar to those in the DSM-IV.

If OCD is indeed more prevalent than schizophrenia, why do we not diagnose it more often? The answer to this question lies in the egodystonic nature of the disorder. Patients will often attempt to disguise their symptoms due to the shame or embarrassment associated with them. Thus, they will not reveal their obsessive-compulsive symptoms unless asked about them specifically and directly. The following five specific questions, presented below, should be asked in every psychiatric interview, in order to improve diagnosis.

1.   Do you wash or clean a lot?
2.   Do you check things a lot?
3.   Is there any thought that keeps bothering you that you would like to get rid of but can't?
4.   Do your daily activities take a lot of time to complete?
5.   Are you concerned about orderliness or symmetry?

If these five questions are not asked, it is likely the diagnosis of OCD patients will elude the clinician, since, unless they are questioned directly, these patients will probably not reveal their symptoms. The crucial importance of diagnosing OCD lies in the fact that with appropriate treatment (to be discussed in Chapter 9) many patients will show substantial improvement in their obsessive compulsive symptoms and in their quality of life (Koran et al., 1996) and will experience a significant decrease in suffering as well.

EPIDEMIOLOGY

In the last decade, the prevalence of OCD symptoms in the general population has been found to be remarkably high. Until 1984, the most quoted figure was 0.05% (Woodruff and Pitts, 1969). However, since 1984, at least three studies carried out in North America found the prevalence of OCD in the general population to be greater than 2%. Robins et al. (1984) found a prevalence figure of 2.5%, Bland et al. (1988) found a figure of 3.0% and Karno et al. (1988) of 2.5% of OCD prevalence in the general population.

The prevalence of OCD in countries other than North America has also been examined. A major study carried out by Weissmann et al. in 1994 over four different continents examined the prevalence of OCD across the globe. This study found OCD prevalence to be approximately 2% in the United States, Canada, Latin America and Puerto Rico. The findings were the same in Europe and New Zealand, while in Asia and Korea, OCD prevalence was found to be 1.9%, and in Taiwan 0.7%. Therefore, with the exception of Taiwan, where the prevalence of all psychiatric disorders is relatively low, OCD prevalence worldwide is approximately 2%. This finding defines OCD as a global problem, as the estimated total number of patients who suffer from the disorder worldwide appears to be at least 50 million.

Additional demographic findings from this study—the Cross National Collaborative Study (Weissmann et al., 1994)—show the mean age of onset of OCD to be roughly in the twenties; female-to-male ratio to be roughly 1:2; and the course of OCD to be usually chronic.

The high prevalence of OCD has been confirmed across different cultures in additional studies, including in the United States, Canada, Puerto Rico, Finland, Germany, Israel, Hong Kong, Taiwan, Korea and New Zealand (Table 8.1). The prevalence of OCD among children and adolescents appears to be as high as among adults (Flament et al., 1988).

However, it should be noted that not all the authors agree with these figures. For example, Nelson and Rice (1997) and Stein et al. (1997) have suggested that diagnosis of OCD by the Diagnostic Interview Schedule and by laypersons leads to over-diagnosis, and proposed lower prevalence rates of 1–2%.

A further question which may be examined regards the influence of culture on the content of obsessions in different countries. Various studies carried out in the United States, India, England, Japan, Denmark and Israel, among OCD sufferers, revealed the content of obsessions to be relatively similar across locations. The most common

TABLE 8.1   OCD prevalence worldwide

Study	Location	Prevalence %
Robins et al., 1984	USA	2.5
Bland et al., 1988	Canada	3.0
Karno et al., 1988	USA	2.5
Zohar et al., 1993	Israel	3.6*
Reinherz et al., 1993	USA	2.1*
Chen et al., 1993	Hong Kong	2.1
Lindal and Stefannson, 1993	Iceland	2.0
Weissman et al., 1994	USA,	2.3
	Canada,	2.3
	Puerto Rico,	2.5
	Germany,	2.1
	Taiwan,	0.7
	Korea,	1.9
	New Zealand	2.2
Valleni-Basile et al., 1994	USA	3.0

*Note: adolescent population.

TABLE 8.2   Content of obsessions in different countries (%)

	Dirt/ contamination	Harm/ aggression	Somatic	Religious	Sexual
USA (N = 425)	38	24	7	6	6
India (N = 410)	32	20	14	5	6
UK (N = 86)	47	27	—	5	10
Japan (N = 61)	39	12	13	—	5
Denmark (N = 61)	34	23	18	8	6
Israel (N = 34)	50	20	3	9	6

obsession across these six countries, regardless of cultural background, appears to be the obsession with dirt or contamination. The second most common obsession is harm or aggression, the third is somatic, the fourth, religious and the last being sexual obsessions. It appears, therefore, that the content of obsessions is remarkably similar regardless of cultural or geographic location. The commonly occurring obsessions, according to country are presented in Table 8.2.

Table 8.3 presents the various obsessions and compulsions, according to their general prevalence.

TABLE 8.3 Commonly occurring obsessions and compulsions

Obsessions	%	Compulsions	%
Contamination	45	Checking	60
Pathological doubt	42	Washing	50
Somatic	36	Counting	36
Need for symmetry	31	Need to ask or confess	31
Aggressive impulse	28	Symmetry/precision	28
Sexual impulse	26	Hoarding	18
Other	13	Multiple compulsions	48
Multiple obsessions	60		

Source: Reproduced by permission of Rasmussen and Tsuang (1986).

COMORBIDITY

Coexisting Axis I diagnoses in primary OCD are major depressive disorder (67%) (3,14), simple phobia (22%), social phobia (18%) and eating disorder (17%) (Rasmussen and Eisen, 1990). Major depressive disorder, which as we have noted, is the most prevalent coexisting Axis I diagnosis with primary OCD, can clearly develop as a secondary disorder among individuals who find themselves wasting long hours each day washing or checking or obsessing on a persistently recurring thought, which prevents them from leading fully productive lives.

OCD and Tic Disorder

The comorbidity with tic disorders suggests interesting pathophysiological and therapeutic implications. In juvenile OCD the rate of tic disorders affects up to 40% of cases and there is a substantial increase in the prevalence of Tourette's syndrome (TS) among relatives of OCD patients (Pauls, 1992). Tic-related OCD may constitute a separate OCD phenotype, on the basis of symptom profiles, sex ratio, age of onset, family and genetic data, neurochemical and neuroendocrine findings, and patterns of response to treatment.

OCD and Depression

Depression is the most common complication of OCD and by recognizing this relationship, DSM-IV no longer excludes a diagnosis of OCD if depression is present. Instead, it stipulates that the obsession may not be related in content to the guilt-ridden rumination of major depression. However, a precise definition of the relationship between OCD and depression remains elusive. At the clinical level, the illnesses often seem inseparable—one worsening or improving in synchrony with the other.

However, in other clinical cases, OCD symptoms may remain in remission while depression recurs. Although researchers have reported some similarities in the biological markers for depression and OCD, the differences between the two outweigh their similarities (see Zohar and Insel, 1987b for review).

The most striking difference is that antidepressants with excellent efficacy, such as the noradrenergic re-uptake inhibitor desipramine, appear to be totally ineffective in the treatment of OCD (Goodman et al., 1990). Only medications possessing serotonergic properties, such as clomipramine, fluoxetine, fluvoxamine, paroxetine, sertraline and citalopram, have consistent efficacy in reducing OCD symptoms. Other differences relate again to the lack of therapeutic effect of electroconvulsive therapy (ECT) or lithium augmentation in OCD, as compared with their proven efficacy in depression (McDougle et al., 1991; Jenicke and Rauch, 1994).

OCD and Other Anxiety Disorders

Despite the DSM-IV classification of OCD as an anxiety disorder, there are some important differences between OCD and other anxiety disorders. These include: age of onset (younger in OCD patients as compared with those with panic disorder), sex distribution (equal distribution of males and females among OCD patients as compared with greater prevalence among females of other anxiety disorders), responses to anxiogenic and anxiolytic compounds (Zohar et al., 1987b; Gross et al., 1998) and selective responsivity of serotonergic medications (cf. Zohar and Pato, 1991).

OCD and Phobia

Phobias are distinguished from OCD by the absence of a relation between the phobic objects and the obsessive thoughts or compulsive behaviors. The fears in OCD often involve harm to others rather than harm to oneself. In addition, the OCD patient when "phobic" is usually afraid of a stimulus that is unavoidable (i.e. virus, germs or dirt) as opposed to the classic phobic objects, like tunnels, bridges or crowds.

OCD and OCPD

The relationship between OCD and obsessive-compulsive personality disorder (OCPD) has been a focus of debate. This is due to the presence of certain similarities in the diagnosis of OCD, an Axis I disorder in DSM-IV, and of obsessive-compulsive personality disorder, an Axis II disorder in DSM-IV. Both disorders reveal a preoccupation with aggression and control, both use the defenses of reaction formation, undoing, intellectualization, denial and isolation of affect. The psychoanalytic formulation suggests that OCD develops when these defenses fail to contain the obsessional character's anxiety. In this view, OCD is often considered to be on a continuum with OCPD pathology.

Epidemiologic evidence, however, reveals that a concurrent diagnosis of OCPD is neither necessary nor sufficient for the development of OCD on Axis I, in most OCD patients. Moreover, while prospective research is lacking, it appears that OCPD is not a risk factor for developing OCD, as the prevalence of OCPD among OCD patients is not that different from its prevalence in other psychiatric disorders (Mavissakalian et al., 1993). This observation raises an interesting theoretical perspective which is divergent from the continuum hypothesis for OCPD and OCD. Diagnostic confusion can be lessened if one remembers that OCD symptoms are usually ego-dystonic, while compulsive character traits are ego-syntonic and rarely provoke resistance. Moreover, OCPD does not have the degree of functional impairment characteristic of OCD.

OCD and Schizophrenia

About 10% to 25% of chronic schizophrenia patients may also present with OCD symptoms (range 5–45%) (Leckman et al., 1997), and 15% may qualify for the diagnosis of OCD. As in OCD, the OCD symptoms in these patients will not necessarily surface unless specific questions are asked. Many patients with schizophrenia can distinguish the ego-dystonic OC symptoms, perceived as coming from within, from the ego-syntonic delusions perceived as intruding from the outside. Follow-up studies demonstrate diagnostic stability over time and it seems that the presence of OCD in schizophrenia predicts a poor prognosis (Leckman et al., 1997). Several studies among patients with schizophrenia and OCD reported an improvement in OCD symptomatology after the addition of a specific antiobsessive medication (ibid.).

Due to the different (poorer) prognosis of patients with schizo-obsessive symptoms, as well as preliminary data regarding their response to specific therapeutic intervention (i.e., the combination of antipsychotic and antiobsessive medications), and taking into account the high prevalence of this presentation, several researchers have suggested that a "schizo-obsessive" category may be considered (Leckman et al., 1997).

COURSE AND PROGNOSIS

OCD is characterized by a slow onset of symptoms and it may take years for symptoms to become full-blown. However, a rapid onset of symptoms may occur, sometimes associated with a traumatic event, such as pregnancy or loss. Due to the secretive nature of the disorder, there is often a delay of more than 10 years before patients come to psychiatric attention (Hollander et al., 1996). However, this delay may be shortened by the increasing public awareness regarding the disorder, through a proliferation of articles, books and movies on the subject. The course is usually long, with most patients experiencing a chronic course, while others experience a fluctuating one (Sasson et al., 1997).

A poor prognosis is indicated by yielding to (rather than resisting) compulsions. Further indications include childhood onset, bizarre compulsions, the need for hospitalization, coexisting MDD, delusional beliefs, the presence of overvalued ideas (that is, some acceptance of the obsessions and compulsions), and the presence of a personality disorder (especially schizotypal personality disorder). A good prognosis is indicated by good social and occupational adjustment, the presence of a precipitating event, and an episodic nature to the symptoms. Obsessional content does not appear to be related to prognosis. However, further research is needed in order to examine the nature and determinants of prognosis in OCD.

REFERENCES

American Psychiatric Association (1995) *Diagnostic and Statistical Manual of Mental Disorders* 4th edition. Washington, DC: American Psychiatric Association.

Bland RC, Newman SC, Orn H (1988) Age of onset of psychiatric disorders. *Acta Psychiatr Scand* **77** Suppl 338: 43–49.

Chen CN, Wong J, Lee N, Chan-Ho MW, Lau JT, Fung M (1993) The Satin Community Mental Health Survey in Hong Kong II. Major findings. *Arch Gen Psychiatry* **50**: 279–284.

Flament MF, Whitaker A, Rapoport JL et al. (1988) Obsessive compulsive disorder in adolescence: An epidemiological study. *J Am Acad Child Adolesc Psychiat* **27**: 764–771.

Goodman WK, Price LH, Delgado PL, Palumbo J, Krystal JH, Nagy LM, Rasmussen SA, Heninger GR, Charney DS (1990) Specificity of serotonin reuptake inhibitors in the treatment of obsessive compulsive disorder: Comparison of fluvoxamine and desipramine. *Arch Gen Psychiatry* **47**: 577–585.

Gross R, Sasson Y, Chopra M, Zohar J (1998) Biological models of obsessive compulsive disorder: The serotonin hypothesis. In RP Swinson, MM Antony, S Rachman, MA Richter (eds) *Obsessive Compulsive Disorder: Theory, Research and Treatment*. New York: Guilford Publications, pp. 141–153.

Hollander E, Greenwald S, Neville D et al. (1996) Uncomplicated and comorbid obsessive-compulsive disorder in epidemiological sample. *Depression and Anxiety* **4**: 111–119.

Jenicke MA, Rauch SL (1994) Managing the patient with treatment-resistant obsessive compulsive disorder. *J Clin Psychiatry* **55**: 1–17.

Karno M, Golding JM, Sorenson SB et al. (1988) The epidemiology of obsessive-compulsive disorder in five US communities. *Arch Gen Psychiat* **45**: 1094–1099.

Koran LM, Thienemann ML, Davenport R (1996) Quality of life for patients with obsessive-compulsive disorder. *Am J Psychiatry* **153**: 783–788.

Leckman JF, Grice DE, Boardman J, et al. (1997) Symptoms of OCD. *Am J Psychiat* **154**: 911–917.

Lindal E, Stefansson JG (1993) The lifetime prevalence of anxiety disorders in Iceland as estimated by the US National Institute of Mental Health Diagnostic Interview Schedule. *Acta Psychiatr Scand* 29–34.

Mavissakalian MR, Hamann MS, Haidar SA, deGroot CM (1993) DSM-III personality disorders in generalized anxiety, panic/agoraphobia, and obsessive-compulsive disorders. *Comprehensive Psychiatry* **34**: 243–248.

McDougle CJ, Price LH, Goodman WK et al. (1991) A controlled trial of lithium augmentation in fluvoxamine-refractory obsessive-compulsive disorder: Lack of efficacy. *J Clin Psychopharmacol* **11**: 175–181.

Nelson E, Rice J (1997) Stability of diagnosis of obsessive compulsive disorder in the epidemiologic catchment area study. *Am J Psychiat* **154**: 826–831.

Pauls, D (1992) The genetics of OCD and Gilles de la Tourette's syndrome. *Psychiatr Clin North Am* **15**: 759–766.

Rasmussen SA, Eisen JL (1990) Epidemiology of obsessive-compulsive disorder. *J Clin Psychiatry* **51** Suppl: 10–13.

Rasmussen SA, Eisen JL (1992) Epidemiology and clinical features of obsessive-compulsive disorder. In Jenike MA, Baer L, Minichiello WE (eds) *Obsessive Compulsive Disorders: Theory and Management.* Chicago: Year Book Medical Publishers, 10–27.

Rasmussen SA, Tsuang MT (1986) The epidemiology of obsessive compulsive disorder. *J Clin Psychiatry* **45**: 450–457.

Reinherz HZ, Gianconia RM, Lefkowitz ES, Pakiz B, Frost AK (1993) Prevalence of psychiatric disorders in a community population of older adolescents. *J Am Academy Child and Adolescent Psychiatry* **32**: 369–377.

Robins LN, Helzer JE, Weissman MM et al. (1984) Lifetime prevalence of specific psychiatric disorders in three sites. *Arch Gen Psychiat* **41**: 949–958.

Sasson Y, Zohar J, Chopra M, Lustig M, Iancu I, Hendler T (1997) Epidemiology of OCD: A world view. *J Clin Psychiatr* Suppl 58: 1–5.

Stein MB, Forde DR, Anderson G, Walker JR (1997) Obsessive compulsive disorder in the community: An epidemiologic survey with clinical reappraisal. *Am J Psychiat* **154**: 1120–1126.

Valleni-Basile LA, Garrison CZ, Jackson KL, Waller JL, McKeown RE, Addy CL, Cuffe SP (1994) Frequency of obsessive-compulsive disorder in a community sample of young adolescents. *J Am Academy Child and Adolescent Psychiatry* **33**: 782–791.

Weissman MM, Bland RC, Canino GJ et al. (1994) The cross-national epidemiology of obsessive compulsive disorder. *J Clin Psychiat* **55** Suppl 13: 5–10.

Woodruff R, Pitts F (1969) Monozygotic twins with obsessional illness. *Am J Psychiatry* **120**: 1075–1080.

Zohar J, Insel TR (1987) Obsessive-compulsive disorder: Psychological approaches to diagnosis, treatment and pathophysiology. *Biol Psychiatry* **22**: 667–687.

Zohar J, Mueller EA, Insel TR, Zohar-Kadouch RC, Murphy DL (1987b) Serotonergic responsivity in obsessive-compulsive disorder: Comparison of patients and healthy controls. *Arch Gen Psychiatry* **446**: 946–951.

Zohar J, Pato MT (1991) Diagnostic considerations. In Pato MT, Zoahr J (eds) *Current Treatments of Obsessive Compulsive Disorder.* Washington, DC: American Psychiatric Press.

Zohar AH, Ratzosin G, Pauls DL, Apter A, Bleich A, Kron S, Rappaport M, Weizman A, Cohen DJ (1992) An epidemiological study of obsessive-compulsive disorder and related disorders in Israeli adolescents. *J Am Acad Child Adolesc Psychiatry* **31**: 1057–1061.

9

Obsessive-Compulsive Disorder: Biology and Treatment, A Generation of Progress

I. Iancu, Y. Sasson, N. Nakash, M. Chopra and J. Zohar

Sheba Medical Center, Tel Hashomer and Sackler School of Medicine, Tel Aviv University, Tel Aviv, Israel

INTRODUCTION

Until about thirty years ago, OCD was considered to be a treatment-refractory disorder. Dynamic psychotherapy was of little benefit and several pharmacological treatments were attempted without much success (Salzman and Thaler, 1981). The introduction of clomipramine (CMI) in the 1960s and of the selective serotonin re-uptake inhibitors (SSRIs) in the late 1980s and early 1990s has significantly improved the prognosis of patients with this disorder. Numerous studies have reported on the efficacy of various serotonin re-uptake inhibitors (SRIs) in OCD, paving the way to a better understanding of the pathophysiology of this disorder, and helping to clarify its biological basis.

The sizeable progress in OCD may provide an example of the fruitful integration between studies on selective treatments, together with specific pharmacological challenges combined with advanced methodologies of imaging studies (both before and after treatment), and the integration of the neurological aspects (Salzman and Thaler, 1981; Robins et al., 1984; Weissman et al., 1994; Renynghe de Voxrie, 1968; Fernandez-Cordoba and Lopez-Ibor, 1967). This section will discuss each of these aspects further.

ETIOLOGY

Specific Clinical Response

Reports that clomipramine (CMI), a tricyclic antidepressant with a serotonergic profile, is effective in treating symptoms of OCD (Renynghe de Voxrie, 1968; Fernandez-Cordoba and Lopez-Ibor, 1967) has directed researchers' interest in the relationship between serotonin and OCD. Moreover, OCD is currently unique

Anxiety Disorders: An Introduction to Clinical Management and Research. Edited by E. J. L. Griez, C. Faravelli, D. Nutt and J. Zohar. © 2001 John Wiley & Sons, Ltd.

among psychiatric disorders, as only serotonergic medications appear to be effective in this disorder (Dolberg et al., 1996). For example, non-serotonergic drugs, such as desipramine (DMI), which are effective in depression and panic disorder, are entirely ineffective in OCD (Zohar and Insel, 1987; Goodman et al., 1990; Leonard et al., 1991).

While this does not necessarily reflect on pathogenesis, the specific response to serotonergic drugs has paved the way for further research on the role of serotonin in the pathogenesis of OCD in particular, and in OCD-related disorders in general. As yet, abnormality of the serotonergic system and particularly hypersensitivity of post-synaptic 5-HT (hydroxy tryptamine) receptors, constitute the leading hypothesis for the underlying pathophysiology of OCD (Zohar and Insel, 1987; Thoren et al., 1980; Insel et al., 1985; Weizman et al., 1986; Marazziti et al., 1992; Vitiello et al., 1991; Kim et al., 1998; Marazziti et al., 1997; Flament et al., 1987; Charney et al., 1988; Hollander et al., 1992; Lesch et al., 1991; Bastani et al., 1990; Sasson and Zohar, 1996; Benkelfat et al., 1989).

CSF Indices

Clinical studies have assayed CSF levels of serotonin metabolites, for example, 5-HIAA (Thoren et al., 1980; Insel et al., 1985), and affinities of platelet binding sites of tritiated imipramine (which binds to serotonin reuptake sites) (Weizman et al., 1986; Marazziti et al., 1992; Vitiello et al., 1991; Kim et al., 1991) and have reported variable findings of those measures in OCD patients. One study supported the relationship between decreased function of the serotonergic system and positive response to SSRIs, demonstrating normalization of the number of platelet 5-HT transporters following treatment with different SSRIs (Marazziti et al., 1997). In an earlier study, patients who responded to CMI had higher pretreatment levels of 5-hydroxyindole-acetic acid (5-HIAA, a metabolite of 5-HT serving as an index of 5-HT turnover) than the nonresponders (Thoren et al., 1980). Moreover, clinical improvement was positively correlated with the decrease in CSF concentration of 5-HIAA (ibid.).

Peripheral Indices

Another approach is to examine peripheral measures of serotonergic and noradrenergic function in OCD. In one study, clinical improvement during CMI therapy closely correlated with pretreatment platelet serotonin concentration and monoamine oxidase (MAO) activity, as well as with the decrease in both measures during CMI administration (Flament et al., 1987). Moreover, only the plasma levels of CMI, a potent 5-HT re-uptake inhibitor, but not the plasma levels of its primary metabolite, desmethyl CMI, which has noradrenergic properties, correlated significantly with improvement in OCD symptoms. These findings suggest that the effects of antiobsessive medications, CMI in this study, on serotonin function are pertinent to the antiobsessional action observed.

Serotonin Antagonists

Support for the importance of serotonin in the therapeutic response to SRIs in OCD was provided by a study in which the investigators administered the serotonin receptor antagonist, metergoline and placebo to 10 patients with OCD in a double-blind crossover study (Berkelfat et al., 1989). Patients receiving CMI on a long-term basis responded with greater anxiety to a four-day administration of metergoline when compared with the placebo phase.

Pharmacological Challenges

Additional evidence for the pathogenesis of the serotonergic system in OCD was provided by challenge studies. Obsessive-compulsive (OC) symptoms can be induced specifically by either behavioral or pharmacological challenge (Hollander et al., 1992; Pigott et al., 1991; Rauch et al., 1999). Behavioral challenge is individually tailored according to a known stressful stimulus for the patient, while pharmacological challenge is directed towards a specific receptor subsystem in the brain. Inducing symptoms via challenge can reveal state-dependent features of pathological brain mechanisms (Goodman et al, 1991). The typical design for a challenge test consists of within-subject and across-states repeated measures of several dependent variables, such as behavioral, physiological or brain measures.

Exacerbation of OC symptoms has been described in challenge studies applying methyl-chlorophenylpiperazine (mCPP)—a serotonergic agonist of 5HT1D, 5HT2/5HT1C and 5HT1A (Zohar et al., 1987; Hollander et al., 1988). This exacerbation was blocked by pre-treatment with metergoline, a non-specific 5HT antagonist (Pigott et al., 1991), and down-regulated by chronic treatment with clomipramine (Zohar et al., 1988).

Others, however, have failed to show that mCPP challenge induces exacerbation of OC symptoms (Charney et al., 1988). In a detailed review of the literature it has been demonstrated that about 50% of OCD patients challenged by mCPP had some OC symptom exacerbation. However, no OC symptom exacerbation has been demonstrated, following challenge with either ipsapirone or MK-212 (specific agonists of 5HT1A and 5HT2/5HT1C, respectively). Based on such observation, OC symptom provocation following mCPP challenge was related specifically to the 5HT1D receptor subtype (Gross-Isseroff et al., 1995). We have examined this assumption by using sumatriptan, a 5HT1D agonist, as a pharmacological challenge in comparison to placebo in OCD patients (Stern et al., 1998). OC symptom exacerbation was demonstrated in about 50% of the patients with sumatriptan and none with placebo.

Challenges with L-Tryptophan (Charney et al., 1988), mCPP (Zohar and Insel, 1987; Hollander et al., 1992), sumatriptan (5-HT1D agonist-(6)), ipsapirone (a 5HT1A receptor ligand-(28)) and MK-212 (affecting 5HT1A and 5HT2C-(29)) among others were used to evaluate whether they worsen obsessive-compulsive symptoms or whether they have other differentiating physiologic responses (thermal or neuroendocrine) in OCD patients, as compared with controls. Only two compounds (mCPP and sumatriptan) have shown behavioral hypersensitivity and neuro-endocrine hyposensitivity to be characteristic of the OCD challenge response. These studies have the potential to pinpoint the receptor subtype involved in OCD, raising the possibility that 5HT2C and 5HT1D receptors, but not 5HT1A, may be involved in OCD (Sasson and Zohar, 1996).

Dopamine

The most compelling evidence for dopaminergic involvement in OCD comes from the abundance of OCD symptoms in basal ganglia disorders, such as TS, Sydenham's chorea and post-encephalitic Parkinsonism. The therapeutic benefits obtained through the co-administration of dopamine blockers and SRIs in a subset of OCD patients with tic disorders (McDougle et al., 1990) has also suggested a role for dopamine dysfunction. A study evaluating levels of platelet sulphotransferase, an enzyme involved in the catabolism of catecholamines (providing a marker of presynaptic dopamine function), reported a decreased level of platelet H3-imipramine binding and a parallel increase in the level of sulphotransferase activity in OCD as compared with controls. This provides further support for the hypothesis of reduced 5-HT activity and increased dopamine transmission in OCD (Marazziti et al., 1992).

Immune Factors

Study of autoimmune factors has been prompted by the association of OCD and the autoimmune disease of the basal ganglia, Sydenham's chorea. This complication of rheumatic fever is accompanied by obsessive-compulsive symptoms in over 70% of cases (Swedo et al., 1994). Ten out of 11 children had antibodies directed against the caudate (ibid.). These children had a history of obsessive-compulsive symptoms which began prior to the onset of the chorea, reached a peak in line with the motor symptoms and declined with their resolution. This is consistent with the hypothesis of basal ganglia dysfunction in OCD.

Antibodies against two peptides of the basal ganglia have also been found (Roy et al., 1994). A strong connection was reported between OCD/Tourette syndrome and the B cell antibody D8/17, another anti-brain antibody (Swedo et al., 1994). The specificity of these antibodies to OCD is as yet unclear. Cell-mediated immune function alterations were reported in OCD, however, replication studies are needed.

Brain Imaging Studies

Positron emission tomography (PET) has displayed increased activity (i.e. metabolism and blood flow) in the frontal lobes, the basal ganglia (especially the caudate nucleus), and the cingulum of OCD patients (Rauch, 1998). Pharmacological and behavioral treatments reportedly reverse those abnormalities (Baxter et al., 1992). The data from functional imaging studies are consistent with the data from structural brain-imaging studies. Both computed tomographic and magnetic resonance imaging studies have found decreased sizes of caudates bilaterally. Both functional and structural imaging procedures are consistent with the observation that neurological procedures involving the cingulum are sometimes effective in the treatment of OCD patients.

Overall, the brain imaging research suggests a role for the prefrontal cortex-basal ganglia thalamic circuitry. Dysfunction of these circuits can be explored by neuropsychological testing and evoked potentials. A recent study of OCD patients showed that they are slower in performing tasks involving frontocortical systems, suggesting alterations at this level (Galderisi et al., 1995). An evoked potential study showed enhanced processing negativity in the frontal cortex consistent with prefrontal hyperactivity shown in brain imaging studies (Towey et al., 1994).

Genetics

A significantly higher concordance rate was found for monozygotic twins than for dizygotic twins (Rasmussen and Tsuang, 1986). Some 35% of the first-degree relatives of childhood-onset OCD patients are also afflicted with the disorder (Lenane et al., 1990). Although this high rate is possibly related to the early onset subtype, it nevertheless suggests a genetic component in OCD. Genetic research has yet to find abnormalities at the 5-HT transporter gene level. A study exploring the polymorphism of the promoter region of the gene for the 5-HT transporter failed to identify any differences between OCD patients and controls (Billet et al., 1997).

Other Biological Data

Sleep EEG and neuroendocrine studies have found several abnormalities similar to those seen in depression, such as decreased REM latency, non-suppression on the dexamethasone-suppression test and decreased growth hormone secretion with clonidine infusions (Insel et al., 1982a,b). Only a part of the biological markers found in depression was found relevant in OCD, and their specificity and importance are still unclear.

Behavioral Factors

According to learning theory, obsessions are conditioned stimuli. When a relatively neutral stimulus is coupled with an anxiety-provoking one, through conditioning it will produce anxiety, even when presented alone. Compulsions reduce anxiety and the patient repeats and learns them in order to avoid anxiety. Avoidance strategies are learned and become fixed, eventually becoming a source of disability.

Psychosocial Factors

The dynamic aspects of OCD were first described by Sigmund Freud, who coined the term "obsessional neurosis". The disorder was thought to be the result of a regression from the oedipal to the anal phase, with its characteristic ambivalence. The coexistence of hatred and love towards the same person was believed to leave the patient paralyzed with doubt and indecision. Freud originally suggested that obsessive symptoms result from unconscious impulses of an aggressive or sexual nature. These impulses, he maintained, cause extreme anxiety which is avoided via the defense mechanisms. One of the striking features among OCD patients is the degree to which they are preoccupied with aggression or cleanliness (anal phase), either overtly in the content of their symptoms or in the underlying associations.

Freud described three major psychological defense mechanisms that are important in OCD: isolation, undoing and reaction formation. According to the psychoanalytic formulation, OCD develops when these defenses fail to contain the anxiety. Isolation is the separation of the idea and the affect that it arouses, when the patient is only aware of the affectless idea. Undoing is a secondary defense in order to combat the impulse and quiet the anxiety that its imminent eruption into consciousness arouses. Undoing is a compulsive act, performed in order to prevent or undo the results that the patient irrationally anticipates from a frightening obsessional thought or impulse. Reaction formation is related to the production of character traits rather than symptom formation (characteristic of the above defenses). This trait seems highly exaggerated and inappropriate (i.e. the transformation of anger and hate into exaggerated love and dedication).

Etiology: A Summary

The efficacy of the SSRIs for OCD, together with the lack of efficacy of adrenergic antidepressants, has suggested that serotonin is involved in the pathophysiology of OCD. This relationship was validated by research on serotonergic markers in OCD and by the challenge paradigm (Dolberg et al., 1996). It is still unclear which type of serotonergic receptor is involved in the pathogenesis and mechanism of action of antiobsessional drugs. Further studies of the serotonergic system in OCD may clarify the role of serotonin in the pathophysiology and management of OCD.

THE PHARMACOLOGICAL TREATMENT OF OCD

Since the early 1980s, several potent serotonin re-uptake inhibitors (SRIs) have been studied extensively in OCD. Aggregate statistics for all SRIs suggest that 70% of treatment-naive patients will improve at least moderately (Rasmussen et al., 1993).

Efficacy of Serotonergic vs. Adrenergic Antidepressants

While anecdotal reports have suggested that clinical benefit can be obtained with a range of antidepressant medications, consistent efficacy has only been demonstrated for SRIs and SSRIs. Studies have directly compared CMI with other antidepressants and a consistent pattern emerges: antidepressant drugs that are less potent serotonin reuptake inhibitors than CMI are generally ineffective in OCD (Thoren et al., 1980; Zohar and Insel, 1987; Goodman et al., 1990; Leonard et al., 1991).

Clomipramine (CMI) was the first effective medication reported for OCD, in the late 1960s (Renynghe de Voxrie, 1968; Fernandez-Cordoba and Lopez-Ibor, 1967). Since then, numerous placebo-controlled studies have clearly shown CMI's effectiveness. This culminated in the multi-center, controlled US trial (N = 520) that confirmed CMI's effectiveness (Clomipramine Collaborative Study Group, 1991). In this study, after 10 weeks of treatment, 58% of patients treated with CMI rated themselves much or very much improved, versus 3% of placebo-treated patients.

Beside CMI, other non-tricyclic SRIs, such as fluoxetine, fluvoxamine, paroxetine, sertraline and citalopram are gaining acceptance as effective alternatives for the treatment of OCD in controlled studies.

Onset of Treatment Response

It has been suggested that a relatively long period up to 8 or even 12 weeks is needed before one can consider the specific pharmacological intervention to be ineffective. Often, several months are required to achieve maximum response.

Long-term Treatment of OCD

It has been demonstrated that the length of treatment should be considerable and that most patients relapse after premature discontinuation. Pato et al. (1988) reported that 16 out of 18 patients with OCD relapsed within seven weeks after discontinuing CMI, although some had been treated for more than a year (mean = 10.7 months). All patients regained therapeutic effects when CMI was reintroduced. Leonard et al. (1991) examined the effect of CMI substitution during long-term CMI treatment in 26 children and adolescents with OCD (mean duration of treatment was 17 months).

Half of the patients were blindly assigned to two months of desipramine (DMI) treatment, and then CMI was reintroduced. Almost 90% relapsed during the two-month substitution period in comparison with only 18% of those kept on CMI. It seems advisable for OCD patients to be maintained on antiobsessive medications for more than a year before a very gradual attempt to discontinue the treatment is carried out.

The required maintenance dose in OCD is also unclear. In a study that examined this issue, Mundo et al. (1997) investigated the effect of dose reduction in 30 patients previously treated successfully with CMI or fluoxetine. Patients were randomized to receive the same drug dosage, to receive a reduced dose or a very reduced dose. There was no difference found between the groups during the 102 days of the study.

Drug Dosage

Higher doses of SSRIs and SRIs have been used in the treatment of OCD as compared to depression, but empirical data supporting this practice are scant. Two fixed-dose studies using fluoxetine and one Pan-European study with paroxetine found some advantage with using higher doses, while one fixed-dose study with sertraline has not (Dolberg et al., 1996; Sasson and Zohar 1996). It seems reasonable to use higher doses in non-responders or when only partial relief is attained.

Comparative Studies of CMI vs. SSRIs

The introduction of SSRIs has raised a question regarding the comparative efficacy of CMI versus that of the SSRIs. SSRIs are important alternatives to CMI, since their range of side-effects is clearly different (lacking anticholinergic side-effects, sedation, safety with overdose, to name some). Although SSRIs may provoke nausea, headaches and sleep disturbances, these side-effects are usually less troublesome to most patients.

Fluoxetine was compared with CMI in 11 OCD patients in a 10-week crossover study (Pigott et al., 1990). Although no significant differences were noted regarding clinical efficacy, the proportion of fluoxetine non-responders who responded later on to CMI tended to be higher in comparison with CMI non-responders who were switched to fluoxetine. Patients reported significantly fewer side-effects while on fluoxetine. Freeman et al. (1994) compared the efficacy of fluvoxamine and CMI in a multi-center, randomized, double-blind, parallel group comparison in 66 patients. Both drugs were equally effective and well tolerated, but fluvoxamine produced fewer anticholinergic side-effects and caused less sexual dysfunction than CMI, and more reports of headache and insomnia. Paroxetine was of comparable efficacy to CMI and both were significantly more effective than placebo in a multinational double-blind placebo-controlled, parallel-group study with 399 OCD patients (Zohar and Judge, 1996). Bisserbe et al. (1997) reported that sertraline (50–200 mg/day) was significantly more effective than CMI (50–200 mg/day) in a double-blind study (N = 160). A summary of comparison studies with SRIs and CMI is presented in Table 9.1.

TABLE 9.1 Comparisons of SRIs with Clomipramine

Study	N	SSRI	Comparator	Result
Pigott et al., 1990	11	Fluoxetine ≤ 80 mg	Clomipramine ≤ 250 mg	No difference
Lopez-Ibor et al., 1996	55	Fluoxetine 40 mg	Clomipramine ≤ 150 mg	No difference
Smereldi et al., 1992	10	Fluvoxamine ≤ 200 mg	Clomipramine ≤ 200 mg	No difference
Freeman et al., 1994	66	Fluvoxamine ≤ 200 mg	Clomipramine ≤ 250 mg	No difference
Koran et al., 1996	79	Fluoxamine 100–200 mg	Clomipramine 100–250 mg	No difference
Milanfranchi et al., 1997	26	Fluvoxamine ≤ 300 mg	Clomipramine ≤ 300 mg	No difference
Zohar and Judge, 1996	399	Paroxetime ≤ 60 mg	Clomipramine ≤ 250 mg	No difference
Bisserbe et al., 1997	168	Sertraline ≤ 200 mg	Clomipramine ≤ 200 mg	SRI more effective

Psychological Approaches

The role of a psychodynamic approach in OCD is limited, whereas modern interventions like cognitive and behavioral therapy show promising results (Van Balkom et al., 1998; Marks et al., 1975). Behavioral therapy (BT) is as effective as pharmacotherapy in OCD (Van Balkom et al., 1998), and some data indicate that the beneficial effects are longer-lasting with behavior therapy (Greist, 1996). About two-thirds of patients with moderately severe rituals can be expected to improve substantially, but not completely. A combination of BT and pharmacotherapy might constitute the optimal treatment for OCD. Two recent neuroimaging studies found that patients with OCD who are successfully treated with BT show changes in cerebral metabolism similar to those produced by successful treatment with SRIs (Galderisi et al., 1995; Schwartz et al., 1996).

BT can be conducted in inpatient and outpatient settings. The principal behavioral approaches in OCD are exposure for obsessions and response prevention for rituals. Desensitization, thought stopping, flooding, implosion therapy, and aversion conditioning have also been used with OCD patients. In BT the patient must collaborate and carry out assignments. In a study with 18 OCD patients, patients receiving exposure and response prevention showed significant improvement, whereas patients on a general anxiety management intervention (control) showed no improvement from baseline (Lindsay et al., 1997). Direct comparisons of BT and pharmacotherapy are few and are limited by methodological issues. However, Cox et al. (1993) reported equal efficacy in a meta-analysis.

Despite the fact that biological interventions are more efficacious for OCD patients, psychodynamic factors might be of considerable benefit in understanding what precipitates exacerbations of the disorder and in treating various forms of resistance to treatment, such as noncompliance to medications or to homework assignments. Symptoms may hold important psychological meanings that make patients reluctant to give them up. Therefore, a psychological assessment of the patient's resistance to treatment may improve compliance.

In the absence of controlled studies of insight-oriented psychotherapy for OCD, the anecdotal reports reporting lasting change do not enable a generalization of its efficacy. Also, the efficacy of medications in producing rapid improvement has rendered slow and long-term psychotherapy out of favor.

Non-specific approaches, such as supportive psychotherapy, have a place in OCD and may help patients improve their functioning and adjustment. Management should also include attention to family members through the provision of emotional support, reassurance, education, and advice on how to cope with and respond to the patient. Family therapy may reduce marital discord and build a treatment alliance, also to help in the resistance to compulsions. Group therapy is useful for providing a support system for some patients.

TREATMENT-RESISTANT OCD

Despite the abundance of reports concerning the efficacy of various agents in OCD, about 20–30% of patients do not respond at all and another 20–30% display only partial response. Possible reasons for treatment refractoriness in OCD are presented below, according to Goodman et al. (1993).

- Inadequacy of trial
  - duration too short?
  - dose too low?
  - impaired absorption/increased metabolism?
  - noncompliance?
- Coexisting condition limits drug efficacy
- Incorrect diagnosis?
- Exogenous countertherapeutic influences
  - family environment?
  - antiexposure instructions?
- Underlying biological heterogeneity
  - OCD as a syndrome with multiple etiologies
- Search for putative subtypes

In treating these partial or complete non-responders, sound clinical choices are called for. However, as well-controlled, double-blind studies are lacking, many of these clinical decisions are based on case reports and uncontrolled studies, and therefore, these recommendations should be treated cautiously.

Athough the focus here is on the pharmacological approach, we suggest that in cases of partial or non-response, an attempt should be made to combine behavioral therapy (BT) with the pharmacological treatments. BT involves imaginary flooding and *in vivo* exposure and response prevention. In cases of non-response, family therapy, too, should be suggested, in order to assess the family dynamics and to determine whether there is a family member who cooperates with the patient's disorder—for example, impedes exposure trials—hence preventing any improvement.

Switching Medications

If the patient could not tolerate adequate doses of SSRIs or has not responded to SSRI administered in the upper range of the relevant dose, a trial of CMI is recommended (and vice versa). CMI should be given after an adequate work-up that includes an ECG and ruling out ophthamological problems (i.e. closed angle glaucoma). Although no fixed dose studies were carried out, it seems that high doses of CMI are needed in order to attain responses in OCD patients. The titration to these doses should last for 1–3 weeks. If possible, therapeutic drug monitoring should be performed in order to ascertain blood levels (200–500 ng/ml) for the parent drug plus the desmethyl derivative and to avoid side-effects that result from very high (or even toxic) blood levels. If tolerated, a dose of 200–300 mg/day is considered efficacious in OCD, and this dose would be administered for 10 weeks before determining a lack of response.

Caution is necessary if CMI is administered immediately after fluoxetine; in this case, lower initial doses of CMI should be the rule, due to fluoxetine's long half-life and the fact that it inhibits cytochrome P450 enzymes (thus increasing the availability of CMI). Switching from SSRIs, with shorter half-lives and less inhibition of cytochrome P450 enzymes (such as fluvoxamine and sertraline) to CMI is less problematic. However, the common procedure of slow titration is recommended.

Neuroleptics

If the diagnosis is OCD and a tic disorder, small doses of pimozide or haloperidol, in addition to the serotonergic drug are associated with a higher therapeutic response.

Augmentation

Augmentation is called for when there is partial or no response to the above-mentioned approaches, i.e. combination of SSRIs (or SRIs) with other medications.

To date, only two augmenting agents have been found to be effective in double-blind studies, i.e., risperidone and pindolol, which will be discussed below. However, many other augmenting agents have been tried and may be effective for some refractory patients. These include buspirone, lithium, trazodone, tryptophan and thyroid hormones.

Risperidone

Risperidone in small doses—one to two mg twice a day—was found in one double-blind and three open studies to be effective in alleviating OC symptoms in some partial or non-responders (Ravizza et al., 1996).

Pindolol

Pindolol augmentation (2.5 mg of pindolol, three times daily) with SSRIs is the second augmenting agent which has been found in double-blind studies to be effective and thus might be placed quite high on the list of augmenting agents (Dannon et al., 2000). However, it appears to give an extra "push" to partial responders rather than actually turning non-responders into responders.

Other Options

As OCD is considered an anxiety disorder by the DSM-IV (but not by the ICD-10), it is not surprising that anxiolitics have been suggested in the treatment of OCD patients. Thus, alprazolam and clonazepam have been reported as efficient in several uncontrolled studies and case series, and even in a small double-blind randomized, multiple cross-over study. However, since OCD is a chronic disorder, the use of anxiolitics for long periods raises questions of dependency brought about by long-term use of benzodiazepines.

Despite reports in open studies regarding the efficacy of trazodone, buspirone and lithium, the results in double-blind studies were negative. Adding drugs affecting dopamine function, especially atypical antipsychotics (risperidone), to SRI therapy in treatment-resistant OCD patients, resulted in improvement in patients with a personal or family history of tics (McDougle et al., 1997).

Thyroid supplementation has been reported to be efficacious in open trials as adjunctive agents to SRIs. However, the efficacy of this agent in OCD was not confirmed in a controlled study (Pigott et al., 1991).

Clonidine, an alpha-2 adrenergic agonist, has been reported to be effective in treating OC symptoms in the context of Tourette's syndrome (Cohen et al., 1980) and there are reports of improvement in typical OCD patients (Hollander et al.,

1988). However, there are no controlled data to support this agent's efficacy and its side-effect profile discourages its use in OCD.

Intravenous Clomipramine

Several studies reported on the efficacy of intravenous CMI with intractable OCD. This strategy includes daily infusions of CMI for circa 14 days, the maximum dose being 325 mg.

Monoamine Oxidase Inhibitors (MAOIs)

A placebo-controlled trial of fluoxetine and phenelzine for OCD provides no evidence to support the use of phenelzine in OCD except possibly for patients with symmetry-related or other atypical obsessions. An earlier controlled, comparative study of CMI and clorgyline, a reversible MAO-A inhibitor, also failed to show any beneficial effect of MAOIs. Only one small, controlled study, which compared phenelzine and CMI (without placebo) suggests that they are similar. Doses of phenelzine up to 90 mg/day should be used for at least 10 weeks.

As some OCD patients may be hypersensitive to the activation of their serotonergic systems, specific attention should be paid, on the one hand, to the dangerous combination of SSRIs and MAOIs, and, on the other hand, to the longer wash-out periods for serotonergic medication needed by OCD patients before initiating MAO treatment. Hence the wash-out period needed for discontinuation of CMI and other SSRIs having a relatively short half-life (such as fluvoxamine and sertraline) for OCD patients should be at least four weeks, whereas with fluoxetine it should be even longer (at least six weeks).

Last-line Therapies

The evidence accumulated so far with regard to Electroconvulsive Therapy (ECT) is not compelling, and altogether, it seems that the pure anti-obsessional effect of ECT is questionable. ECT should probably be reserved for the symptomatic (antidepressive) treatment of severely depressed and suicidal OCD patients.

Neurosurgery has been reported to be effective in some OCD patients, with procedures that disconnect the outflow pathways originating from the orbitofrontal cortex. Cingulotomy can help some intractable patients, but while immediate results may be striking, the long-term prognosis is more reserved (Jenike et al., 1991).

A treatment algorithm for resistant OCD is presented in Figure 9.1.

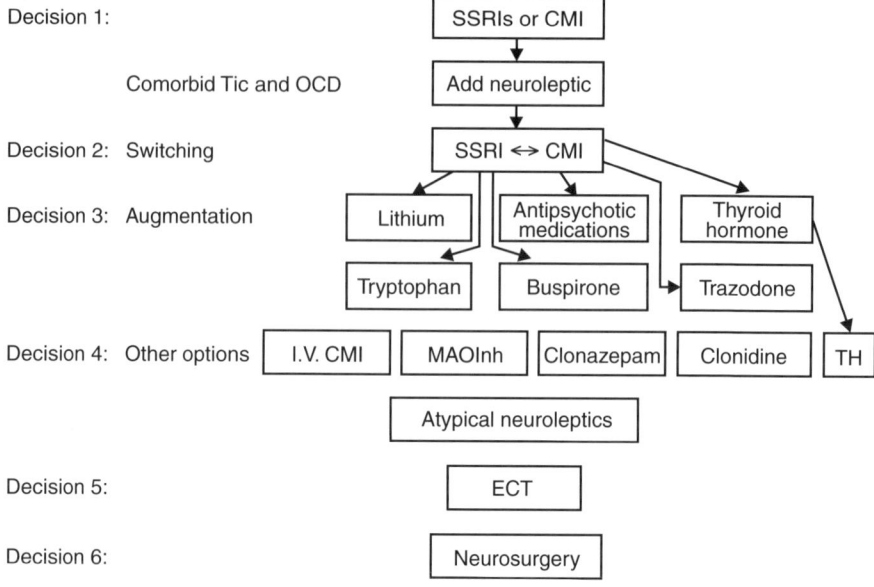

FIGURE 9.1   Treatment decisions for resistant OCD

Review of Treatments in OCD

The first-line treatment consists of either an SSRI or a CMI. One of the five SSRIs provides an effective and safe option. The choice of a particular SSRI depends on the drug's pharmacokinetic profile, as well as on the physician's acquaintance with the drug. The dose should be higher than in depression (40–60 mg fluoxetine, for example) and the trial should last at least 12 weeks. In choosing CMI, cardiovascular problems and closed angle glaucoma should first be ruled out. Doses of 200–300 mg of CMI are needed. Titration should last for 1–3 weeks and this dose should be continued for at least 12 weeks before determining response.

If the patient cannot tolerate the first drug (i.e. SSRI) or did not respond, a trial of a drug from the other group is advised (CMI and vice versa). If the first line was a SSRI, CMI should be administered. The third stage in non-responders and in cases of partial response, includes small doses of antipsychotics (especially in TS), a combination of SRIs and CMI, the addition of lithium or trazodone, buspirone or tryptophan. The fourth stage consists of either atypical neuroleptics, thyroid supplementation, clonidine, MAOIs, I.V. CMI, or clonazepam. In resistant cases, ECT or neurosurgery should be tried.

CONCLUSION

Until 20 years ago, the approach to treating OCD was characterized by pessimism.

Since then, effective treatments have been developed, using BT and the SRIs. Although introduced for OCD in 1967, it was only in the 1980s that double-blind studies confirmed the efficacy of CMI, an SRI. This was followed by the further introduction of the SSRIs, which also proved effective for OCD. The antiobsessive activity of these drugs was found to be independent from the drug's antidepressant effect, as established by efficacy in both depressed and non-depressed patients.

Overall, serotonergic therapies have enabled a better outlook for these patients and have enlarged our understanding of the pathophysiology of OCD (Zohar and Insel, 1987; Dolberg et al., 1996). Previously thought to be a rare and untreatable disorder, OCD is now recognized as common, and there is now good reason to expect that OCD patients will benefit substantially from behavior therapy and potent SRIs. Many OCD patients do not seek treatment and the illness tends to be chronic. There is a 10-year lag between the onset of symptoms and the seeking of professional help, due to feelings of embarrassment. Further delay is often the case until correct diagnosis and treatment are obtained (Hollander, 1997). US census data suggest that over 8 billion dollars are spent each year on the management of OCD, one-fifth of that spent on cardiac disease (DuPont et al., 1995). Because OCD patients often attempt to conceal their symptoms, it is incumbent upon clinicians to screen for OCD in every mental status examination, since appropriate treatment can result in improved quality of life, in reduced OCD chronicity and in reduced costs to the individual and society.

REFERENCES

Bastani B, Nash JF, Meltzer HY (1990) Prolactin and cortisol responses to MK-212, a serotonin agonist, in obsessive-compulsive disorder. *Arch Gen Psychiat* 47: 833–839.

Baxter LR Jr, Schwartz JM, Bergman KS, et al (1992) Caudate glucose metabolic rate changes with both drug and behavior therapy for OCD. *Arch Gen Psychiat* 49: 681–689.

Benkelfat C, Murphy DL, Zohar J et al. (1989) Clomipramine in obsessive compulsive disorder: Further evidence for a serotonergic mechanism of action. *Arch Gen Psychiat* 46: 23–28.

Berman I, Sapers BL, Chang HHJ, Losonczy MF, Schmilder Z, Green AI (1995) Treatment of obsessive-compulsive symptoms in schizophrenic patients with clomipramine. *J Clin Psychopharmacol* 15: 206–210.

Billet EA, Richter MA, King N et al (1997) Obsessive compulsive disorder, response to serotonin reuptake inhibitors and the serotonin transporter gene. *Molecul Psychiat* 2: 403–406.

Bisserbe JC, Lane RM, Flament MF et al. (1997) A double-blind comparison of sertraline and clomipramine in outpatients with obsessive-compulsive disorder. *Eur Psychiat* 153: 1450–1454.

Charney DS, Goodman WK, Price LH et al. (1988) Serotonin function in obsessive-compulsive disorder: A comparison of the effects of tryptophan and m-chlorophenylpyperazine in patients and healthy subjects. *Arch Gen Psychiat* 45: 177–185.

Cox BJ, Swinson RP, Morrison B et al. (1993) Clomipramine, fluoxetine, and behavior therapy in the treatment of OCD: A meta-analysis. *J Behav Ther Exp Psychiat* 24: 149–153.

Clomipramine Collaborative Study Group (1991) Clomipramine in the treatment of patients with obsessive-compulsive disorder. *Arch Gen Psychiat* **48**: 730–738.

Dannon PN, Sasson Y, Hirschmann S, Iancu I, Grunhars LJ, Zohar J (2000) Pindolol augmentation in treatment-resistant obsessive-compulsive disorder: a double-blind placebo controlled trial. *Eur Neuropsychopharmacol* **10**: 165–169.

Dolberg OT, Iancu I, Sasson Y et al. (1996) The pathogenesis and treatment of Obsessive-Compulsive Disorder. *Clin Neuropharm* **19**: 129–147.

DuPont RL, Rice DP, Shiraki S et al. (1995) Economic costs of obsessive compulsive disorder. *Medical Interface*. April, 102–109.

Fernandez-Cordoba E, Lopez-Ibor AJ (1967) La monoclorimipramina en enfermos psiquiatricos resistenses a otros tratamientos. *Actas Luso Esp Neurol Psiquiatr* **26**: 119–147.

Flament MF, Rapoport JL, Murphy DL et al. (1987) Biochemical changes during clomipramine treatment of childhood obsessive-compulsive disorder. *Arch Gen Psychiat* **44**: 219–225.

Flament MF, Whitaker A, Rapoport JL et al. (1988) Obsessive compulsive disorder in adolescence: An epidemiological study. *J Am Acad Child Adolesc Psychiat* **27**: 764–771.

Freeman CPL, Trimble MR, Deakin JFW et al. (1994) Fluvoxamine versus clomipramine in the treatment of obsessive compulsive disorder: A multi-center, randomized, double-blind, parallel group comparison. *J Clin Psychiat* **55**: 301–305.

Galderisi S, Mucci A, Catapano F (1995) Neuropsychological slowness in obsessive-compulsive patients: Is it confined to tests involving the fronto-subcortical systems? *Br J Psychiat* **167**: 394–398.

Goodman WK, McDougle CJ, Barr LC et al. (1993) Biological approaches to treatment-resistant obsessive compulsive disorder. *J Clin Psych* **54**: 16–26.

Goodman WK, Price LH, Delgado PL et al. (1990) Specificity of serotonin reuptake inhibitors in the treatment of obsessive compulsive disorder: Comparison of fluvoxamine and desipramine. *Arch Gen Psychiat* **47**: 577–585.

Greist JH (1996) New developments in behavior therapy for obsessive-compulsive disorder. *Int Clin Psychopharmacol* **11** Suppl 5: 63–73.

Hollander E (1997) Obsessive compulsive disorder: The hidden epidemic. *J Clin Psychiat* Suppl **12**: 3–6.

Hollander E, DeCaria CM, Nitescu A et al. (1992) Serotonergic function in obsessive-compulsive disorder: Behavioral and neuroendocrine responses to oral m-chlorphenyl-pyperazine and fenfluramine in patients and healthy volunteers. *Arch Gen Psychiat* **49**: 21–28.

Hollander E, Prohovnik I, Stein DJ (1995) Increased cerebral blood flow during m-CPP exacerbation of obsessive-compulsive disorder. *J Neuropsychiatry* **7**: 485–490.

Insel TR, Gillin JC, Moore A, Mendelson WB, Lowenstein RJ, Murphy DL (1982a) The sleep of patients with OCD. *Arch Gen Psychiat* **39**: 1372–1377.

Insel TR, Kalin NH, Guttmacher LB, Cohen RM, Murphy DL (1982b) The dexamethasone suppression test in patients with primary OCD. *Psychiat Res* **6**: 153–158.

Insel TR, Mueller EA, Alterman I et al. (1985) Obsessive compulsive disorder and serotonin: Is there a connection? *Biol Psychiat* **20**: 1174–1188.

Jenike MA, Baer L, Ballantine T et al. (1991) Cingulotomy for refractory obsessive-compulsive disorder. *Arch Gen Psychiat* **48**: 548–555.

Karno M, Golding JM, Sorenson SB et al. (1988) The epidemiology of obsessive-compulsive disorder in five US communities. *Arch Gen Psychiat* **45**: 1094–1099.

Kim SW, Dysken MW, Pandey GN et al. (1991) Platelet 3H-imipramine binding sites in obsessive compulsive behavior. *Biol Psychiat* **30**: 467–474.

Leckman JF, Grice DE, Boardman J et al. (1997) Symptoms of OCD. *Am J Psychiat* **154**: 911–917.

Lenane MC, Swedo SE, Leonard H et al (1990) Psychiatric disorders in first degree relatives of children and adolescents with obsessive-compulsive disorder. *J Am Acad Child Adolesc Psychiat* **29**: 407–412.

Leonard H, Swedo SE, Lenane MC et al. (1991) A double-blind desipramine substitution during long-term clomipramine treatment in children and adolescents with obsessive-compulsive disorder. *Arch Gen Psychiat* **48**: 922–927.

Lesch KP, Hoh A, Disselkamp-Tietze J et al. (1991) 5-Hydroxytryptamine 1A receptor responsivity in obsessive compulsive disorder: Comparison of patients and controls. *Arch Gen Psychiat* **48**: 540–547.

Lindsay M, Craig R, Andrews G (1997) Controlled trial of exposure and response prevention in obsessive-compulsive disorder. *Br J Psychiat* **171**: 135–139.

Lucey JV, Costa DC, Adshead G, Deahl M, Busatto G, Gacinovic S et al. (1997) Brain blood flow in anxiety disorders: OCD, panic disorder with agoraphobia, and post-traumatic stress disorder on 99m TcHMPAO single photon emission tomography (SPET). *Br J Psychiatry* **171**: 346–350.

Marazziti D, Hollander E, Lensi P et al. (1992) Peripheral markers of serotonin and dopamine function in obsessive-compulsive disorder. *Psychiatr Res* **42**: 41–51.

Marazziti D, Pfanner C, Palego L et al. (1997) Changes in platelet markers of obsessive compulsive patients during a double-blind trial of fluvoxamine versus clomipramine. *Pharmacopsychiatry* **30**: 245–249.

Marks IM, Hodgson R, Rachman S et al. (1975) Treatment of chronic obsessive-compulsive neurosis in vivo exposure: A 2-year follow-up and issues in treatment. *Br J Psychiat* **127**: 349–364.

McDougle J, Goodman WK, Price LH et al. (1990) Neuroleptic addition in fluvoxamine-refractory obsessive-compulsive disorder. *Am J Psychiat* **147**: 652–654.

McDougle JC, Goodman WK, Price LH (1997) Dopamine antagonists in tic-related and psychotic spectrum obsessive-compulsive disorder. *J Clin Psychiat* **55** Suppl 3: 24–31.

Mundo E, Barregi SR, Pirola R et al. (1997) Long-term pharmacotherapy of obsessive-compulsive disorder: A double-blind controlled study. *J Clin Psychopharmacol* **17**: 4–10.

Nelson E, Rice J (1997) Stability of diagnosis of obsessive compulsive disorder in the epidemiologic catchment area study. *Am J Psychiat* **154**: 826–831.

Pato MT, Zohar-Kadouch R, Zohar J et al. (1988) Return of symptoms after discontinuation of clomipramine in patients with obsessive compulsive disorder. *Am J Psychiat* **145**: 1521–1525.

Pauls D (1992) The genetics of OCD and Gilles de la Tourette's syndrome. *Psychiatr Clin North Am* **15**: 759–766.

Pigott TA, Pato MT, Bernstein SE et al. (1990) Controlled comparisons of clomipramine and fluoxetine in the treatment of obsessive-compulsive disorder: Behavioral and biological results. *Arch Gen Psychiat* **47**: 926–932.

Pigott TA, Zohar J, Hill JL et al. (1991) Metergoline blocks behavioral and neuroendocrine effects of orally administered mCPP in patients with obsessive-compulsive disorder. *Biol Psychiatry* **29**: 418–426.

Rasmussen SA, Eisen JL (1992) Epidemiology and clinical features of obsessive-compulsive disorder. In Jenike MA, Baer L, Minichiello WE (eds) *Obsessive Compulsive Disorders: Theory and Management*. Chicago: Year Book Medical Publishers, pp. 10–27.

Rasmussen SA, Eisen JL, Pato MT (1993) Current issues in the pharmacological management of obsessive-compulsive disorder. *J Clin Psychiat* **54**: 4s–9s.

Rasmussen SA, Tsuang MT (1986) Clinical characteristics and family history in DSM-III obsessive-compulsive disorder. *Am J Psychiat* **143**: 317–322.

Rauch SL (1998) Neuroimaging in OCD: clinical implications. CNS Spectrums **3** Suppl 1: 26–29.

Rauch SL, Jenike MA, Alpert NM, Baer L, Breiter HCR, Savage CR et al. (1994) Regional cerebral blood flow measured during symptom provocation in obsessive-compulsive disorder using oxygen 15-labeled carbon dioxide and positron emission tomography. *Arch Gen Psychiatry* **51**: 62–70.

Renynghe de Voxrie GV (1968) Anafranil (G34586) in obsessive compulsive neurosis. *Arch Neurol Belg* **68**: 787–792.

Robins LN, Helzer JE, Weissman MM et al. (1984) Lifetime prevalence of specific psychiatric disorders in three sites. *Arch Gen Psychiat* **41**: 949–958.

Roy BF, Benkelphat C, Hill JL et al. (1994) Serum antibody for somatostatin: 14 and prodynorphin 209–240 in patients with obsessive compulsive disorder, schizophrenia, Alzheimer's disease, multiple sclerosis and advanced HIV infection. *Biol Psychiat* **35**: 335–344.

Salzman L, Thaler FH (1981) Obsessive compulsive disorder: A review of the literature. *Am J Psychiat* **138**: 286–296.

Sasson Y, Zohar J (1996) New developments in obsessive-compulsive disorder research: Implications for clinical management. *Int Clin Psychopharmacol* **11** Suppl 5: 3–12.

Schwartz JM, Stoessel PW, Baxter LR Jr et al. (1996) Systematic changes in cerebral glucose metabolic rate after successful behavior modification treatment of OCD. *Arch Gen Psychiat* **53**: 109–113.

Stein MB, Forde DR, Anderson G, Walker JR (1997) Obsessive compulsive disorder in the community: An epidemiologic survey with clinical reappraisal. *Am J Psychiat* **154**: 1120–1126.

Stern L, Zohar J (1998) The potential role of 5-HT1d receptors in the pathophysiology and treatment of obsessive compulsive disorder. *CNS Spectrums* **3**(8): 46–49.

Swedo SE, Leonard HL, Kiessling LS (1994) Speculations on antineuronal antibody-mediated neuropsychiatric disorders of childhood. *Pediatrics* **93**: 323–326.

Swedo SE, Leonard HL, Mittelman BB et al. (1997) Identification of children with pediatric autoimmune neuropsychiatric disorders associated with streptococcal infections by a marker associated with rheumatic fever. *Am J Psychiat* **154**: 110–112.

Thoren P, Asberg M, Gronholm B et al. (1980) Clomipramine treatment of obsessive compulsive disorder. II. Biochemical aspects. *Arch Gen Psychiat* **27**: 1289–1294.

Towey JP, Tenke CE, Bruder GE et al (1994) Brain event-related potential correlates of over focused attention in obsessive-compulsive disorder. *Psychophysiology* **31**: 535–543.

Van Balkom AJLM, De Haan E, Van Oppen P, Spinhoven P, Hoogduin KAL, Van Dyck R (1998) Cognitive and behavioral therapies alone versus in combination with fluvoxamine in the treatment of Obsessive Compulsive Disorder. *J Nerv Ment Dis* **186**: 492–499.

Vitiello B, Shimon H, Behar D et al. (1991) Platelet imipramine binding and serotonin uptake in obsessive-compulsive patients. *Acta Psychiat Scand* **84**: 29–32.

Weissman MM, Bland RC, Canino GJ et al. (1994) The cross national epidemiology of obsessive compulsive disorder. *J Clin Psychiat* **55** Suppl 3: 5–10.

Weizman A, Carmi M, Hermesh H et al. (1986) High affinity imipramine binding and serotonin uptake in platelets of eight adolescent and ten adult obsessive-compulsive patients. *Am J Psychiat* **143**: 335–339.

Zohar J, Insel T (1987) Obsessive-compulsive disorder: Psychobiological approaches to diagnosis, treatment, and pathophysiology. *Biol Psychiat* **22**: 667–687.

Zohar J, Insel TR, Berman KF, Foa EB, Hill JL et al. (1989) Anxiety and cerebral blood flow during behavioral challenge. *Arch Gen Psychiatry* **46**: 505–510.

Zohar J, Judge R (1996) Paroxetine versus clomipramine in the treatment of obsessive-compulsive disorder. *Br J Psychiat* **169**: 468–474.

10

Generalised Anxiety Disorder

N. Caycedo and E.J.L. Griez

Barcelona, Spain and Maastricht University, Maastricht, The Netherlands

INTRODUCTION: ABOUT A DISPUTED CONCEPT

In 1896, Kraepelin classified the psychiatric disorders into 13 categories. One of them, the "psychogenic neurosis" was the first attempt to classify anxiety disorders. However, common opinion regarded anxiety as an aspecific phenomenon, a mere symptom that was present in a variety of disorders rather than the expression of a disease in itself. The Freudian concept of "anxiety neurosis" may represent the first attempt to consider severe and chronic anxiety as a true medical condition deserving the status of an independent nosologic entity. Later, a distinction was introduced between "anxiety neurosis" and "hysteric anxiety". The first edition of the *Diagnostic and Statistical Manual of Mental Disorders* (DSM-I) in the early 1950s adopted a large part of the Freudian view. Anxiety disorders were classified under "anxious reaction", which concept referred to Freud's anxiety neurosis, and "phobic reaction", which referred to the hysteric neurosis. In 1968, the DSM-II introduced some modifications into the neurosis concept, but remained under the influence of the psychoanalytic system. "Neuroses" were divided into anxiety neurosis, hysteric neurosis, phobic neurosis, obsessive-compulsive neurosis, depressive neurosis, hypochondriac neurosis, neurasthenic neurosis and depersonalisation neurosis (APA, 1968).

Traditional doctrines about pathological anxiety were challenged in the early 1960s, when the first effective psychotropics became available. Klein first noticed that patients with the so-called "anxiety neurosis" appeared to respond in two different ways to treatment with the new psychotropics (Klein, 1964). Indeed, while the first benzodiazepines had proven remarkably effective for anxiety, some patients with "anxiety neurosis" failed to improve with the new anxiolytics. Paradoxically, those patients benefited from imipramine, which had just been introduced as an antidepressant. Klein observed that the patients who failed to benefit from benzodiazepines, but improved with imipramine, were those who reported to have frequent bursts of paroxysmal anxiety, in addition to a chronic background. It appeared that imipramine was able to block their repetitive "attacks" that represented their worse symptoms. In contrast, subjects who did benefit from benzodiazepines failed to report

Anxiety Disorders: An Introduction to Clinical Management and Research. Edited by E.J.L. Griez, C. Faravelli, D. Nutt and J. Zohar. © 2001 John Wiley & Sons, Ltd.

this type of paroxysmal anxiety. Accordingly, Klein proposed a new subdivision in Freud's anxiety neurosis. He coined the vocal "panic" for the bursts of acute anxiety, and introduced the terms of panic attacks (PA) and panic disorder (PD). Based on the different pharmacosensitivity, panic attacks should be considered a separate type of anxiety, qualitatively different from chronic, generalised anxiety. Anxiety neurosis was to be divided into two different disorders. In 1975, the Research Diagnostic Criteria (RDC) started with a new classification system, which formed the precursor of the current DSM classification. Under the influence of Klein's hypothesis, the RDC mentioned for the first time general anxiety disorders (GAD) as a separate entity. Consequently, when the DSM-III (APA, 1980) was published, the subcategory of anxiety neurosis was changed into "anxiety states" and included panic disorder (PD), generalised anxiety disorder (GAD) and obsessive-compulsive disorder (OCD), contrasting with "phobic states", which included simple and social phobia. GAD was defined as a generalised and persistent feeling of anxiety. Persistent was operationalised as complaints of at least one month's duration. The symptoms were divided into four categories, including autonomic hyperactivity, motor tension, apprehensive expectation and vigilance/scanning (APA, 1980). To qualify for the diagnosis, a patient should suffer at least from symptoms out of three of four categories. The GAD diagnosis excluded those patients with criteria for any other axis I mental disorder. However, it was obvious that nearly all patients with a primary diagnosis of an anxiety disorder, except simple phobia, do show symptoms mentioned under the category of GAD. Actually, GAD was to be considered as a residual category among the anxiety disorders.

Nevertheless, some clinical studies indicated that various patients were suffering from GAD regardless of their primary diagnosis. For instance, some patients successfully treated for another anxiety disorder still reported feelings of discomfort, fitting into the category of generalised anxiety (Sanderson and Barlow, 1990). These findings led to a new definition of GAD in DSM III-R (APA, 1987). GAD was to be defined as a primary diagnostic category rather than a residual disorder. It was considered that GAD may be diagnosed when other axis I disorders are present. The new definition assigned a central place to the criteria of "apprehensive expectation", and "worry", as the main characteristic of this disorder. Pathological worrying was operationalised as excessive and/or unrealistic and not circumscribed to one single life circumstance (worry about finances, work, family). In addition, the worries should not be caused by the presence of other mental disorders like the worry about panic attacks in the case of a PD, or about public speaking in the case of social phobia (Barlow et al., 1986). The DSM III-R also revised the somatic symptom criteria. The patient should present with at least six from a list of 18 symptoms, which are divided in three categories: motor tension, autonomic hyperreactivity and vigilance/scanning. The criterion of duration of complaints was extended to at least six months. The exclusion criteria were limited to a current affective disorder or psychotic disorder (Sanderson and Barlow, 1990).

The DSM-IV (APA, 1994) also considers GAD as an independent diagnostic category. It increases the emphasis on "the uncontrollable worry": worry must be excessive (that is, the intensity, duration, and frequency of the worry are out of proportion to the likelihood or impact of the feared event), pervasive (that is, worry occurs about a number of events or activities on more days than not for at least six months), and uncontrollable (that is, the person finds it difficult to control the worry) (APA, 1994). In addition, whereas the associated symptom criterion for DSM-III-R consisted of 18 symptoms grouped into three clusters (motor tension, vigilance and scanning, and autonomic hyperactivity), this criterion has retained only six symptoms in DSM-IV. All symptoms of autonomic hyperactivity have been eliminated (Brown, 1997).

Thus, the diagnosis of GAD has been controversial since its inception (see Figure 10.1). In particular, its right to exist as an independent entity is widely discussed, due to its high comorbidity rates that are repeatedly found in most surveys. GAD has been considered as a prodromal or residual state of other psychiatric disorders. While it is behind any doubt that a generalised anxiety does exist at a symptomatically or syndromal level, the question is still open whether it should be considered as a disease on itself. The main objective of this chapter is to review the current knowledge about GAD, its prevalence, its morbidity and its correlates, in an attempt to clarify some difficulties concerning its current status as an independent nosologic entity.

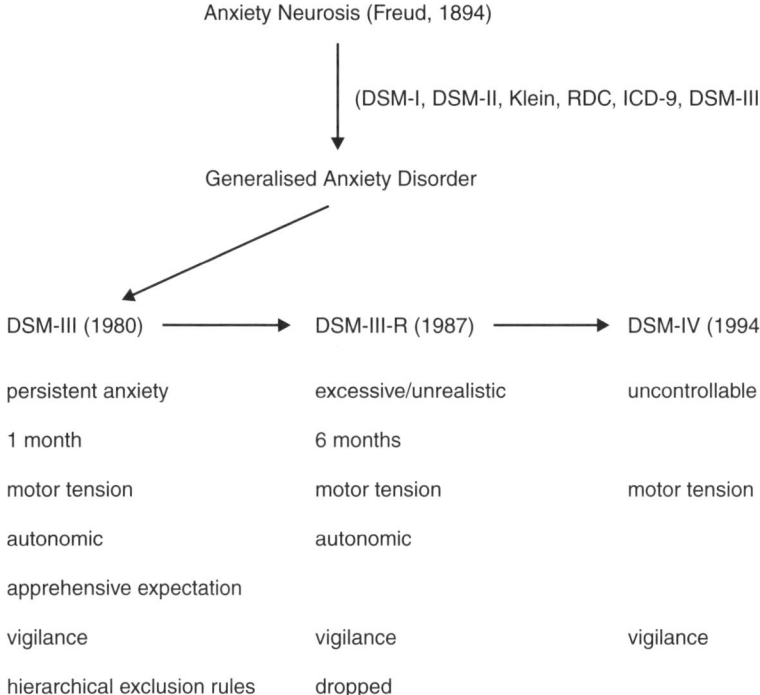

FIGURE 10.1   Changing diagnostic criteria for GAD
Source: Modified by permission of Brawman-Mintzer and Lydiard (1996).

PREVALENCE

Before GAD was given the status of a separate nosological entity in the DSM-III, the overall estimation of the prevalence of anxiety neurosis varied widely. One study gave an estimation of 2.9%, but this study of course, like all others, did not distinguish between panic and GAD (Blazer et al., 1991). Owing to the above reviewed continuing changes in the diagnostic criteria for GAD, the prevalence rates of this disorder have varied accordingly. In fact, DSM-III-R rates are different from the International Classification of Diseases (ICD-10) rates, or even the Research Diagnostic Criteria (RDC) rates. The National Comorbidity Survey of psychiatric disorders (NCS) performed an epidemiological study in the USA about the prevalence of GAD, according to the diagnostic criteria of DSM-III-R. In a representative national sample of 8098 individuals, the prevalence rates were 1.6% for current GAD (defined as the most recent six-month period of anxiety), 3.1% for 12-month period of GAD and 5.1% for lifetime GAD (Wittchen et al., 1994). These rates are definitely higher than rates of panic disorders (Brawman-Mintzer and Lydiard, 1997). These data agree with the Epidemiological Catchment Area Study (ECA). This study reported a 12-month GAD prevalence of 3% and lifetime prevalence of 4–6% (Blazer et al., 1991). According to Anderson et al. (1987), the 12-months prevalence rates of overanxious anxiety disorder (the GAD equivalent for children) are 2.9%. On the other hand, the elderly showed GAD prevalence rates higher than any other anxiety disorder, varying from 0.7% to 7.1% (Flint, 1994).

In primary care centres, the GAD prevalence is approximate. This implies that GAD is the most frequently diagnosed anxiety disorder in primary care centres. Noteworthy in these centres is that the GAD diagnosis is often unrecognised (Barrett et al., 1988). In addition, most GAD diagnoses are in primary care associated with a high rate of psychiatric comorbidity. Contrasting herewith, in mental health centres, the GAD prevalence is one of the lowest compared with other anxiety disorders (Barlow, 1988). Thus, it appears that the bulk of subjects meeting the criteria for a GAD diagnosis are confined to the primary care setting, where GAD should be a very common condition, even though GAD is underdiagnosed. One of the consequences of this situation is the relatively small number of good studies on GAD. Apparently, as a rule, patients with GAD complaints do not seek treatment in specialised care setting. According to Noyes et al. (1987), only 10% of the patients with anxiety disorders who are treated by psychiatrists, have a diagnosis of GAD. Nevertheless, in spite of the changing diagnostic criteria, and in spite of being an underdiagnosed condition, the available data strongly suggest that GAD is one of the most common anxiety disorders. Patients with GAD more often visit primary care centres than mental health centres. In primary care centres, the diagnosis is frequently either incomplete or overlooked at all, probably as a result of the high comorbidity rate with other psychiatric disorders.

COURSE

GAD is a disorder characterised by extreme anxiety and worry. Its age of onset is between the late teens and early twenties. In most studies, the average duration of GAD was 20 years, suggesting a chronic course. Stress seems to play an important role in GAD onset (Barlow et al., 1986). There have been studies showing genetic factors to predispose to its onset (Kendler et al., 1992). GAD can be divided in two subgroups. The early-onset subgroup usually suffers with subclinical anxiety symptoms. These patients have always been anxious, withdrawn, socially sensitive and maladjusted worriers. The late-onset subgroup shows a better social adjustment; unfavourable events provoke the onset of the disorder. However, although the circumstances of onset are different, once the condition has developed, the symptomatology is largely similar in both groups (Hoehn-Saric et al., 1993). This stresses the significance of longitudinal studies to complement cross-sectional studies in analysing the course of the disorder.

The Epidemiologic Catchment Area Study (ECA) found a higher GAD prevalence (DSM-III diagnosis) in women, in persons under 30 years old and in the black population. The prevalence of lifetime GAD was higher in urban areas and in low-income brackets. This study could not find a clear relationship with the level of education (Blazer et al.,1991). Risk factors were also assessed in the National Comorbidity Survey. Like the ECA study, GAD prevalence in women was higher (twice as common as among men). On the contrary, the GAD prevalence in young persons was lower. In persons older than 24 years, being separated, divorced, widowed, unemployed and a homemaker were significant correlates of GAD. Most GAD patients reported a high interference with their lives (49%). Some 66% sought professional help, and 44% had received medical treatment. Approximately half of the GAD patients went to the primary care sector. In contrast, GAD subjects who had comorbid psychiatric disorders sought help in mental health centres. The presence of a more "differentiated mental disorder" being correlated to specialised care has been repeatedly mentioned in other studies (Brawman-Mintzer and Lydiard, 1996). According to a study carried out by Massion et al. (1993), one-third of GAD patients are single, and 1701, of them are separated, widowed or divorced. GAD patients have been found underemployed, while 37% receive public assistance. GAD patients demonstrate difficulties at work, have social adjustment problems, and show a low self-satisfaction with their lives.

Yonkers et al. (1996) found a low GAD remission rate of 0.15 after one year. These data are consistent with Noyes et al. (1980) and Kendler et al. (1992). According to Yonkers, the complete remission rate after two years was 0.25. Most patients' symptoms stood at a stable level. In the rare patients with complete remission, relapse risk was 0.07 after six months and 0.15 one year later. Relapse risk was higher for those patients with partial remission and for those patients who showed comorbidity with other anxiety or depressive disorders. In spite of a complete GAD remission, approximately half of them showed symptoms related to a comorbid psychiatric disorder.

Summarising, GAD is a common and chronic disorder, which frequently leads to significant distress and serious functional impairment. It specially affects women. GAD patients generally visit primary care centres and are in need of medical treatment.

COMORBIDITY

GAD displays high psychiatric comorbidity, mainly with other anxiety and mood disorders. This fact complicates the diagnostic process, its treatment, as well as its prognosis (Kessler et al., 1998). Yonkers et al. (1996) carried out a clinical study with patients from 11 Boston area hospitals. All patients suffered from an anxiety disorder. Within a period of six months before their inclusion, they had not been diagnosed with other types of psychiatric pathology (organic mental disorder, schizophrenia or psychosis). The authors analysed 164 patients with a current diagnosis of GAD; 87% showed a lifetime history of another anxiety disorder and 83% had some other kind of current anxiety disorder. These data agree with a study performed by Brawman-Mintzer et al. (1993). Among the anxiety disorders, panic disorder with agoraphobia (PDA) and social phobia showed the highest GAD comorbidity. As far as mood disorders are concerned, one-third of these GAD patients were suffering with a major depression. Figure 10.2 illustrates another review performed by Brawman-Mintzer and Lydiard. The highest comorbidity rates among anxiety disorders in GAD patients were found to be social phobia (16–59%), simple phobia (21–55%), panic disorder (3–27%) and major depression (8–39%) (Brawman-Mintzer and Lydiard, 1996). The high comorbidity with simple phobia agrees with the results of the study by Noyes et al. published in 1992.

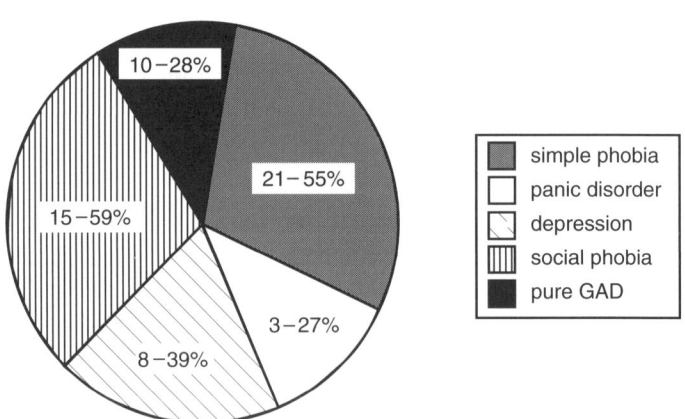

FIGURE 10.2   Psychiatric comorbidity in GAD
Source: Reproduced by permission of Brawman-Mintzer and Lydiard, 1996; (based on data from Sanderson and Barlow, 1990; Angst, 1993).

It might be possible that these high comorbidity rates are a consequence of the study design, since patients sampled for these studies proceeded from clinical cohorts. Large epidemiological surveys have shed some light on the problem of comorbidity in GAD. The ECA study (Blazer et al., 1991) found that between 58% and 65% of subjects who have ever suffered from GAD, also have at least one other disorder. GAD had a very large comorbidity with panic disorder and major depression. In the Zurich study, Angst found a strong association between GAD and major depression, dysthymia, hypomania and panic disorder (Angst, 1993). The National Comorbidity Survey (Wittchen et al., 1994) found that major depression and dysthymia had the highest GAD comorbidity rates followed by alcoholism, phobia, drug abuse and panic disorder. This study shows that 89.9% of subjects with a lifetime diagnosis of GAD had at least one other lifetime psychiatric disorder, whereas 65% of those with a current diagnosis of GAD had another comorbid disorder. On the other hand, 33% of those patients did not show any other recent or present psychiatric diagnosis. Overall, the vast majority of the above-mentioned studies show a strong association between GAD and other anxiety and affective disorders, especially panic disorder, social phobia, major depression and other mood disorders.

IS GAD AN INDEPENDENT NOSOLOGIC ENTITY?

In the light of the above, the validity of GAD as a separate entity has been widely discussed (Breslau and Davis, 1985). The symptomatic profile of GAD fails to make a sharp distinction with other anxiety disorders, especially panic disorders (PD). GAD has been considered as a mild expression of PD. Alternatively, GAD has been said to represent a residual phase of chronic depression, or even a variant of an anxious personality disorder (Nisita et al., 1990). Uhde and co-workers found that, in people who develop PD, generalised anxiety symptoms may appear before the first panic attacks or continue after resolution of these panic attacks (Uhde et al., 1985). Adding to the unsatisfactory delineation of GAD at a cross-sectional level, such findings warrant a closer look at a number of studies on the validity of GAD as an independent disorder. We will briefly report on a number of family, clinical and challenge studies that tried to compare GAD with PD, after a careful exclusion of any lifetime history of PD in the analysed GAD population.

Family Studies

Most family and twin studies suggest a clear difference between PD and GAD. Genetic factors are more significant in PD. In GAD, the environmental factors seem to play a dominant role. Cloninger et al. (1981) found that a relatively high percentage of relatives of PD patients suffered from panic attacks. The relatives of patients suffering from another anxious disorders did not show panic attacks. Crowe et al. (1983) compared the prevalence of panic attacks in PD patients' families and in control families. They found a higher prevalence of panic attacks in PD patients' families than in control families. A twin study carried out by Torgensen (1983), using DSM-III criteria, showed that PD rate was higher in monozygotic than in dizygotic twins. No relationship was found with GAD in any of the monozygotic twins suffering from PD. Thus, PD seems to be influenced by hereditary factors. GAD did not seem to be influenced by these factors. This study also strongly suggests that GAD could be related to life events during early childhood. Noyes et al. (1987) showed that the frequency of GAD was higher among first-degree relatives of probands with GAD than among the relatives of control subjects, but it was not higher among relatives of probands with PD. On the other hand, the frequency of PD was higher among relatives of probands with panic disorder than among control relatives, and was not higher among relatives of GAD probands (see Table 10.1).

In another study, Noyes et al. (1992) compared GAD patients with PD patients. The GAD patients had more often positive family histories of GAD than PD patients. On the other hand, PD patients had more often positive family histories of PD than subjects with GAD (Table 10.2). The authors concluded that GAD patients were different from PD patients.

In general, the family studies support a distinction between GAD and PD. Strong arguments do exist to isolate a diathesis leading to the development of PD. However, in the case of GAD, the result seems to stress the importance of environmental factors.

Clinical Studies

In general, the published clinical studies to support distinguishing between GAD and PD reveal that patients with GAD show often less autonomic and less severe symptoms. Hoehn-Saric observed that GAD patients had less somatic symptoms

TABLE 10.1 Frequency of GAD and PD in first-degree relatives of GAD (N = 20) and PD (N = 20)

	GAD	PD
1st degree relatives of GAD	19.5%	4.1%
1st degree relatives of PD	5.4%	14.9%

Source: Reproduced from data by permission of Noyes et al., 1987.

TABLE 10.2 Frequency of positive family histories in subjects with GAD (N = 41) and subjects with PD (N = 71)

	+ GAD	+ PD
GAD subjects	41.5%	9.8%
PD subjects	18.6%	45.7%

Source: Reproduced from data by permission of Noyes et al., 1992.

than PD patients, and PD patients showed more cardiovascular symptomatology (Hoehn-Saric, 1982; Hoehn-Saric et al., 1989). Anderson and co-workers compared PD and GAD subjects for symptomatology, age of onset, course, and outcome of illness. GAD patients showed less autonomic symptoms. Compared with PD, the GAD onset was earlier and more gradual. GAD patients displayed a chronic course and better outcome than patients with PD (Anderson et al., 1984). These data agree with other study results (Thyer et al., 1985; Cameron et al., 1986).

Noyes et al. (1992) carried out a study in order to analyse the differences between GAD and PD, and Table 10.3 summarises the outcome. The study included 41 subjects with GAD diagnosis (without panic attacks history), and 71 patients with panic disorder diagnosis. Subjects with psychosis, organic mental history and primary mood disorders history were excluded. The median age of onset in the GAD cohort was 20 years (mean 23.6 years). The PD cohort had a median age of 25 years (mean 26.5 years). Subjects with GAD showed a wider range in age of onset than subjects with PD. In the GAD cohort the median illness duration (252.4 months) was longer than the PD group (134.3 months). The social impairment was higher for GAD patients than for PD patients. The GAD patients consulted psychiatric centres less frequently than PD patients.

Chief complaints reported in the GAD group were: difficulty in sleeping (41.1%), restlessness or inability to relax (39%), muscular tension (34.2%), apprehension (19.5%), worry (19.5%) and irritability (19.5%). In comparison, chief complaints reported in the PD group were: apprehension (31%), rapid or pounding heartbeat (25.4%), fear of dying (23.9%), muscular tension (22.5%), dizziness (19.7%), thoracic pain (15.5%), trembling (15.5%) and dyspnea (12.7%). GAD patients reported more symptoms related to vigilance and scanning (difficulty in sleeping, restlessness or inability to relax, to concentrate, irritability and impatience) than subjects with PD. On the other hand, subjects with PD more frequently reported symptoms of autonomic hyperactivity (rapid or pounding heartbeat, thoracic pain, dyspnea, dizziness or imbalance, numbness, choking) than subjects with GAD.

In a similar study, Nisita et al. (1990) found differences in age, time interval between time of onset until the first medical (specialists) consultation, and associated

TABLE 10.3   PD and GAD: onset and course

	GAD, N = 41	PD, N = 71
Onset	Gradual (95%)	Sudden (1–2/3)
	Early median: 20 years	Late median: 25 years
	Mean: 23.6 years	Mean: 26.5 years
	Large variation	Normal variation
Course	Chronic	Episodic
Duration of illness	252.4**	134.3**
Social impairment	1.4*	1.7*

Source: Reproduced from data by permission of Noyes et al., 1992.
Notes: *P < 0.001.
**P < 0.05.

symptomatology. GAD patients started treatment later than PD patients. These findings support the clinical observation that severe symptomatology of PD patients implies an earlier search for treatment. Life events at onset of the actual disorder were reported more often in GAD (30%) than in PD (10%). According to Nisita et al. (1990), GAD patients have always been anxious subjects. In stress periods, they suffer from more symptomatology than the general population. Because of the fact that their anxious traits form part of their daily life, they do not recognise these symptoms as part of a disorder. Complaints arise in periods of symptomatic exacerbation, which they interpret as the onset of illness. This interpretation agrees with Barlow's opinion. He considers GAD as a chronic apprehensive expectation or a chronic worry (Barlow et al., 1986).

In conclusion of the above-mentioned studies, GAD patients report more hyper-arousal symptoms of the central nervous system, whereas PD subjects report more symptoms of autonomic hyperactivity. The onset of GAD symptoms is earlier and more gradual, and its course is generally chronic. Although the mean onset of symptoms is earlier in GAD patients, their first specialist's consultation is usually later than PD patients. This might be related to the fact that the initial symptomatology of GAD patients minimally interferes with their work and social life.

Challenge Studies

Experimental challenges, such as lactate infusion, CO_2 inhalation and 5-HT de-pletion are believed to trigger specific mechanisms related to particular disorders. The response to a challenge in a group of patients with a specific disorder may be considered as a marker for that disorder. Early small-scale studies have suggested that contrary to PD subjects, patients with GAD are not vulnerable to lactate infusion (Cowley et al., 1988). It has been well established that PD patients taking a breath of 35% CO_2 have both a strong autonomic reaction and a definite, brief increase in anxiety, contrary to normals. A group of patients with GAD was selected after careful exclusion of any lifetime history of PA, and underwent the 35% CO_2 challenge. Unlike normals, GAD patients displayed a strong autonomic reaction, but unlike PDs, they failed to report any increase in anxiety (Verburg et al., 1995). Comparable results discriminating between GAD and PD were recently obtained by Perna and coworkers (1999). These data support the theory that GAD and PD are distinct entities based on different underlying processes. The results may also suggest a disturbed autonomic function in GAD.

Summary

Although the basis of distinguishing GAD from PD might still seem unsatisfactory, most available data suggest two separate entities (Hoehn-Saric and McLeod, 1985; Noyes et al., 1987). Family studies, clinical studies and challenge studies generally support that PD is different from GAD. Both disorders show different rates and risk factors in the community, a different family aggregation (Weissman, 1990; Nisita et al., 1990; Noyes et al., 1992), a different pattern of reaction to lactate and CO_2 challenge, and distinct symptomatologies and clinical courses (see Maser, 1998).

TREATMENT

There is evidence that both pharmacological and non-pharmacological procedures, or a combination of these strategies are effective in the treatment of GAD. The pharmacological treatment of GAD includes benzodiazepines, azapirones and anti-depressants. Among psychotherapy, the cognitive-behavioural therapy has been demonstrated to be effective in GAD treatment (Brawman-Mintzer and Lydiard, 1996). Although in some cases of subsyndromal anxiety one course of therapy might be sufficient, anxiety as a rule has a chronic course and repeat interventions will be required. In general, the treatment of GAD should be thought of as being intermittent. However, in spite of hundreds of controlled studies on the therapy of current GAD, remarkably little is known about long-term drug treatment.

Benzodiazepines (BDZs)

The effectiveness of benzodiazepine in generalised anxiety has been well established. (Rickels et al., 1993). This class of drugs represents the treatment of choice for limited generalised anxiety because of its rapid action and the effective reduction of insomnia and somatic/adrenergic symptoms. The BDZ treatment leads in 65% of the cases to a rapid response within one or two weeks. There is evidence that BDZs may be more effective on some specific symptoms, particularly the somatic symptoms of arousal existing of autonomic dysregulation. There should be somewhat less effect for the cluster of psychic symptoms, which includes apprehensive worry and irritability (Rickels et al., 1982). Several studies have shown that irritability may even worsen in conjunction with high-potency BDZs (Rosenbaum et al., 1984). It is also worth noting that subsyndromal depressive symptoms may predict a less favourable response to BDZs. Psychic symptoms may be more responsive to other drugs such as buspirone or imipramine (Rickels et al., 1993).

Overall, BDZs remain a widely used option for GAD. There is little doubt that this situation is influenced by a wide acceptance of both patients and practitioners, an overall excellent tolerance, and a rapid onset of action. However, there is a relative lack of well-controlled data to support continued benefits of BDZs over the long term in GAD. It has been estimated that approximately 70% of patients with GAD will respond well to adequate BDZ treatment, but within one year 65% will suffer from recurrences of symptomatology (Schweizer and Rickels, 1996). Another complicating factor is the changing concept of GAD. Since its first delineation in the DSM-III, the multiple revisions of the diagnostic criteria show a continued tendency to emphasise

the so-called psychic component to the detriment of the autonomic/somatic symptoms. The growing trend is to consider that the core of GAD lies in its being a
"cognitive" condition, mainly characterised by pathological worry and ruminations.
Now we have noted that BDZs are believed to be relatively less effective on that
component of the disorder, compared with the autonomic dysregulation. It is therefore less clear how effective BDZs will appear when GAD is defined according the
latest criteria (Connor and Davidson, 1998).

The use of BDZs includes a serious risk for physical dependence and a withdrawal
reaction. Factors predicting major difficulties in withdrawal are the following
(Schweizer et al., 1996):

- high anxiety and depression levels before treatment
- high dosage of BDZs
- the use of BDZs with a short half-life
- current tobacco dependence
- history of recreational drugs use
- the presence of an axis II pathology
- a history of panic attacks and
- rapid rate of BDZ taper.

The risks for physical dependence and withdrawal problems at the end of the
treatment have resulted in a relative limitation of BDZ use. There are pharmacological alternatives to BDZs even though the effectiveness, feasibility and long-term
effects of these alternatives have been less documented. A treatment with buspirone
or an antidepressant may be a good choice (Schweizer and Rickels, 1996).

Azapirones

Although the *buspirone* spectrum is not as broad as the BDZs, buspirone has been
shown to be effective in numerous patients suffering from current GAD. The first
results of drug action usually appear in the range of two to four weeks (Schweizer and
Rickels, 1996). Buspirone may be seen as an effective anxiolytic in treatment of GAD.
According to some authors, buspirone may yield a slight antidepressant activity,
making it probably an very valuable option in those cases of GAD with depressive
features or high levels of "psychic symptoms", i.e. worry and ruminations. There is,
for instance, evidence that buspirone is effective in the treatment of psychic symptoms
of anxiety with obsessive ideas (Rickels et al., 1982). Buspirone should be taken into
account when problems related to drug abuse and drug discontinuation have been
identified, and where the importance of avoiding withdrawal symptoms is considered
to be high (Connor and Davidson, 1998). Gammans et al. (1992) analysed the pooled
data from eight randomised, double-blind, placebo-controlled studies and indicated
that buspirone offers effective treatment for patients with GAD, irrespective of the
presence or absence of coexisting depressive symptoms. When depressive symptoms

are present, buspirone is effective regardless of the intensity of those symptoms. The available evidence is that certain factors may predict a more favourable response to one class of drugs over another. The presence of prominent somatic symptoms will predict a better response to benzodiazepines. Prominent psychic symptoms seem to predict a more favourable response to buspirone (Schweizer, 1995).

Antidepressants

Although *antidepressants* are now well-established treatments in several anxiety disorders, their role in the treatment of GAD remains less documented. Controlled trials by Hoehn-Saric et al. (1988) and Rickels et al. (1993) have provided evidence for the benefit of imipramine and trazodone in GAD. *Imipramine* was more effective than diazepam on psychic anxiety symptoms, with the benefit of an additional significant antidepressant effect. *Trazodone* was also found to be effective. It remains a little used, but potentially useful drug for GAD. Its hypnotic properties may be welcome where insomnia is a major problem. Rickels et al. (1993) found that both imipramine and trazodone resulted in acute efficacy in GAD within two to four weeks after the start of treatment. These drugs were effective regardless of a history of depression or panic. The antidepressant *nefazodone* enjoys the advantage of greater patient acceptability and tolerability than trazodone (Connor and Davidson, 1998). Other antidepressants are being tested in GAD. There has been recent evidence in favour of the effectiveness of *venlafaxine* in GAD.

Other Drugs

The development of partial agonists at the GABA/BDZ receptor complex opens up the possibility of BDZ-like compounds that are effective anxiolytics, but less likely to produce sedation, withdrawal, and memory impairment. *Partial BDZ agonists* have been developed, the most comprehensively studied being abecarnil. Abecarnil displays affinity for BDZ receptors and shows promising anxiolytic effects in initial clinical studies. Although the data are encouraging, the question remains whether, at well-tolerated doses that are unlikely to produce significant withdrawal, the drug is clinically adequate in GAD (Connor and Davidson, 1998).

Psychotherapy

Uhlenhuth et al. (1995) carried out a study among internationally recognised experts in treating anxiety and depression; 67% of the expert panel selected *pharmacotherapy combined with psychotherapy*. The role for psychotherapy in the treatment of moderate GAD is promising (Rickels and Schweizer, 1990). Some studies confirm that *cognitive therapy* might be an interesting alternative in GAD treatment (Power et al., 1990; Chambless and Gillis, 1993; Schweizer and Rickels, 1996).

The aim of *cognitive-behaviour therapy* is to help the patient recognise and alter patterns of distorted thinking and dysfunctional behaviour and, by these processes, to alleviate the suffering and interference that the disorder causes (Harvey and Rapee, 1995). Cognitive-behaviour treatment includes cognitive therapy, behaviour therapy and relaxation. A range of relaxation techniques are available, among others Schultz's autogenic training, Jacobson's progressive relaxation, Caycedian sophrology (Chéné, 1996). Relaxation has to be presented as a skill to be learned through repeated daily practice (Barlow and Rapee, 1991).

An important trend emerging in studies that provide long-term outcome data is the substantial reduction in the use of anxiolytic medication in treated patients with GAD (Beck et al., 1985; Butler et al., 1991). As a result, Brown et al. (1993) have suggested that cognitive-behaviour therapy may offer an approach for discontinuing these medications in the long-term treatment of patients with GAD. Because the benefits of cognitive-behaviour treatment appear to be maintained at long-term follow-up assessment, cognitive-behaviour treatment may provide a long-term and cost-effective solution to GAD (Harvey and Rapee, 1995). Controlled studies of cognitive-behavioural treatments for GAD have found these techniques to produce greater improvement than no treatment and to yield maintained gains up to two years later, despite chronicities of several years (Borkovec and Costello, 1993).

Comorbidity

A last word of caution relates to the treating GAD with its comorbidity in mind. Long-term treatment planning cannot be undertaken except on the assumption that the majority of patients suffering from a principal anxiety disorder also suffer from another disorder, or will suffer from one in the near future (Schweizer, 1995). This is particularly true in the case of GAD, where comorbidity is present in the vast majority of cases. As mentioned before, social phobia, panic disorder, major depression and dysthymia are very frequently diagnosed in patients with GAD. The presence of *social phobia* might suggest the efficacy of a monoamine-oxidase inhibitor (MAOI). This only will be an inferred treatment preference, based on the efficiency of MAOIs in generalised social phobia drug treatment without GAD comorbidity (Liebowitz et al., 1988). If both GAD and *panic disorder* are present, good clinical practice recommends an antidepressant with established effectiveness in PD.

Preliminary data (Rickels et al., 1993) confirm that the presence of *depressive symptomatology* in GAD patients predicts a better response to antidepressant medication. As already mentioned, the apparently antidepressant properties of buspirone suggest that these components offer better treatment results than BDZs in GAD patients with depressive symptoms.

The clinicians, treating GAD in the long term, must be alert to emergent comorbidity that may well require significant modifications in the maintenance treatment strategy. Due to few research data, the long-term pharmacological treatment still is largely unexplored (Schweizer and Rickels, 1996).

CONCLUSION

The concept of GAD emerged progressively after the original delineation of PD by Klein in the early 1960s. Almost half a century later, the concept of PD has become one of the best validated diagnostic categories in psychiatry. On the other hand, the category of GAD was left behind in the shadow of PD. Most of the performed work to contrast PD and GAD succeeded in converting the construct of PD, but failed to establish GAD as an entity on its own. It is beyond any doubt that anxiety does exist; the question is whether a disorder, let aside a disease, characterised by "pure" anxiety, exists. The progressive shaping of diagnostic criteria focusing on cognitive symptoms may have produced a concept with some construct validity (Brown, 1997), but says nothing about possible underlying mechanisms and the exact status of GAD. An essential issue is to know whether GAD is a prodromal phase of severe psycho-pathology. Only well-conducted longitudinal studies will tell us. However, if that is the case, GAD, once thought of as a residual category, may emerge as a condition of key importance to both the clinician and the investigator. Particularly in the primary care setting, the identification of GAD might help clinicians in recognising early stages of potentially severe mental disorders and taking preventive action by starting early treatment well before invalidating conditions develop. On the other hand, the investigator should become particularly interested in the underlying mechanisms and the factors of development of a condition that represents the forerunner of major psychopathologies.

ACKNOWLEDGEMENT

We would like to thank Koen van Rangelrooij, MD, for his contribution to the preparation of this chapter.

REFERENCES

American Psychiatric Association (1952) *Diagnostic and Statistical Manual of Mental Disorders.* Washington, DC: American Psychiatric Association.
American Psychiatric Association (1968) *Diagnostic and Statistical Manual of Mental Disorders* 2nd edition. Washington, DC: American Psychiatric Association.
American Psychiatric Association (1980) *Diagnostic and Statistical Manual of Mental Disorders* 3rd edition. Washington, DC: American Psychiatric Association.
American Psychiatric Association (1987) *Diagnostic and Statistical Manual of Mental Disorders* 3rd revised edition. Washington, DC: American Psychiatric Association.
American Psychiatric Association (1994) *Diagnostic and Statistical Manual of Mental Disorders* 4th

edition. Washington, DC: American Psychiatric Association.

Anderson DJ, Noyes R, Crowe RR (1984) A comparison of panic disorder and generalized anxiety disorder. *Am J Psychiatry* **141**: 572–575.

Anderson JC, Williams S, McGee R (1987) DSM-III disorders in preadolescent children: Prevalence in a large sample from the general population. *Arch Gen Psychiatry* **44**: 67–76.

Angst J (1993) Comorbidity of anxiety, phobia, compulsion and depression. *Int Clin Psychopharmacol* **8** Suppl 2: 21–25.

Barlow DH (1988) *Anxiety and its Disorders: The Nature and Treatment of Anxiety and Panic.* New York: Guilford.

Barlow DH, Blanchard EB, Vermilyea JA et al. (1986) Generalized anxiety and generalized anxiety disorder: Description and reconceptualisation. *Am J Psychiatry* **143**(1): 40–44.

Barlow DH, Rapee RM (1991) *Mastering Stress: A Lifestyle Approach.* Dallas, TX: American Health Publishing.

Barrett JE, Barrett JA, Oxman TE et al. (1988) The prevalence of psychiatric disorders in a primary care practice. *Arch Gen Psychiatry* **45**: 1100–1106.

Beck AT, Emery G, Greenberg R (1985) *Anxiety Disorders and Phobias: A Cognitive Perspective.* New York: Basic Books.

Blazer DG, Hughes D, George LK, et al. (1991) Generalized anxiety disorder. In Robins LN, Regier DA (eds) *Psychiatric Disorders in America: The Epidemiologic Catchment Area Study.* New York: The Free Press.

Borkovec TD, Costello E (1993) Efficacy of applied relaxation and cognitive-behavioral therapy in the treatment of generalized anxiety disorder. *Int Consult Clin Psychol* **61**: 611–619.

Brawman-Mintzer O, Lydiard RB (1996) Generalized anxiety disorder: Issues in epidemiology. *J Clin Psychiatry* **57** Suppl 7: 3–8.

Brawman-Mintzer O, Lydiard RB (1997) Biological basis of generalized anxiety disorder. *J Clin Psychiatry* **58** Suppl 3: 16–25.

Brawman-Mintzer O, Lydiard RB, Emmanuel N et al. (1993) Psychiatric comorbidity in patients with generalized anxiety disorders. *Am J Psychiatry* **150**: 1216–1218.

Breslau N, Davis GC (1985) Further evidence on the doubtful validity of generalized anxiety disorder. *Psychiatry Res* **16**: 177–179.

Brown TA (1997) The nature of generalized anxiety disorder and pathological worry: current evidence and conceptual models. *Can J Psychiatry* **42**: 817–825.

Brown TA, O'Leary TA, Barlow DH (1993) Generalized anxiety disorder. In Barlow DH (ed.) *Clinical Handbook of Psychological Disorders: A Step by Step Treatment Manual* (2nd edition). New York: Guilford Press.

Butler G, Fennell M, Robson P et al. (1991) Comparison of behaviour therapy and cognitive behavior therapy in the treatment of generalized anxiety disorder. *J Consult Clin Psychol* **59**: 167–175.

Cameron OG, Thyer BA, Nesse RM et al. (1986) Symptom profiles of patients with DSM-III anxiety disorders. *Am J Psychiatry* **143**: 1132.

Chambless DL, Gillis MM (1993) Cognitive therapy of anxiety disorders. *J Consult Clin Psychol* **61**: 248–260.

Chéné PA (1996) *Sophrologie: fondements et methodologie* (3rd edition). Paris: Ellebore.

Cloninger CR, Martin RL, Clayton P et al. (1981) A blind follow-up and family study of anxiety neurosis: Preliminary analysis of the St Louis 500. In De Kein DF, Rabkin J (eds) *Anxiety: New Research and Changing Concepts.* New York: Raven Press.

Connor KM, Davidson RT (1998) Generalized anxiety disorder: Neurobiological and pharmacotherapeutic perspectives. *Biol Psychiatry* **44**: 1286–1294.

Cowley DS, Dager SR, McCellan J, Roy-Byrne DL (1988) Response to lactate infusion in generalized anxiety disorder. *Biol Psychiatry* **24**: 409–414.

Crowe RR, Noyes R, Pauls DL et al. (1983) A family study of panic disorder. *Arch Gen Psychiatry* **40**: 1065–1069.

Flint AJ (1994) Epidemiology and comorbidity of anxiety disorders in the elderly. *Am J Psychiatry* **151**: 640–649.

Gammans RE, Stringfellow JC, Hvizdos AJ et al. (1992) Use of buspirone in patients with generalized anxiety disorder and coexisting depressive symptoms. *Neuropsychobiol* **25**: 193–201.

Harvey AG, Rapee RM (1995) Cognitive behaviour therapy for generalized anxiety disorder. *Psychiatric Clin North Am* **18**: 859–870.

Hoehn-Saric R (1982) Comparison of generalized anxiety disorder with panic disorder patients. *Psychopharmacol Bull* **18**: 104–108.

Hoehn-Saric R, Hazlett RL, McLeod DR (1993) Generalized anxiety disorder with early and late onset of anxiety symptoms. *Compr Psychiatry* **34**(5): 291–298.

Hoehn-Saric R, McLeod DR (1985) Generalized anxiety disorder. *Psychiatr Clin North Am* **8**: 73–88.

Hoehn-Saric R, McLeod DR, Zimmerli WD (1988) Differential effects of alprazolam and imipramine in generalized anxiety disorder: somatic versus psychic symptoms. *J Clin Psychiatry* **49**: 293–301.

Hoehn-Saric R, McLeod DR, Zimmerli WD (1989) Somatic manifestations in women with generalized anxiety disorder: Psychophysiological responses to psychological stress. *Arch Gen Psychiatry* **46**: 1113–1119.

Kendler KS, Neagle MC, Kessler RC et al. (1992) Generalized anxiety disorder in women: A population-based twin study. *Arch Gen Psychiatry* **49**: 290–296.

Kessler RC, Stang PE, Wittchen HU, Ustun TB, Roy-Burne PP, Walters EE (1998) Lifetime depression comorbidity in the National Comorbidity Survey. *Arch Gen Psychiatry* **55**(9): 801–808.

Klein DF (1964) Delineation of drug responsive anxiety syndromes. *Psychopharmacologia* **5**: 397–408.

Liebowitz MR, Gorman JM, Fyer AJ et al. (1988) Pharmacotherapy of social phobia: An interim report of a placebo-controlled comparison of phenelzine and atenolol. *J Clin Psychiatry* **49**: 252–257.

Lydiard RB, Brawman-Mintzer O, Ballenger JC (1996) Recent developments in the psychopharmacology of anxiety disorders. *J Consult Clin Psychol* **64**: 660–668.

Maser JD (1998) Generalized anxiety disorder and its comorbidities: Disputes at the boundaries. *Acta Psychiatr Scand* **98** Suppl 393: 11–22.

Massion A, Warshaw M, Keler M (1993) Quality of life and psychiatric morbidity in panic disorder versus generalized anxiety disorder. *Am J Psychiatry* **49**: 267–272.

Nisita C, Petracca A, Akiskal HS et al. (1990) Delimitation of generalized anxiety disorder: Clinical comparisons with panic and major depressive disorders. *Compr Psychiatry* **31**(5): 409–415.

Noyes R, Clancey J, Hoenk PR et al. (1980) The prognosis of anxiety neurosis. *Arch Gen Psychiatry* **37**: 133–138.

Noyes R, Clarkson C, Crowe RR et al. (1987) A family study of generalized anxiety disorder. *Am J Psychiatry* **144**: 1019–1024.

Noyes R Jr, Woodman C, Garvey MJ et al. (1992) Generalized anxiety disorder vs panic disorder. *J Nerv Ment Dis* **180**: 369–379.

Ornel J, Van den Brink W, Koeter MWJ et al. (1990) Recognition, management and outcome of psychological disorders in primary care: A naturalistic follow-up study. *Psychol Med* **20**: 909–923.

Perna G, Bussi R, Allevi L, Bellodi L (1999) Sensitivity to 35% CO_2 in patients with generalized anxiety disorder. *J Clin Psychiatry* **60**: 379–384.

Power KG, Simpson RJ, Swanson V et al. (1990) A controlled comparison of cognitive-behaviour therapy, diazepam, and placebo, alone and in combination for the treatment of generalized anxiety disorder. *J Anxiety Disorders* **4**: 267–292.

Rickels K, Downing G, Schweizer E et al. (1993) Antidepressants for the treatment of generalized anxiety disorder: A placebo-controlled comparison of imipramine, trazodone and diazepam. *Arch Gen Psychiatry* **50**: 884–895.

Rickels K, Schweizer E (1990) The clinical course and long term management of generalized anxiety disorder. *J Clin Psychopharmacol* **10**: 101S–110S.

Rickels K, Wiseman K, Norstad N et al. (1982) Buspirone and diazepam in anxiety: A controlled study. *J Clin Psychiatry* **43**(12): 81–86.

Rosenbaum JE, Woods SW, Groves JE et al. (1984) Emergence of hostility during alprazolam treatment. *Am J Psychiatry* **141**: 792–793.

Sanderson WC, Barlow DH (1990) A description of patients diagnosed with DSM-III-R Generalized anxiety disorder. *J Nerv Ment Dis* **178**: 588–591.

Schweizer E (1995) Generalized anxiety disorder: Longitudinal course and pharmacologic treatment. *Psychiatry Clin North Am* **18**: 843–857.

Schweizer E, Rickels K (1996) The long-term management of generalized disorder: Issues and dilemmas. *J Clin Psychiatry* **57** Suppl 7: 9–12.

Schweizer E, Rickels K (1997) Strategies for treatment of generalized anxiety in the primary care setting. *J Clin Psychiatry* **58** Suppl 3: 27–31.

Thyer BA, Parrish RT, Curtis GC et al. (1985) Ages of onset of DSM-III anxiety disorders. *Compr Psychiatry* **26**: 113–122.

Torgensen S (1983) Genetic factor in anxiety disorders. *Arch Gen Psychiatry* **40**: 1085–1089.

Torgensen S (1986) Childhood and family characteristics in panic and generalized anxiety disorders. *Am J Psychiatry* **143**: 630–632.

Uhde TW, Boulenger J, Roy-Byrne PP et al. (1985) Longitudinal course of panic disorder: Clinical and biological considerations. *Progr Neuro-Psychopharmacol Biol Psychiatry* **9**: 39–50.

Uhlenhuth EH, Mitchel BB, Ban TA et al. (1995) International study of expert judgement on therapeutic use of benzodiazepines and other psychotherapeutic medications: II. Pharmacotherapy of anxiety disorders. *J Affective Dis* **35**: 153–162.

Verburg K, Griez E, Meijer J, Pols H (1995) Discrimination between panic disorders and generalized anxiety disorder by 35% CO_2 challenge. *Am J Psychiatry* **152**: 1081–1086.

Weissman MM (1990) Panic and generalized anxiety: Are they separate disorders? *J Psychiat. Res* **24**: 157–162.

Wittchen HU, Zhao S, Kessler RC et al. (1994) DSM-III-R generalized anxiety disorder in the National Comorbidity Survey. *Arch Gen Psychiatry* **51**: 355–364.

Yonkers KA, Warshaw MG, Massion AO, Keller MB (1996) Phenomenology and course of generalized anxiety disorder. *Br J Psychiatry* **168**(3): 308–313.

11

Post-traumatic Syndromes: Comparative Biology and Psychology

W.S. de Loos

Central Military Hospital, Utrecht, The Netherlands

INTRODUCTION

The concept of post-traumatic stress disorder (PTSD) is well known nowadays, after it was introduced into DSM-III in 1980 (APA, 1980). The problems US society had with its Vietnam veterans were a strong incentive for its development and recognition. However, many names and concepts have preceded it (Kinzie and Goetz, 1996), and it is becoming ever more obvious that other well-known syndromes can also be the consequence of traumatic experience. The clinical manifestation of PTSD can occur a long time, even decades, after the initial traumatic experience (Van Dyke et al., 1985; Herrmann and Eryavec, 1994). It may be triggered by associations (symbols of retraumatisation) and by other challenges to a state of psychosocial compensation that could only be attained by considerable mental effort. It is also striking how, for many years, some patients have been able to conceal their suffering from horrible nightmares from their immediate environment, e.g. their spouses.

Psychotraumatic disturbances have their roots in a combination of three elements, which are the perception of threat, the inability to control such a threat and the consequent disruption of existential stability and expectancy. Although anxiety is supposedly an overwhelming sensation during such a threat, it is not always reported as such, afterwards; this may be related to peri-traumatic dissociation (Shalev et al., 1996) or numbing.

THE SPECTRUM OF POST-TRAUMATIC SYNDROMES

What kind of syndromes can be considered as post-traumatic? When, in 1871, Jacob Mendez Da Costa, an American army physician, described the syndrome of *irritable heart* (Da Costa, 1871; Paul, 1987), he described a post-traumatic syndrome within the cultural context of his time (Gersons and Carlier, 1992; Kinzie and Goetz, 1996). The

Anxiety Disorders: An Introduction to Clinical Management and Research. Edited by E. J. L. Griez, C. Faravelli, D. Nutt and J. Zohar. © 2001 John Wiley & Sons, Ltd.

earlier description of *railway spine* (Ericksen, 1867; Trimble, 1981) relating to the many railway accidents of that time, may have been a varying mixture of neurological damage, psychological arousal and conversion symptoms. The military have offered us other diagnostic entities, which were culturally acceptable presentations of a post-traumatic syndrome, like weakness of the heart, disordered action of the heart, valvular disease of the heart, trench syndrome, shell shock syndrome and combat fatigue (Skerritt, 1983; Paul, 1987). The observation of the inseparable presence of physical symptoms in psychotraumatic disorders led Kardiner, an American army psychiatrist treating many veterans from World War I, in 1941, to designate post-traumatic neurosis as a *physioneurosis* (Kardiner, 1941). In military life, a notion of psychological distress was not acceptable in general until very recently. In the case of *traumatic neurosis*, the negative connotation in the sense of secondary gain, in both the Anglo-Saxon and the German ambit, is exemplary in this respect. The Vietnam War has pulled the wall, in a way, leading to the acceptance of *post-traumatic stress disorder* (PTSD) as a formal diagnosis.

The psychotraumatic syndromes depend in their phenomenology on the developmental stage in which they are induced in any person and by the duration of traumatisation and of the syndrome itself in the individual. The clinical diagnoses we can arrange within this spectrum are:

1. Borderline personality disorder (Gunderson and Sabo, 1993; Lonie, 1993; Van der Kolk et al., 1994).
2. Behavioural hyperactivity (Haddad and Garralda, 1992).
3. Dissociative disorders (Putnam et al., 1986; Van der Hart and Horst, 1989; Van der Kolk et al., 1989; Van der Kolk and Van der Hart, 1989).
4. Somatoform (Cheung, 1993; Barsky et al., 1994; Labbate et al., 1998) and "functional" disorders (Scarinci et al., 1994).
5. Post-traumatic stress disorder.
6. Post-traumatic personality change or disorder (Herman, 1992; Southwick et al., 1993; Jongedijk et al., 1996).

The place of attention-deficit/hyperactivity disorder (ADHD) will be discussed below. Variants and combinations can occur, e.g. chronic pain syndromes (Benedikt and Kolb, 1986) or self-destructive behaviour in the form of self-cutting or suicide attempts (Van der Kolk et al., 1991). For borderline personality disorder diagnosed during childhood, it has been argued that it, in fact, constitutes PTSD of early childhood (Famularo et al., 1991), but more scrutiny reveals that probably several causes or conditions can each contribute to its development (Zanarini et al., 1998). The diagnosis of PTSD in childhood is indeed somewhat different from that of adolescence or adulthood with more emphasis on observable behaviours, such as playing, games and drawings, and developmental progress (McFarlane, 1987; Haddad and Garralda, 1992).

THE BIOLOGICAL BASIS OF POST-TRAUMATIC RESPONSES

The Basic Stress Responses: Defence and Inhibition

When trying to understand stress response syndromes it is useful to consider comparative physiology and behaviour and trace the roots of human adaptation in its phylogenic development. The ontogeny of the human individual reflects this also to a great extent. The literature on behavioural and psychological physiology describes two important responses to adaptational challenges. Both can be seen as efforts to survive confrontations with members of their own species, predators, or physical dangers.

The first is the *defence reaction*, described in 1915 by Walter B. Cannon as a preparation for fight or flight (Cannon, 1915). It consists of both behavioural and physiological components. The behavioural components are species-specific; the physiological are more general, such as: pupillodilation; pilo-erection; increase of muscle tone (Hunsperger, 1969), ventilation, cardiac output (Stebbins and Smith, 1964), oxygen consumption and muscle blood flow (Smith et al., 1979); decrease of blood flow in the skin, intestine and kidneys; bladder and bowel emptying; and many others like neurohumoral, hormonal, immunological and haemostatic changes. The functional anatomy of the defence system has its organisational centre in the amygdala (Hilton and Zbrozyna, 1963; Stock et al., 1978; Kapp et al., 1981), particularly its central nucleus (Iwata et al., 1987), but the central or peri-aquaductal grey matter is also involved (Hilton and Redfern, 1986). Outflow is mainly through the sympathetic system and the adrenal medulla. Understanding of the ethology and comparative physiology of the defence reaction permits excellent understanding of the psychophysiology of alarm and anxiety in humans. From a biological point of view, there are good reasons why, so often, physical symptoms are the first signals of post-traumatic syndromes. The core of the response to any form of existential menace is the inborn repertoire for survival behaviour present in all mammals.

The other important survival response is the *general adaptation syndrome* described by Hans Selye later in the century (Selye, 1946). It is characterised by behavioural inhibition when all possible active ways of surviving a challenge are being blocked off. It can be compared to the psychodynamic concept of unsolvable conflict or to Martin P. Seligman's behavioural model of *learned helplessness* (Seligman, 1975; Maier and Seligman, 1976; Abramson et al., 1978), while James P. Henry described it from a comparative physiological and ethological point of view as *conservation-withdrawal* (Henry, 1976; Henry, 1992). The corresponding neuroanatomical organisation is centralised in the septo-hippocampal system. It produces its physiological outflow through the anterior pituitary and the vagal motor system, and activates glucocorticoid hormone release. The physiology of inhibition in the human has much resemblance to what is known in ethology as subordinate behaviour.

Somatic Stress Syndromes

When considering the psychophysiology of the defence reaction, the symptoms of many functional syndromes can be understood as forms of recurrent or persistent alarm. Examples known in the literature are hyperventilation, hyperdynamic beta-adrenergic circulation, adrenal exhaustion, hyperkinetic heart syndrome, circulatory neurasthenia, effort syndrome (Cohen et al., 1948), autonomic dysfunction syndrome, neurasthenia, epidemic neuromyasthenia, benign myalgic encephalomyelitis, irritable bowel syndrome, chronic pelvic pain (CPP), "allergic to everything", sugar intolerance, reactive hypoglycaemia. More modern connotations are fibromyalgia, post-viral fatigue, chronic fatigue (and immune deficiency) syndrome (CFS/CFIDS), yuppie flu, etc. These functional syndromes basically consist of the psychophysiological arousal symptoms of the defence reaction. In none of these, a pathological basis, i.e. a histological or physiological defect, has been found. In addition, on close examination, these so-called syndromes show considerable overlap (McKell and Sullivan, 1947; Prior et al., 1989).

I have noted already that *somatoform disorders* can be considered as post-traumatic syndromes and this has been substantiated by some evidence for somatisation disorder (Cheung, 1993) and *hypochondriasis* (Barsky et al., 1994). It is even more evident as one notices that the basis of the physical complaints of these patients is actually largely made up by the psychophysiology of the defence reaction. The patient's interpretation and illness behaviour make it hypochondriasis. Also in somatisation disorder, the basis of the physical complaints is in the psychophysiology of alarm (defence) and may be combined with conversion symptoms. The behavioural presentation is different from hypochondriasis; there may be more variation over time and very often patients are subject to multiple interventions, which may cause new problems of a pathological kind. Sexual or physical abuse in early life is the typical history of such patients.

About a century ago, the French psychologist Pierre Janet has laid the basis for our understanding of *conversion disorder* as a post-traumatic syndrome (Van der Kolk et al., 1989). One of his famous examples was a case of behavioural repetition, a re-enactment of a traumatic memory (Janet, 1928). Conversion in its present usual meaning can be well understood as a sensory or motoric avoidance symptom, upon which relational behaviour becomes superimposed.

Finally, among the somatoform disorders we have *pain disorder associated with psychological factors or with both these and a general medical condition* (DSM-IV), which is one of the most difficult problems in health care. In my personal experience, psychophysiological or pathological causes of pain can usually be found in a patient with chronic pain but it can take much time and effort to discover either of these, or both. The patient's behaviour can be an important reason for this and it reflects the description in the DSM-IV (APA, 1994), which points out that psychological factors are associated with the pain disorder. It may be a matter of interpretation whether a psychophysiological substrate, e.g. oesophageal or intestinal muscle contractions or stretching, voluntary muscle hypertonia etc., is such a psychological factor. In such cases a physical substrate, with activation of peripheral pain receptors and circuitry, is undoubtedly present and this coincides with the patient's own perceptions. In fact, I have never met a case where pain or dysaesthesia could only and with certainty be understood as a memory, which is the implication and consequence of the absence of any substrate outside the central nervous system.

The Generation of Somatic Symptoms

The three core groups of symptoms of post-traumatic syndromes are functions of memory, of avoidance and of alarm with its behavioural and physiological signs. With respect to the physical complaints, it is important to realise how physical signs and symptoms can be generated, see Box 1.

Box 1: The Generation of Physical Signs and Symptoms

1. Biological source
   a. Psychophysiological
   b. Pathophysiological
2. Amplification
   a. Positive
      (1) normal (psychophysiological) responses
      (2) mild pathophysiological symptoms
   b. Negative: denial of major pathophysiological signs
3. Voluntary control
   a. Adaptation to irreparable defect
   b. Autonomic nervous system reactions
   c. Conversion (sensory/motoric)
      Simulation (fantasy)
   e. Malingering (illegal gain)

A biological substrate is the rule. Amplification and voluntary control determine the presentation. As we have seen above, this is especially important in the somatoform disorders. The biological substrate may be either psychophysiological or pathological but its occurrence does not bring the patient to the doctor by itself. Epidemiological surveys have clearly demonstrated that this is a result of psychological variables (Drossman et al., 1988).

Amplification can be negative which is named dissimulation. It can make patients with serious pathology postpone seeing a doctor for unreasonably long times. It is a phenomenon that can also be observed in patients with post-traumatic syndromes. It may seem paradoxical in comparison to the frequent medical consultations of many of such patients but it can be understood when considering a number of circumstances. Firstly, workaholism is a defence strategy, which is employed by many traumatised people with considerable success over periods of decades. Breakdown of this psychological defence can occur due to a serious disease. Secondly, alexithymia, which is so common among traumatised persons (Sifneos, 1973; Krystal, 1988; Hyer et al., 1990) not only implies inability to "read", that is to verbalise one's emotions from the psychophysiological reactions of the body. It implies a more general inefficiency in judging the signals of the body, also in pathology.

Then, voluntary control over physical symptoms can help a patient to live with an irreparable defect like asthma or either with symptoms of a pounding heart, a dry mouth, trembling and sweating, etc. in cases of stage fright or even panic (Beitman et al., 1987). Voluntary control also plays a role in the therapy of conversion disorder with respect to a patient's regaining responsibility for his symptoms. Finally, cases of simulation and malingering can also be headed under voluntary control but in a different way. In practice, these occur less often in traumatised persons than was originally suggested within the connotations of *compensation neurosis* as described by Strümpell in 1895 (Fischer-Homberger, 1975), *traumatic neurosis*, or *accident neurosis* (Bonhoeffer, 1927; Miller, 1961). Mayou (1996) has indeed underscored the dismissal of these prejudiced concepts.

DIAGNOSTIC INTEGRATION

Diagnostic Taxonomy: Matrix Diagnosis

The conceptual difficulties of describing the functional and somatoform syndromes listed in the previous paragraph have also caused problems in arranging them in the disease taxonomies that are commonly in use. The DSM tries to integrate the somatic, psychological, and social dimensions at the price of creating comorbidity (Van Praag, 1990; Van Praag, 1995; Van Praag, 1996). I see only one way to reach integration, that is by constructing a matrix of dimensions that follows the natural development of the human species (phylogeny) and individuals (ontogeny). All the observable aspects of an individual's functioning should then be broken down into dimensions based on these developmental lines. It is a matrix constructed for the full integrity of the individual patient. Semantically, it corresponds to the meaning of a matrix in mathematics.

The genetically determined, unchangeable biological properties are at the basis of this system. Imprinting and learning are processes directly based on the genetic make-up of an individual. Imprinting is the creation of read-only-memories (ROMs), a biological parallel of computer "firmware". Learning is the adaptation and neural plasticity of functional circuits in response to repeated activation. Associative memory is another aspect of learning. Associations are acquired and, then, automated programmes. Acquisition of this dimension starts during ontogeny as the first layer over

POST-TRAUMATIC SYNDROMES

POST-TRAUMATIC SYNDROMES 211

Box 2: Diagnostic Matrix of Dimensions

1. Genetic floorplan
    a. structural floorplan (embryology/anatomy)
    b. homeostatic physiology
    c. psychophysiology (inborn responses to adaptational challenges)
2. Acquired automated mechanisms (neuromotor/neurohumoral output, sensory input)
    a. organising effects
    b. imprinting (Read Only Memory)
    c. long-term potentiation/dendritic plasticity
    d. association
3. Declarative faculty
    a. reflexive consciousness
    b. emotional development
4. Complex language dependent systems
    a. cognition: science, logic, mathematics, philosophy
    b. groups/systems: politics

---

the inborn properties. Intrusive memory of sensory input and imprinted or amplified physiological memory belong to this dimension, as well as impulsiveness or temperament.

From a heuristic point of view, it seems logical to separate linguistic development from the second dimension, considering the phylogeny of *homo sapiens sapiens*. Reflexive consciousness and the development of emotional expression are representations of the declarative faculty including relational behaviour, literature, etc. Alexithymia is a description of incomplete or inhibited emotional development at the declarative level. It is characteristic of somatoform disorders and functional or psychophysiological syndromes. Psycho-physiological syndromes as listed in the paragraph on somatic stress syndromes can thus be seen as phylogenic and ontogenic precursors of more differentiated psychiatric syndromes.

Complex language-dependent systems can be seen as the present ultimate development of phylogeny and ontogeny. They constitute what we use to call human "civilisation" including all aspects of science, philosophy and political systems, structures that are based on semantically explicit cognition. Although scientific theory development requires economy in calling in assumptions or abstractions, it seems appropriate and efficacious to categorise this level of development in a separate dimension, making a link with sociology.

This diagnostic matrix is a dimensional analysis slightly different from Van Praag's proposal for functionalisation, verticalisation or "two-tier" diagnosing (Van Praag, 1990) and more extensive but permits inclusion of his idea. It allows us to break down pathology at the level of the genome (Bell, 1998) or allostatic physiology (McEwen, 1998), and phenotypical expressions or changes by organising effects of hormones and stressors, long-term potentiation, imprinting, plasticity, apoptosis, learning in all its aspects, deviant behaviour and irresponsible use of scientific progress or political power, genocide, etc.

Application to Syndromal Diagnosis

In the case of the somatoform disorders as syndromal diagnoses, these dimensional diagnostics would produce results as given in Box 3. The dimensions of the matrix are compared with the memory (B), avoidance (C) and arousal (D) criteria for PTSD in the DSM.

Box 3: Somatoform Disorders as Post-traumatic Syndromes

Hypochondriasis
   psychophysiology of alarm defence   D   1
   catastrophic interpretation   □   2
   alexithymia*   C   3
Somatisation disorder
   psychophysiology of alarm defence   D   1
   conversion   C   2
   alexithymia   C   3
   illness behaviour   □   3
Pain disorder associated with psychological factors
   a.   memory, no physiological substrate outside the CNS   B   2
   b.   psychophysiology of alarm   D   1
        attributed to a psychodynamic factor   B   3
   c.   pathophysiological cause, unrecognised   □   1
   d.   illness behaviour (iatrogenic?)   □   3
Conversion disorder
   motoric or sensory avoidance   C   2
   alexithymia   C   3
   illness behaviour   □   3

Key:

DSM criterion		Matrix dimension	
A	Trauma	1	Genetic floorplan
B	Memory	2	Acquired automated mechanisms
C	Avoidance and numbing	3	Declarative faculty
D	Arousal/hypervigilance	4	Complex, language dependent systems

Note: *i.e. inability to verbalise psychophysiology as emotion.

Psychophysiology is a component of the biological dimension, which is common to all species across their phylogenic development. It is the physiology of adaptation that occurs in all normal individuals. Pathophysiology is defective functioning and is irreversible. Interpretation of a symptom can be an associative process. Conversion is avoidance associated with certain memories. Dissociation is also a process at the level of this dimension. It seems a logical assumption that different species, animals and man, could share it. This is different for the third level, the semantic or declarative dimension. Humans learn to declare their emotions and they learn from their own psychophysiological sensations, which become incorporated in associative pro- grammes. Incomplete emotional declaration is known as alexithymia and is a basic phenomenon in somatoform and functional disorders (Sifneos, 1973). Breaking down syndromal diagnoses or classifications into their constituents allows recognition of the characteristic elements of psychological traumatisation.

PSYCHOLOGICAL AND BEHAVIOURAL ASPECTS

Predictors and Risk Factors

Genetic Factors

There are indications that genetic factors may contribute to the susceptibility to PTSD symptomatology. Comparison of monozygotic (MZ) with dizygotic (DZ) twins in order to determine the effects of heredity, shared environment and unique environment demonstrated that heredity indeed contributes substantially to the susceptibility to nearly all symptoms, taking into account differences in concordance for combat exposure between MZ and DZ twins. The level of combat exposure itself predicted mainly the re-experiencing symptoms and the avoided activities, not the numbing. Interestingly, shared family-life experiences did not contribute to the susceptibility to PTSD symptoms (True et al., 1993). In an earlier study, a specific effect of the level of combat exposure on the occurrence and intensity of the same PTSD symptoms had been shown, demonstrating a dose–response relationship within a genetically homogeneous population on a paired observations basis (Gold- berg et al., 1990). Also in other studies, a dose–response relationship of duration and intensity of combat exposure was demonstrated (Buydens-Branchey et al., 1990).

Polymorphism of the dopamine D_2-receptor gene, the occurrence of the D_2A1 allele, has been found associated with PTSD although PTSD can certainly not be thought of as a single gene disorder (Comings et al., 1996). It is inferred that the D_2A1 allele is in linkage desequilibrium with a mutation of a non-transcribed portion of the DRD2 gene causing receptor dysfunction. The statistical significance was very high and highest for the hyperarousal ("D") criterion. Increased prevalence of the same allele had previously been found in attention-deficit/hyperactivity disorder (ADHD), Gilles de la Tourette's syndrome, conduct disorder and substance-related disorder, e.g. alcoholism. This suggests that genetically determined differences in the dopaminergic system may have an important role in pathological development of human stress responses and that this transcends DSM diagnostic groups as a pathogenic dimension at the molecular level, the biological floorplan. The existence and influence of this type of susceptibility traits might also explain why only a limited number of exposed individuals develop a post-traumatic disorder. In the case of ADHD, specifically, it could clarify the confusion about ADHD as a post-traumatic syndrome versus independent familial predisposition for ADHD (Wozniak et al., 1999). At the same time this implies that for the development of a psychiatric disorder that can be classified as one of the above, additional factors, genetic, developmental or environmental, are needed to produce them.

Psychological Factors and Interactions

Prospectively, neuroticism and extroversion were factors that could predict the exposure to traumatic events *per se*, but early misconduct or a family history of a psychiatric disorder could not do so and educational level was only marginally significant in this study of exposure (Breslau et al., 1995). With respect to development of PTSD, cognitive variables may well affect the ability to cope with trauma, thereby influencing whether a person develops the chronic condition (McNally and Shin, 1995). Linked to this, education was indeed found to influence the development of PTSD.

A prospective study in World War II veterans provides an indication of the specificity of PTSD symptoms. Combat exposure and number of physiological symptoms during combat stress predicted PTSD symptoms at one and at 41 years after the war. On the other hand, psychosocial vulnerability during adolescence and at age 65, and the display of physiological symptoms during civil life stress predicted trait neuroticism at age 65. Thus, combat exposure proved more specific for the development of PTSD, and premorbid vulnerability more specific for psychoneurotic pathology (Lee et al., 1995).

Interestingly but not unexpected, characteristics of the individual and his or her behaviour also influence the likelihood of exposure to traumatic events. Correlation for volunteering for military service in Vietnam, for actual service in South-East Asia, for self-reported combat experiences, and for being awarded combat decorations were higher within MZ than in DZ twins (Lyons et al., 1993).

Gender is another factor that influences susceptibility to traumatic experiences in developing PTSD. More women than men develop PTSD after exposure to major trauma and duration of symptoms in women is longer (Yonkers and Ellison, 1996; Seeman, 1997; Breslau et al., 1997). In veterans this held true after adjustment for pre-combat physical or sexual abuse and pre-combat psychiatric history (Engel et al., 1993). However, such abuse itself seemed to promote the development of PTSD after combat exposure (Bremner et al., 1993).

Early Signs as Predictors

A much better predictor of the development of PTSD has been found in peri-traumatic dissociation, even better and stronger than depression, anxiety and intrusive symptoms (Shalev et al., 1996). This might help clinicians to identify subjects at risk for development of the disorder. Heart rate in the peri-traumatic phase, i.e. in the emergency room after traffic accidents, etc., was also positively correlated to the development of PTSD (Shalev et al., 1998a). In an extension of the study, again peri-traumatic dissociation and heart rate predicted the development of PTSD and were associated with more intrusive symptoms and with exaggerated startle (Shalev et al., 1998b). Comorbid depression occurred in more than 40% at one and four months but was stated to be an independent consequence and to be associated with prior depression.

A negative correlation between serum cortisol immediately after traumatisation and the development of PTSD was found in two different settings, namely sexual assault and motor vehicle accidents (Resnick et al., 1995; McFarlane et al., 1997). These psychophysiological factors raise the issue of pre-traumatic vulnerability in the development of PTSD (Yehuda et al., 1998), which would discard the notion that this disorder is a normal reaction to abnormal events as has been proposed by some experts in the field during the last two decades.

The *acute stress response*, a classification newly introduced in the DSM-IV, has been shown to have internal coherence and can strongly predict the development of PTSD (Brewin et al., 1999). Although the development of PTSD could indeed be predicted in road traffic accident victims on the basis of the existence and severity of early PTSD-related symptoms one week after the accident, the following three months appeared to be the critical period for the development of the full disorder (Koren et al., 1999).

Lifetime Development

In retrospect, the long-term development of PTSD may show several patterns. An acute PTSD may gradually develop into a chronic condition. A delayed form may manifest itself clinically after a considerable number of years up to three or four decades (Van Dyke et al., 1985; Herrmann and Eryavec, 1994). A first and early manifestation may be followed by a symptom-free interval of years to decades and then relapse. A study in Dutch resistance veterans has revealed no differences at all between veterans who had or had not been in German concentration camps (Op den Velde et al., 1993). It is clinical experience, also of my own, that PTSD of substantial duration is not the immediate consequence of one single event. If that would appear to be the case, it usually becomes clear after some time that significant earlier traumatisation has occurred. The said single event, then, will probably have triggered memories that had been unconscious ("forgotten") for a longer time.

Any individual who has significantly been traumatised may and almost certainly will meet circumstances or events during later life that symbolise the trauma and trigger the syndrome (Ørner and De Loos, 1998). Conditions that can trigger or exacerbate PTSD more or less acutely are intrusive medical treatments (Kutz et al.,

1988; Hamner, 1994; Doerfler et al., 1994) or other medical illness (e.g. with a stay in hospital acting as a memory of the concentration camp sick barrack), retirement or other reasons for drop-out from work (ending workaholism as a defence mechanism), general anaesthesia (an accidental, unwanted narco-analysis procedure), trains (association with the concentration camp transports), etc. Before the manifestation of their PTSD such patients may have had precursors of an aspecific type like *surménage* or "exhaustion" syndromes (*adjustment disorders* in DSM-IV terminology), functional syndromes (which are probably best described as undifferentiated somatoform disorders) or unspecified psychiatric syndromes. They also may have been given entirely different psychiatric diagnoses because the trauma criterion had not been recognised or because the flashbacks had been taken for delusions or hallucinations (Mueser and Butler, 1987; Spivak et al., 1992), a problem that is also known in dissociative identity disorder.

A retrospective attempt to follow the longitudinal course of chronic PTSD showed that hyperarousal symptoms developed first, followed by avoidance symptoms, and finally by symptoms of the intrusive cluster. Symptoms plateaued within a few years after the Vietnam War, which was the stressor under study. Recording of alcohol and substance abuse revealed a course grossly parallel to PTSD symptoms (Bremner et al., 1996). Prospectively, it has been confirmed that it takes some time for the consequences of traumatic exposure to become apparent. During a two-year follow-up of veterans after Operation Desert Storm (the Gulf War), hyperarousal symptoms were more severe than symptoms of re-experiencing or avoidance. Only two years after exposure to combat, its level was significantly associated with the score on the Mississippi trauma scale (Southwick et al., 1995).

Comorbidity

Both in veterans (Green et al., 1989; Hovens et al., 1994) and in civilian survivors of disaster (Green et al., 1992), PTSD is often found in conjunction with other DSM diagnoses, such as major depression (Shalev et al., 1998b), dysthymia, panic, phobia, alcohol abuse, generalised anxiety disorder, obsessive compulsive disorder (OCD) and somatisation, either at a current or a lifetime base. In clinical samples, PTSD rarely develops as a single syndrome. It is questionable whether panic, phobia and dysthymia are essentially independent diagnoses with respect to PTSD or, in fact, dimensional morbidity units fitting into broader syndromes. I refer to my remarks on dimensional diagnosis in which I feel supported by Van Praag's scepticism about traditional comorbidity conceptions (Van Praag, 1990). However, PTSD did occur as an isolated diagnosis in the above-mentioned studies, a phenomenon which existence I can confirm from personal clinical experience.

Thus, the question comes back to what the essential functional elements in psychotraumatic syndromes are. To my opinion, these are, first, persistently increased vigilance and, second, the mnemonic elements of what caused this increased vigilance. These are intricately connected to the neurobiological processes of startle, defence, long-term potentiation, imprinting, kindling and memory intrusion (Post et al., 1995; Sanes and Lichtman, 1999).

REFERENCES

Abramson LY, Seligman MEP, Teasdale JD (1978) Learned helplessness in humans: critique and reformulation. *J Abnorm Psychol* **87**: 49–74.

American Psychiatric Association (1980) *Diagnostic and Statistical Manual of Mental Disorders* 3rd edition. Washington, DC: American Psychiatric Association.

American Psychiatric Association (1994) *Diagnostic and Statistical Manual of Mental Disorders* 4th edition, Washington, DC: America Psychiatric Association.

Barsky AJ, Wool C, Barnett MC, Cleary PD (1994) Histories of childhood trauma in adult hypochondriacal patients. *Am J Psychiatry* **151**: 397–401.

Beitman BD, Basa I, Flaka G, DeRosear L, Mukerji V, Lamberti J (1987) Non-fearful panic disorder: Panic attacks without fear. *Behav Res Ther* **25**: 487–492.

Bell J (1998) The new genetics in clinical practice. *Br Med J* **316**: 618–620.

Benedikt RA, Kolb LC (1986) Preliminary findings on chronic pain and posttraumatic stress disorder. *Am J Psychiatry* **143**: 908–910.

Bonnhoeffer K (1927) Bemerkungen zur "Unfallneurose" an der Hand einiger neuer Arbeiten ("Accident neurosis" based on several new articles). *Dtsch Med Wochenschr* **53**: 14–16.

Bremner JD, Southwick SM, Darnell A, Charney DS (1996) Chronic PTSD in Vietnam combat veterans: Course of illness and substance abuse. *Am J Psychiatry* **153**: 369–375.

Bremner DJ, Southwick SM, Johnson DR, Yehuda R, Charney DS (1993) Childhood physical abuse and combat-related posttraumatic stress disorder in Vietnam veterans. *Am J Psychiatry* **150**: 235–239.

Breslau N, Davis GC, Andreski P (1995) Risk factors for PTSD-related events: A prospective analysis. *Am J Psychiatry* **152**: 529–535.

Breslau N, Davis GC, Andreski P, Peterson EL, Schultz LR (1997) Sex differences in posttraumatic stress disorder. *Arch Gen Psychiatry* **54**: 1044–1048.

Brewin CR, Andrews B, Rose S, Kirk M (1999) Acute stress disorder and posttraumatic stress disorder in victims of violent crime. *Am J Psychiatry* **156**: 360–366.

Buydens-Branchey L, Noumair D, Branchey M (1990) Duration and intensity of combat exposure and posttraumatic stress disorder in Vietnam veterans. *J Nerv Ment Dis* **178**: 582–587.

Cannon WB (1915) *Bodily Changes in Pain, Hunger, Fear and Rage.* New York: Appleton Press.

Cheung P (1993) Somatisation as a presentation in depression and post-traumatic stress disorder among Cambodian refugees. *Aust N Z J Psychiatry* **27**: 422–428.

Cohen ME, White PD, Johnson RE (1948) Neurocirculatory asthenia, anxiety neurosis or the effort syndrome. *Arch Intern Med* **81**: 260–281.

Comings DE, Muhleman D, Gysin R (1996) Dopamine D_2 receptor (DRD_2) gene and susceptability to posttraumatic stress disorder: A study and replication. *Biol Psychiatry* **40**: 368–372.

Da Costa JM (1871) On irritable heart: A clinical study of functional cardiac disorder and its consequences. *Am J Med Sci* **61**: 17–52.

Doerfler LA, Pbert L, DeCosimo D (1994) Symptoms of posttraumatic stress disorder following myocardial infarction and coronary artery bypass surgery. *Gen Hosp Psychiatry* **16**: 193–199.

Drossman DA, McKee DC, Sandler RS, Mitchell CM, Cramer EM, Lowman BC, Burger AL (1988) Psychosocial factors in the irritable bowel syndrome: A multivariate study of patients and non-patients with irritable bowel syndrome. *Gastroenterology* **95**: 701–708.

Engel CC, Engel AI, Campbell SJ, McFall ME, Russo J, Katon W (1993) Posttraumatic stress disorder symptoms and precombat sexual and physical abuse in Desert Storm veterans. *J Nerv Ment Dis* **181**: 683–688.

Ericksen JE (1867) *On Railway Spine and Other Injuries of the Nervous System.* Philadelphia: Henry C. Lea.

Famularo R, Kinscherff R, Fenton T (1991) Posttraumatic stress disorder among children clinically diagnosed as borderline personality disorder. *J Nerv Ment Dis* **179**: 428–431.

Fischer-Homberger E (1975) Die traumatische Neurose: vom somatischen zum sozialen Leiden (Traumatic neurosis: from somatic to social suffering). Berlin: Verlag Hans Huber.

Gersons BPR, Carlier IVE (1992) Post-traumatic stress disorder: The history of a recent concept. *Br J Psychiatry* **161**: 742–748.

Goldberg J, True WR, Eisen SA, Henderson WG (1990) A twin study of the effects of the Vietnam war on posttraumatic stress disorder. *JAMA* **263**: 1227–1232.

Green BL, Lindy JD, Grace MC, Gleser GC (1989) Multiple diagnosis in posttraumatic stress disorder: The role of war stressors. *J Nerv Ment Dis* **177**: 329–335.

Green BL, Lindy JD, Grace MC, Leonard AC (1992) Chronic posttraumatic stress disorder and diagnostic comorbidity in a disaster sample. *J Nerv Ment Dis* **180**: 760–766.

Gunderson JG, Sabo AN (1993) The phenomenological and conceptual interface between borderline personality disorder and PTSD. *Am J Psychiatry* **150**: 19–27.

Haddad PM, Garralda ME (1992) Hyperkinetic syndrome and disruptive early experiences. *Br J Psychiatry* **161**: 700–703.

Hamner MB (1994) Exacerbation of posttraumatic stress disorder symptoms with medical illness. *Gen Hosp Psychiatry* **16**: 135–137.

Henry JP (1976) Mechanisms of psychosomatic disease in animals. *Adv Vet Sci Compar Med* **20**: 115–145.

Henry JP (1992) Biological basis of the stress response. *Integr Physiol Behav Sci* **27**: 66–83.

Herman JL (1992) Complex PTSD: A syndrome in survivors of prolonged and repeated trauma. *J Trauma Stress* **5**: 377–391.

Herrmann N, Eryavec G (1994) Delayed onset post-traumatic stress disorder in World War II veterans. *Can J Psychiatry* **39**: 439–441.

Hilton SM, Redfern WS (1986) A search for brain stem cell groups integrating the defence reaction in the rat. *J Physiol (London)* **378**: 213–228.

Hilton SM, Zbroyna AW (1963) Amygdaloid region for defence reactions and its efferent pathway to the brain stem. *J Physiol (London)* **165**: 160–173.

Hovens JE, Falger PRJ, Op den Velde W, De Groen JHM, Van Duijn H (1994) Posttraumatic stress disorder in male and female Dutch resistance veterans of World War II in relation to trait anxiety and depression. *Psychol Rep* **74**: 275–285.

Hunsperger RW (1969) Postural tonus and cardiac activity during centrally elicited affective reactions in the cat. *Ann N Y Acad Sci* **159**: 1013–1024.

Hyer L, Woods MG, Summers MN, Boudewyns P, Harrison WR (1990) Alexithymia among Vietnam veterans with posttraumatic stress disorder. *J Clin Psychiatry* **51**: 243–247.

Iwata J, Chida K, LeDoux JE (1987) Cardiovascular responses elicited by stimulation of neurons in the central amygdaloid nucleus in awake but not anesthetized rats resemble conditioned emotional responses. *Brain Res* **418**: 183–188.

Janet P (1928) *L'évolution de la mémoire et de la notion du temps: Compte-rendu intégral des conférences d'après les notes sténographiques.* Paris: A. Cahine, pp. 205–225.

Jongedijk RA, Carlier IVE, Schreuder JN, Gersons BPR (1996) Complex posttraumatic stress disorder: An exploratory investigation of PTSD and DESNOS among Dutch war veterans. *J Trauma Stress* **9**: 577–586.

Kapp BS, Gallagher M, Frysinger RC, Applegate CD (1981) The amygdala, emotion and cardiovascular conditioning. In Ben-Ari Y (ed.) *The Amygdaloid Complex.* New York/Amsterdam: Elsevier/North-Holland Biomedical, pp. 355–366.

Kardiner A (1941) *The Traumatic Neurosis of War*. New York: Paul B. Hoebner Inc.

Kinzie JD, Goetz RR (1996) A century of controversy surrounding posttraumatic stress-spectrum syndromes: The impact on DSM-III and DSM-IV. *J Trauma Stress* **9**: 159–179.

Koren D, Arnon I, Klein E (1999) Acute stress response and posttraumatic stress disorder in traffic accident victims: A one-year prospective, follow-up study. *Am J Psychiatry* **156**: 367–373.

Krystal H (1988) *Integration and Self-healing: Affect, Trauma, Alexithymia*. With a contribution from J.H. Krystal. Hillsdale, NJ: Lawrence Erlbaum Associates, Inc.

Kutz I, Garb R, David D (1988) Post-traumatic stress disorder following myocardial infarction. *Gen Hosp Psychiatry* **10**: 169–176.

Labbate LA, Cardena E, Dimitreva J, Roy M, Engel CC (1998) Psychiatric syndromes in Persian Gulf War veterans: An association of handling dead bodies with somatoform disorders. *Psychother Psychosom* **67**: 275–279.

Lee KA, Vaillant GE, Torrey WC, Elder GH (1995) A 50-year prospective study of the psychological sequelae of World War II combat. *Am J Psychiatry* **152**: 516–522.

Lonie I (1993) Borderline disorder and post-traumatic stress disorder: An equivalence? *Austr N Z J Psychiatry* **27**: 233–245.

Lyons MJ, Goldberg J, Eisen SA, True W, Tsuang MT, Meyer JM, Henderson WG (1993) Do genes influence exposure to trauma? A twin study of combat. *Am J Med Gen (Neuropsychiat Gen)* **48**: 22–27.

Maier SF, Seligman MEP (1976) Learned helplessness: theory and evidence. *J Exp Psychiat Gen* **105**: 3–46.

Mayou R (1996) Accident neurosis revisited. (Editorial) *Br J Psychiatry* **168**: 399–403.

McEwen BS (1998) Protective and damaging effects of stress mediators. *N Engl J Med* **338**: 171–179.

McFarlane AC (1987) Posttraumatic phenomena in a longitudinal study of children following a natural disaster. *J Am Acad Child Adolesc Psychiatry* **26**: 764–769.

McFarlane AC, Atchison M, Yehuda R (1997) The acute stress response following motor vehicle accidents and its relation to PTSD. In Yehuda R, McFarlane AC (eds) *Psychobiology of Posttraumatic Stress Disorder. Ann N Y Acad Sci* **821**: 437–441.

McKell TE, Sullivan AJ (1947) The hyperventilation syndrome in gastroenterology. *Gastroenterology* **9**: 6–16.

McNally RJ and Shin LM (1995) Association of intelligence with severity of posttraumatic stress disorder symptoms in Vietnam combat veterans. *Am J Psychiatry* **152**: 936–938.

Miller H (1961) Accident neurosis; I, II. *Br Med J* **i**: 919–925, 992–998.

Mueser KT, Butler RW (1987) Auditory hallucinations in combat-related chronic posttraumatic stress disorder. *Am J Psychiatry* **144**: 299–302.

Op den Velde W, Falger PRJ, Hovens JE, De Groen JHM, Lasschut LJ, Van Duin H, Schouten EGW (1993) Post-traumatic stress disorder in Dutch resistance veterans from World War II. In Wilson JP, Raphael B (eds) *International Handbook of Traumatic Stress Syndromes*. New York: Plenum Press, pp. 219–230.

Ørner RJ, De Loos WS (1998) Second World War veterans with chronic post-traumatic stress disorder. *Adv Psychiat Treatment* **4**: 211–218.

Paul O (1987) Da Costa's syndrome or neurocirculatory asthenia. *Br Heart J* **58**: 306–315.

Post RM, Weiss SMB, Smith M (1995) Sensitization and kindling: Implications for the evolving neural substrate of PTSD. In Friedman MJ, Charney DS, Deutsch AJ (eds) *Neurobiology and Clinical Consequences of Stress: From Normal Adaptation to PTSD*. Philadelphia: Lippincott-Raven Publishers, pp. 203–224.

Prior A, Wilson K, Whorwell PJ, Faragher EB (1989) Irritable bowel syndrome in the gynaecological clinic. *Dig Dis Sci* **34**: 1820–1824.

Putnam FW, Guroff JJ, Silberman EK, Barban L, Post RM (1986) The clinical phenomenology of multiple personality disorder: Review of 100 recent cases. *J Clin Psychiatry* **47**:

285–293.

Resnick HS, Yehuda R, Pitman RK, Foy DW (1995) Effect of previous trauma on acute plasma cortisol level following rape. *Am J Psychiatry* **152**: 1675–1677.

Sanes JR, Lichtman JW (1999) Can molecules explain long-term potentiation? *Nature Neuroscience* **2**: 597–604.

Scarinci IC, McDonald-Haile J, Bradley LA, Richter JE (1994) Altered pain perception and psychological features among women with gastrointestinal disorders and history of abuse: A preliminary model. *Am J Med* **97**: 108–118.

Seeman MV (1997) Psychopathology in women and men: focus on female hormones. *Am J Psychiatry* **154**: 1641–1647.

Seligman MEP (1975) *Helplessness: On Depression, Development, and Death.* San Francisco: WH Freeman & Co.

Selye H (1946) The general adaptation syndrome and the diseases of adaptation. *J Clin Endocrinol* **6**: 117–230.

Shalev AY, Freedman S, Peri T, Brandes D, Sahar T, Orr SP, Pitman RK (1998b) Prospective study of posttraumatic stress disorder and depression following trauma. *Am J Psychiatry* **155**: 630–637.

Shalev AY, Peri T, Canettti L, Schreiber S (1996) Predictors of PTSD in injured trauma survivors: A prospective study. *Am J Psychiatry* **153**: 219–225.

Shalev AY, Sahar T, Freedman S, Peri T, Glick N, Brandes D, Orr SP, Pittman RK (1998a) A prospective study of heart rate response following trauma and the subsequent development of posttraumatic stress disorder. *Arch Gen Psychiatry* **55**: 553–559.

Sifneos PE (1973) The prevalence of "alexithymia" characteristics in psychosomatic patients. *Psychother Psychosom* **22**: 255–262.

Skerritt PW (1983) Anxiety and the heart: A historical review. *Psychol Med* **13**: 17–25.

Smith OA, Hohimer AR, Astley CA, Taylor DJ (1979) Renal and hindlimb vascular control during acute emotion in the baboon. *Am J Physiol* **236**: R198–205.

Southwick SM, Morgan CA, Darnell A, Bremner D, Nicolaou AL, Nagy LM, Charney DS (1995) Trauma-related symptoms in veterans of Operation Desert Storm: A 2-year follow-up. *Am J Psychiatry* **152**: 1150–1155.

Southwick SM, Yehuda R, Giller EL (1993) Personality disorders in treatment seeking combat veterans with posttraumatic stress disorder. *Am J Psychiatry* **150**: 1020–1023.

Spivak B, Trottern SF, Mark M, Bleich A, Weizman A (1992) Acute transient stress-induced hallucinations in soldiers. *Br J Psychiatry* **160**: 412–414.

Stebbins WC, Smith OA (1964) Cardiovascular concomitants of the conditioned emotional response in the monkey. *Science* **144**: 881–883.

Stock G, Schlör KH, Heidt H, Buss J (1978) Psychomotor behaviour and cardiovascular patterns during stimulation of the amygdala. *Pflügers Archiv (Eur J Physiol)* **376**: 177–184.

Trimble MR (1981) *Post-traumatic Neurosis. From Railway Spine to the Whiplash.* Chichester: John Wiley & Sons.

True WR, Rice J, Eisen SA, Heath AC, Goldberg J, Lyons MJ (1993) A twin study of genetic and environmental contributions to liability for posttraumatic stress symptoms. *Am J Psychiatry* **50**: 257–264.

Van Dyke C, Zilberg NJ, McKinnon J (1985) Posttraumatic stress disorder: A thirty year delay in a World War II veteran. *Am J Psychiatry* **142**: 1070–1073.

Van der Hart O, Horst R (1989) The dissociation theory of Pierre Janet. *J Trauma Stress* **2**: 397–412.

Van der Kolk BA, Brown P, Van der Hart O (1989) Pierre Janet on post-traumatic stress. *J Trauma Stress* **2**: 365–376.

Van der Kolk BA, Hostetler A, Herron N, Fisler RE (1994) Trauma and the development of borderline personality disorder. *Psychiatr Clin North Am* **17**: 715–729.

Van der Kolk BA, Perry C, Herman JL (1991) Childhood origins of self-destructive behavior.

Am J Psychiatry **148**: 1665–1671.

Van der Kolk BA, Van der Hart O (1989) Pierre Janet and the breakdown of adaptation in psychological trauma. *Am J Psychiatry* **146**: 1530–1540.

Van Praag HM (1990) Two-tier diagnosing in psychiatry. *Psychiatr Res* **34**: 1–11.

Van Praag HM (1995) Functional psychopathology: An essential step in biological psychiatric research. In Goekoop JG, Hengeveld MW, Spinhoven Ph (eds) *Multidimensionele benaderingen in de psychiatrie. (Multidimensional Approaches in Psychiatry)*. Leiden: Boerhaave Commissie voor Postacademisch Onderwijs in de Geneeskunde, Rijksuniversiteit Leiden, pp. 29–38.

Van Praag HM (1996) Serotonin-related, anxiety/aggression-driven, stressor-precipitated depression: A psycho-biological hypothesis. *Eur Psychiatry* **11**: 57–67.

Wozniak J, Harding Crawford M, Biederman J, Faraone SV, Spencer TJ, Taylor, Blier HK (1999) Antecedents and complications of trauma in boys with ADHD: Findings from a longitudinal study. *J Am Acad Child Adolesc Psychiatry* **38**: 48–55.

Yehuda R, McFarlane AC, Shalev AY (1998) Predicting the development of posttraumatic stress disorder from the acute response to a traumatic event. *Biol Psychiatry* **44**: 1305–1313.

Yonkers KA, Ellison JM (1996) Anxiety disorders in women and their pharmacological treament. In Jensvold MF, Halbreich U, Hamilton JA (eds) *Psychopharmacology and Women*. Washington, DC: American Psychiatric Press, pp. 261–285.

Zanarini MC, Frankenburg FR, Dubo ED, Sickel AE, Trikha A, Levin A, Reynolds V (1998) Axis I comorbidity of borderline personality disorder. *Am J Psychiatry* **155**: 1733–1739.

12

The Psychobiology of Post-Traumatic Stress Disorder

W.S. de Loos

Central Military Hospital, Utrecht, The Netherlands

NEUROANATOMY AND BRAIN AREA FUNCTION

Important findings on the psychobiology of post-traumatic stress disorder (PTSD) reported in the literature during the past 10 years cover a wide range of subjects. The limbic system and especially the amygdala have a critical role in the process of comparing sensory imput to stored memory and organising psychological processes and motor and physiological output (LeDoux, 1998). It has become clear that traumatic experience changes the limbic system and other parts of the brain not only functionally, but also anatomically at a submicroscopic, microscopic and even gross anatomical level. It seems that severe and overwhelming input into the system may cause loss of connections and even cell death (McEwen et al., 1992). Several studies have reported decreased hippocampal volume on the right side (Bremner et al., 1995) and functional studies have shown increased activity in the amygdala of the right hemisphere and decreased activation of Broca's area, suggesting a decreased capacity to put experiences into communicable language (Van der Kolk et al., 1995). This seems to support the more or less obligatory observation of alexithymia in PTSD patients, their inability to express emotions effectively (Sifneos, 1973; Krystal, 1988). Decreased hippocampal volume is also associated with functional deficits in verbal (declarative) memory (Yehuda et al., 1995a). Left hippocampal volume reduction has been found after childhood abuse without the reported correlation with short-term verbal memory deficits (Bremner et al., 1997a; Stein et al., 1997). The explanation offered for this discrepancy is that neuronal plasticity in the very young has the effect that short-term memory functions normally mediated by the hippocampus are partially taken over by other brain structures. A decrease in hippocampal volume has not been found in all studies of this kind but other gross anatomical differences were then found in a study of traumatised children, e.g. smaller intracranial and cerebral volumes negatively correlating with abuse duration. More specifically, a gender by diagnosis effect revealed greater corpus callosum area (middle and posterior regions)

Anxiety Disorders: An Introduction to Clinical Management and Research. Edited by E. J. L. Griez, C. Faravelli, D. Nutt and J. Zohar. © 2001 John Wiley & Sons, Ltd.

reduction in males (De Bellis et al., 1999b) which also suggests a link with the problem of lateralisation in PTSD for which evidence has been found at a neurophysiological level (Brende, 1992; Schiffer et al., 1995; Spivak et al., 1998).

The results of functional anatomical studies using positron or single photon emission are not very conclusive either. They point to involvement of the ventral anterior cingulate gyrus and the right amygdala (increased regional blood flow during exposure to combat-related stimuli) and suppression of Broca's area function (also reported by others (Van der Kolk et al., 1995) in one study (Shin et al., 1997), activation of the left amygdala and nucleus accumbens during trauma-related stimulation in another (Liberzon et al., 1999a), while a third found a decrease in blood flow in the medial prefrontal cortex (area 25), which is relevant for inhibiting amygdala function and extinction of fear conditioning (see LeDoux, 1998), and a less than normal activation of the anterior cingulate (area 24) contrasting with the finding mentioned before (Bremner et al., 1999).

NEUROPHYSIOLOGY

Kindling

A basic neurophysiological concept for the understanding of the phenomena of intrusive memory, traumatic nightmares, acoustic startle, etc. is long-term potentation (Teyler and DiScenna, 1987; Lynch et al., 1988) or the kindling model of epilepsia (Racine, 1978; Adamec, 1990; Wolf et al., 1990; Post et al., 1995). In fact, traumatic dissociative or intrusive memory phenomena have many features in common with complex behavioural attacks or temporal epilepsy. Although speculative, it is conceivable that under certain conditions very strong sensory input may develop into limbic seizures. In panic disorder with agoraphobia some support has been found to link this condition to complex partial epilepsy under the hypothesis that there may be a common neurophysiological substrate (Toni et al., 1996).

Event-related Potentials

Scalp-recorded event-related potentials (ERPs) are the reflections of patterned neural activity associated with information processing in the brain. Subjects are told to detect infrequent, target (task-relevant) stimuli and ignore other, non-target stimuli. The P3 or P300 component is recorded as a positive deflection typically occurring between 300 and 900 msec. and reflects the selective perceptual process used in identifying stimulus relevance. The P300 is affected by the personal meaningfulness of the stimulus to the subject. In a study comparing veterans with and without PTSD, combat-related pictures as non-target stimuli enhanced P300 deflections in PTSD subjects while P300 latencies and reaction times to target stimuli were prolonged. It points to an altered state of early and late cognitive selective attention and confirms the vulnerability to traumatic reminiscences (Attias et al., 1996a). It even proved possible to discriminate PTSD patients and controls, classifying 90% of the patients and 85% of the controls correctly (Attias et al., 1996b). In addition, in survivors of road traffic accident with mild head injury, accident-related words produced a P300 that was very significantly higher in PTSD patients and that correlated well with state of anxiety (Granovsky et al., 1998). Non-target traumatic pictorial stimuli initially produced earlier and approximately five times greater P300 amplitudes but showed amplitude reduction and latency prolongation on repetition. This effect was not observed for target stimuli. It points to the activation of an inhibitory mechanism related to the cognitive processing of traumatic stimuli (Bleich et al., 1996).

In an attempt to resolve the conflicting results, with respect to whether the abnormal physiologic responses in PTSD reflect a general abnormality or are restrictively linked to trauma-related stimuli, a differential analysis was made in survivors of a ship fire with and without PTSD and other manifest or subclinical psychiatric diagnoses for word and non-word (complex) stimuli with respect to intrusion, arousal and avoidance. The complex (non-word) stimuli were thought to be causing attenuated amplitudes at an early stage after stimulus onset (100–150 msec.), a higher positive amplitude in the 200–300 msec. time period and to be related to intrusion. Arousal and avoidance were related to emotionally meaningful words and correlated independently to P300 amplitude, suggesting that avoidance and arousal have another neurobiological basis than intrusion (Blomhoff et al., 1998). The findings of this study in ERP abnormalities preceding the P300 seem to correspond with findings in sexually assaulted women with PTSD in whom the ERP phase at 50–300 msec., described as mismatch negativity, in response to auditory non-word (tone) stimuli was found to be increased. It was concluded that there should be abnormalities in preconscious auditory sensory memory in PTSD (Morgan and Grillon, 1999) in addition to the abnormalities in conscious processing reported in earlier studies. It thus seems as if this is a general abnormality not linked to trauma-related stimuli.

STARTLE

Acoustic startle is an oligo-synaptic response mediated through the cochlear root neurons to the nucleus reticularis pontis caudalis in the brain stem, where pre-pulse inhibition by higher structures via the pedunculopontine tegmental nucleus can occur, to spinal and facial motor neurons resulting in eye-blink and body movements. It occurs at about 300 msec., well within conscious reaction time. Pre-pulse inhibition and habituation of the startle response are stable neurobiological properties of the normal population (Ornitz and Guthrie, 1989; Cadenhead et al., 1999), even in periods of war stress (Shalev et al., 1996). Deficiency of pre-pulse inhibition has been reported for numerous psychiatric disorders (Ornitz et al., 1999). Both clinically and in the laboratory, acoustic startle is a striking phenomenon in post-traumatic syn-dromes (Butler et al., 1990; Paige et al., 1990; Shalev et al., 1992; Shalev and

Rogel-Fuchs, 1992; Orr et al., 1995; Morgan et al., 1996; Orr et al., 1997). Also in children with PTSD, acoustic startle shows little tendency to habituation and shows decreased pre-pulse inhibition (Ornitz and Pynoos, 1989). Conflicting results in the demonstration of increased startle in PTSD patients may be a consequence of different baseline conditions at experimentation. Increased startle is perhaps not a chronic condition in PTSD but the consequence of a greater conditioned emotional response triggered by anticipation of the test situation. Hence, emotionally charged test procedures can be especially informative in distinguishing PTSD patients from other diagnostic groups (Morgan et al., 1995; Grillon et al., 1998a). However, some test circumstances may result in specific aversively conditioned reactions that are independent from PTSD, such as darkness increasing startle responses in all combat veterans independently (Grillon et al., 1998b). An interesting result was obtained when the increased startle response was replicated in right-handed women with sexual assault trauma one to 27 years previously. In addition to the expected result, asymmetry was found with greater responses for the left orbicularis oculi EMG confirming a laterality effect that has been found with different methods as well (Brende, 1992; Schiffer et al., 1995; Spivak et al., 1998). The adrenergic α_2-receptor is thought to play a role in the generation of the startle response, especially its α_{2C}-subtype as has been found in transgenic mice (Sallinen et al., 1998). The increase of PTSD symptomatology by yohimbine, an α_2-receptor antagonist (Southwick et al., 1993a; Southwick et al., 1999), and the decrease of startle responses in a child by clonidine, an α_2-receptor agonist (Ornitz and Pynoos, 1989), are concordant with this finding.

OLFACTORY STIMULI

Another interesting limbic phenomenon is the EEG response to odours significantly associated with traumatic experience (McCaffrey et al., 1993). As is the case in acoustic startle, the alarm centre of the central nervous system cannot be shut off from olfactory input. Mammals do have eyelids but no ear lids or nose lids. Also clinically, odours prove to be very strong triggers for conditioned emotional responses.

CIRCULATORY, SYMPATHETIC AND MOTOR RESPONSES

Base-line Blood Pressure and Heart Rate

The development of physical disease after and caused by emotional experience or traumatic life events has always been intriguing, to the public even more so than to clinical medicine. It is a domain of complex interactions and the much needed prospective follow-up studies have rarely been possible to carry out. Raised blood pressure or hypertension is outstandingly such a domain. It has been shown, now, that veterans with PTSD and no premorbid or familial burden with hypertension who were compared with veterans without PTSD, had significantly higher heart rate and diastolic blood pressure to a degree that is substantial in epidemiological terms (Muraoka et al., 1998). Orthostatic challenging yielded a more or less comparable result. Diastolic blood pressure failed to decrease over time after standing up in medication-free combat veterans with PTSD studied at their homes (Orr et al., 1998a). Analysis of heart rate variability by means of power spectrum analysis again showed higher heart rates and lower heart rate variability at rest. This was interpreted as an indication of lower cardiac parasympathetic tone and elevated sympathetic activity (Cohen et al., 1997).

Psychophysiological Testing (HR, GSR, EMG)

In laboratory settings cardiovascular and other psychophysiological responses, mainly galvanic skin response (GSR) and electromyography (EMG), to stimuli of various kind have been studied extensively. Many studies have demonstrated strong specific responses of blood pressure and especially heart rate to startling aspecific noises and to individually significant sensory input in subjects with PTSD, combat veterans from various war theatres (Pallmeyer et al., 1986; Pitman et al., 1989; Blanchard, 1990; Blanchard et al., 1991a), and in other populations of trauma survivors (Shalev et al., 1993; Shalev et al., 1997). In addition, in Rorschach testing, the projection of traumatic content elicited significant increases in skin conductance (sympathetic activation) and heart rate (Goldfinger et al., 1998).

Vasopressin and oxytocin are two hormones of the central nervous system (neuropeptides) that are of special importance in memory processing. Behavioural and cardiovascular conditioning in animals has shown that vasopressin increases the retention of, both appetitive and aversive memory while oxytocin in low doses has the opposite effect (Bohus et al., 1978; Wan et al., 1992). Similar results have been demonstrated in humans with PTSD with respect to psychophysiological parameters in relation to personal traumatic imagery, most specifically exerted by vasopressin on EMG (Pitman et al., 1993).

Yohimbine, an α_2-adrenergic receptor antagonist that activates noradrenergic neurons, e.g. in the locus coeruleus, hippocampus and amygdala, increased systolic blood pressure significantly more in PTSD subjects than in healthy controls, especially when they had a flashback and/ or a panic reaction after administration of this drug. The same occurred with heart rate which showed no significant response in the controls (Southwick et al., 1993a).

Psychophysiological responses to specific stimuli have been shown to discriminate PTSD from non-PTSD subjects but not to an extent to make it feasible for clinical diagnosis, let alone for medico-legal purposes (Blanchard et al., 1986; Pitman et al., 1987; Keane et al., 1998; Orr et al., 1998b). Response specificity has always been an intriguing issue in psychophysiology and psychotraumatology has not failed us in this respect. Comparison of stimuli related to the diagnosis of PTSD (combat sounds) with the threat of painful electric shocks during a memory task and the presentation of standardised emotionally negative visual stimulation produced the expected result of hyperresponsivity of PTSD subjects to trauma-specific stimuli (Casada et al., 1998). The analysis of heart rate variability as an assessment of differential autonomic activation did not confirm the hypothesis of specific responsiveness unconditionally. PTSD patients demonstrated a degree of autonomic dysregulation at rest that was comparable to that seen in the control subjects' reactions to stress and they seemed unable to marshal a further and more differentiated stress response (Cohen et al., 1998).

OPIOIDS

Addiction to the trauma is a clinical phenomenon in many PTSD patients that was poorly understood until the role of the opioid peptides was discovered. Pain-induced analgesia was known as an experimental model in pharmacology for a considerable time and has been extended, later, to stress-induced analgesia (Van der Kolk and Saporta, 1991; Glover, 1992). It can be blocked with the classical morphine antagonist naloxone. There are indications that flashbacks and other dissociative phenomena in PTSD patients and emotional numbing are opioid-mediated phenomena that can be blocked by naloxone (Van der Kolk et al., 1989; Pitman et al., 1990). Improvement of many PTSD symptoms has been reported after the administration of nalmefene (Glover, 1993), a relative pure opioid -receptor antagonist more potent than naloxone (Reisine and Pasternak, 1996). It is possible although speculative at this moment that clinical phenomena like dissociation, auto-mutilation and conditioned or self-induced analgesia like the fakir syndrome are mental states in which the opioids play an important role. A puzzling finding is that plasma levels of -endorphin, both in the morning and the evening, were found in one study to be lower than in controls (Hoffman et al., 1989). In this same study morning cortisol levels in PTSD subjects were higher than in controls which is at variance with most later findings (see below). The above reported opioid responses to traumatic flashbacks were not accompanied in that study by detectable changes of opioids in the general circulation (B.A. van der Kolk, personal communication). The effects may well be confined to the CNS compartment exclusively. Again, the connection to the hypothalamic-pituitary-adrenal axis is to be considered in the light of its inhibition by opioids at the hypothalamic level (Hockings et al., 1994).

NIGHTMARES

Traumatic nightmares belong to the core symptoms of PTSD. The differential diagnosis of parasomnias (Driver and Shapiro, 1993) in PTSD includes three relevant categories:

1. Night terrors (*pavor nocturnus* and *incubus*) occur during slow wave sleep, predominantly during the first few sleep cycles when slow wave sleep phases are longer; the person does not report to have been dreaming but very suddenly awakens in terror.
2. Anxious dreams or rapid eye movement (REM) sleep nightmares occur during the longer stretches of REM sleep, typically during the last few sleep cycles; these dreams may contain fantasy material and all aspects of condensation characteristic of normal dreaming.
3. Post-traumatic nightmares, or better nightly flashbacks, are not related to any specific sleep stage and occur during all stages of sleep, even slumber sleep. Characteristically, they represent a true memory in which the subject is the actor, not an observer (Schreuder, 1996). They are accompanied by autonomic and motoric arousal like sweating, a pounding heart, hyperventilation (breathlessness), teeth grinding (bruxism), groaning and other vocalisations, gross body movements and even fighting. Awakening is not obligatory and, if it occurs, it does not prevent the nightmare from continuing when the person stays in bed to sleep again. On a phenomenological basis, it is not possible to distinguish between these and flashbacks during daytime; they may be the same from a neurophysiological point of view.

An increasing body of evidence points to disturbances in the electrophysiology of sleep in PTSD, as expressed by REM sleep, slow wave sleep, nightly awakenings, etc. REM sleep is increased in percentage, density, average activity and period duration, not in cycle length, suggesting changes in phasic event generation (Ross et al.,1994), while REM sleep significantly precedes symptomatic awakenings (Mellman et al., 1995). Consistent with this, slow wave sleep is decreased (Fuller et al., 1994).

NEUROENDOCRINOLOGY AND NEUROTRANSMITTERS

Feedback Systems

Many studies have addressed the complex interplay between the sympatho-adrenomedullary system and the hypothalamic-pituitary-adrenocortical (HPA) axis. In most studies, PTSD is characterised by increased norepinephrine (NE) release (Kosten et al., 1987; Blanchard et al., 1991b) on the one hand, but decreased total daily cortisol production (Mason et al., 1986; Yehuda et al., 1990a; Yehunda et al., 1995b) and circulating cortisol levels on the other (Yehuda et al., 1996a; Boscarino, 1996). In one study, lower serum cortisol was paralleled by lowered serum prolactin (Kocijan-Hercigonja et al., 1996). Daily free cortisol excretion was found to be normal at group level but to correlate inversely with intrusive PTSD symptoms in one study (Baker et al., 1999), while it was increased similar to patients with major depression and without any correlation to symptoms in another (Maes et al., 1998). One difference of the last study with the previous one is that it was done in civilians with a majority of females without control for menstrual cycle phase while most of the previous studies were done in male combat veterans. It was also argued that single traumatic events might cause an increased HPA-axis response while repetitive and prolonged trauma might do the opposite. Some support for this view can be found in other research but this problem has not been solved satisfactorily.

In concordance to the release rates reported above, α_2-adrenergic receptors are down-regulated (Perry et al., 1987; Yehuda et al., 1990b) and glucocorticoid receptors are up-regulated (Yehuda et al., 1991; Yehuda et al, 1995c). Norepinephrine release and the up-regulation of glucocorticoid receptors correlate with the severity of PTSD symptomatology (Kellner et al., 1997).

Comorbidity: PTSD and Depression

In PTSD the efficacy of glucocorticoid feedback is increased as demonstrated by a significantly enhanced dexamethasone suppression in comparison to normals (Kudler et al., 1987; Yehuda et al., 1993; Heim et al., 1998) and it is opposite to depression (which is known for its dexamethasone non-suppression). One would even conclude that PTSD and biological depression as defined in this neuro-endocrine way exclude one another. However, many studies describe comorbidity of PTSD and major depressive disorder (MDD) (Shalev et al., 1998), not merely dysthymia. It should be kept in mind that a biological definition of depression is not fully concordant with a psychological one. Individuals with PTSD and comorbid depression are still better-than-normal suppressors but less than having PTSD alone (Yehuda et al., 1993). The enhanced negative feedback of cortisol is not reflected by lower levels of circulating adrenocorticotropic hormone (ACTH), but the pituitary capacity to release ACTH is markedly enhanced which excludes pituitary insufficiency and confirms the increased feedback sensitivity (Yehuda et al., 1996b).

The comorbidity of PTSD and depression seems to influence circulating plasma levels of NE, but not 3-methoxy-4-hydroxyphenylglycol (MHPG or MOPEG) (Yehuda et al., 1998a), which can be considered as a metabolic parameter of central NE turnover, reflecting spillover from the CSF compartment into the systemic circulation (Webster, 1989). Nevertheless, increases in plasma MHPG after administration of yohimbine (see section Circulatory Responses) have been found in subjects with PTSD to exceed the increases in healthy controls. The effect was stronger in PTSD subjects experiencing panic (14 out of 20) and flashbacks (8 of these) induced by the drug (Southwick et al., 1993a). The paralleling differences in circulatory response (systolic blood pressure and heart rate) have been mentioned above. Yohimbine is also reported to induce marked exacerbation of anxiety/panic and PTSD-specific symptoms immediately after ingestion in a natural setting (Southwick et al., 1999), which confirms my clinical experience in veterans with PTSD to whom this medication was prescribed by the urologist for erection problems.

The high levels of NE in PTSD are interpreted as reflecting high sympathetic activity, which corresponds with many findings on cardiovascular stimulation and galvanic skin response (GSR) reactivity. A positive correlation between intrusive PTSD symptoms and urinary excretion of the catecholamines dopamine and epinephrine points in the same direction (Yehuda et al., 1992). Thus, on one hand, post-traumatic stress disorder with or without accompanying symptoms of depression seems to be characterised by sympatho-adrenal arousal, which is reflected by increased cardiovascular responsiveness and sweat gland activation as signs of the defence reaction, the paradigm of active survival strategy; on the other hand, it is characterised by a decrease in the conservation-withdrawal response and its catabolic survival hormone cortisol that induces the organism to consume its intrinsic resources, while waiting for better times.

CRH Testing

The response of ACTH to CRH has been found to be blunted in PTSD as in depression, panic disorder and anorexia nervosa, and to result in slightly but not significantly lower cortisol responses (Smith et al., 1989). This cannot be understood as a feedback effect of functional hypercortisolism as in depression (Gold et al., 1988).

Children: CRH Testing and Urine Sampling

The neuroendocrine pattern in children has not been investigated as intensively as in adults. In one study CRH testing was performed in children aged seven to 15 years old who were living in a stable and safe environment but who had been sexually abused one to 12 years earlier. Some of them had concurrent dysthymia and suicidal ideation and had attempted suicide but none of them was reported to have PTSD. They showed smaller than normal ACTH responses but nonetheless normal cortisol responses to this (De Bellis et al., 1994), which resembles the result found in adults.

A very different finding is the increased ACTH response to CRH in abused children who experienced ongoing chronic adversity and were rated as depressed. They differed from abused depressive children living in a stable environment, depressive non-abused controls and healthy children who all showed the same ACTH response. The increased ACTH response in the first group was not followed by an increased cortisol response, which thereby was the same in all four groups (Kaufman et al., 1997).

A group of children of the same age (8-13) with PTSD was compared with normal controls and children with overanxious disorder. Childhood PTSD was associated with greater comorbid psychopathology including depressive and dissociative symptoms, lower global assessment of functioning and increased suicidal ideation and suicide attempts. The children in this group excreted significantly greater amounts of urinary dopamine and norepinephrine per day than in both comparison groups. Their free cortisol excretion was equal to that of the overanxious group but exceeded the controls. Catecholamine and cortisol excretion was correlated to the duration of traumatisation and to PTSD symptoms (De Bellis et al., 1999a).

It is unclear what the discrepancies between these studies and the results found in adults imply. One of the possibilities is that the psychobiological development stage is a critical factor. Also in a broader sense, age may be a factor influencing the HPA-axis response to challenge (Seeman and Robbins, 1994). Repetition or perseverance of traumatisation is likely to influence the neurohumoral response to it as has been observed in rape victims (Resnick et al., 1995). Other possibilities accounting for the discrepancies are that the studies were done on non-patients and patients with different diagnoses (diagnosing PTSD in young children poses its own difficulties), sample sizes, time of the day and baseline values.

Systems Integration

No convincing correlation has been found between HPA-axis activity in the morning, when it is as high in PTSD patients as in controls, and circulating catecholamines or psychophysiologic parameters like GSR (which reflects sympathetic activity), heart rate or frontalis EMG (Liberzon et al., 1999b). The conclusion was drawn, then, that no integrated multisystem stress response occurred in PTSD, and this conclusion is supported by other findings when the HPA-axis response was studied in connection with CNS noradrenergic activity as represented by MHPG spillover (Goenjian et al., 1996; Yehuda et al., 1998b). This may seem but is not necessarily at variance with the above-described findings on the HPA-axis and catecholamine activity. It means that within an individual these systems are not being coupled per single event. This conclusion is in concordance with the insight that the sympatho-adrenal response system and the HPA-axis are not connected to each other through the activation of CRH, as this neurohormone or neuromodulator acts at different locations in the CNS independently, in different circuits and functions (Schulkin et al., 1998). CRH gene expression in the central nucleus of the amygdala and the bed nucleus of the stria terminalis (BNST) is dissociated from that of the paraventricular nucleus of the hypothalamus which is the classical top of the HPA-axis organisation. Direct application of CRH by infusion into the third ventricle induces multiple physiological stress responses like increase of plasma epinephrine, norepinephrine, glucose and glucagon, of mean arterial blood pressure and heart rate, and inhibition of gastric acid production, all by autonomic nervous system activation (Lenz et al., 1987). Naloxone or a vasopressin antagonist could in part, inhibit the gastric inhibition. This implies involvement of an opioid neuropeptide as a neuromodulator, e.g. a pro-opiomelanocortin (POMC) derived endorphin (De Wied, 1999). The possibility of a relation with dissociation and flashback-related analgesia is intriguing within this context (Pitman et al., 1990). The role of vasopressin is interesting from the viewpoint of its role in the consolidation of memory (Bohus et al., 1978; Chepkova et al., 1995), including the psychophysiologic concomitants of emotional memory (Bohus et al., 1983; Pitman et al., 1993) and its role in the potentiation of CRH-induced ACTH release (Scott et al., 1999).

The Role of CRH

The question of the specificity of CRH activity in the CNS is of special importance in the case of PTSD as higher levels of this neurohormone have been found in the cerebrospinal fluid of patients compared to controls, which may seem paradoxical at first sight given the increased feedback sensitivity of the system (Bremner et al., 1997b; Baker et al., 1999). CRH in the CSF is mainly of extrahypothalamic origin, not related to HPA-axis activity (Garrick et al., 1987). Interestingly, this was accompanied in patients, but not in controls, by positively correlated CSF levels of somatostatin, which often acts as an inhibitory hormone or neuromodulator both in the CNS and peripherally, but its role in these particular circumstances is unclear. It is also unclear, at this point, what actually causes the increased feedback sensitivity within the HPA-axis and whether stimulation of this axis at the level of CRH production by the paraventricular nucleus (PVN) of the hypothalamus is decreased. As mentioned above, the elevated CRH levels in the cerebrospinal fluid are not likely to be generated by the PVN but to be due to spillover from the central amygdala, the bed nucleus of the stria terminalis and possibly also the locus coeruleus. The latter three nuclei have important roles in organising or mediating vigilance, arousal and anxiety reactions and they activate both the central norepinephric system and the sympathetic nervous system (Lenz et al., 1987). Central norepinephric system activation has not systematically been demonstrated (Yehuda et al., 1998b). However, frequently repeated activation of the sympathetic nervous system is a general feature of chronic PTSD. Next to PTSD symptoms, panic and flashbacks, yohimbine challenge has indeed produced increases in systolic blood pressure and heart rate, but also MHPG as a putative parameter of central norepinehrine activation (Southwick et al., 1993a).

HPA-axis Regulation

One of the options for increased HPA feedback sensitivity is increased glucocorticoid receptor function in the hippocampus, which is an important centre for control over the HPA-axis function (Meaney et al., 1989). The hippocampus with its dense population of glucocorticoid receptors is now broadly recognised as the top of the system by exerting inhibitory control over hypothalamic CRH production (Jacobson and Sapolsky, 1991). Glucocorticoid receptors may have been up-regulated, conforming to a theory derived from the model of neonatal handling in rats, in which attenuation of stress responses in adulthood has been observed (Levine, 1957; Denenberg, 1964). This model has been differentiated by more recent studies that individual differences in caring behaviour by the mother animal after separation from the litter are responsible for differential effects of such handling. The better the caring attention of the mother after replacement of the pup into the litter, the higher the glucocorticoid receptor density in the hippocampus and the more efficacious the feedback of circulating glucocorticoid hormone (Liu et al., 1997; Sapolsky, 1997). This process is thought to have a protective effect on the hippocampus against later damage by high glucocorticoid responses under environmental stress, "allostasis" as it was named by Charles Kahn (see: Sterling and Eyer, 1988) or the "allostatic load" (McEwen, 1998). The hippocampal atrophy found in PTSD, as in depression and Cushing's disease (Sapolsky, 1996), is not compatible with such protection if, indeed, the damage is due to high glucocorticoid responses under traumatic circumstances.

Atrophy of the Hippocampus

The smaller volume of the hippocampus, found in several PTSD studies (see section Neuroanatomy), is enigmatic in the light of the above-mentioned atrophy found in MDD and Cushing's disease with their increased levels of cortisol, which is the opposite of what is thought to be happening in PTSD. There is not much doubt about the potential harm of glucocorticoids for the hippocampus, especially the pyramidal cells and dendritic outgrowth and sprouting. It has been postulated that the impact of the initial aversive experience may trigger damaging levels of glucocorticoid release thus causing the observed atrophy in PTSD (Bremner, 1999). Other causes of neuronal damage are excitatory amino acid neurotransmitters, especially glutamate, via its N-methyl-D-aspartate (NMDA) receptor and possibly also its kanainate type feedforward autoreceptor, and serotonin which may also potentate the NMDA receptor (McEwen and Magariños, 1997). Neuroprotection by GABA-ergic inhibition or by neurotrophins (NT) such as brain-derived neurotrophic factor (BDNF) and NT-3 may decrease under certain stressful circumstances.

A postulated consequence of hippocampal atrophy with respect to the striking down-tuning of the HPA-axis, is the putative disinhibition of CRH release from the PVN, which then should result in CRH receptor down-regulation in the pituitary and thereby cause a decrease of ACTH stimulation. From the viewpoint of classical endocrinology, however, it seems improbable that this would result in an absolute decrease of ACTH release from the pituitary, instead of an attenuated increase, and hence produce a decrease of cortisol release from the adrenal and, finally, an enhanced glucocorticoid feedback effect. Continuous hormonal overstimulation at a pharmacological level does produce receptor down-regulation and a sharp and almost complete decline of end-organ activity. This is applied in the treatment of prostate cancer by the use of a long-acting LHRH agonist that down-regulates testosterone production to almost zero, but in physiological circumstances it is not known to occur and the neuroendocrinology of major depression with its increased activity of the HPA-axis does not confirm this either. Moreover, experiments in primates examining the effects of lesions of the hippocampus and other related structures produced chronic glucocorticoid hypersecretion lasting six to 15 months (Sapolsky et al., 1991).

Somatostatin, Vasopressin and the HPA-axis

Thus, there must be other reasons for the opposite characteristics of PTSD and MDD with respect to the HPA-axis. The inhibitory neuropeptide somatostatin has already been mentioned and in the CSF, its levels were found to be correlated with CRH levels in PTSD patients but not in controls (Bremner et al., 1997b). Vasopressin is another candidate for discriminating PTSD and MDD, although this may be part of a very complex pattern of interaction. Vasopressin potentates the release of ACTH (Antoni, 1993; Aguilera, 1998) and it has been shown to co-occur with CRH in the median eminence in a way modulated by neonatal handling and stress (Bhatnagar and Meaney, 1995). It also has an important role in the consolidation of memory (De Wied, 1999) and could play a role in the conditioned physiologic responses found in PTSD (Pitman et al., 1993). Arginine vasopressin (AVP) is secreted into the median eminence where it enters the portal blood circulation that brings it to the pituitary. Experiments in rats have shown that this is controlled indepently from CRH by axonal transport through AVP containing versus AVP deficient CRH neurons, and that under conditions of chronic or repeated stress plastic changes in hypothalamic CRH neurons evolve, resulting in increased AVP stores and co-localization in CRH nerve terminals (De Goeij et al., 1991). Also under conditions of chronic or intermittent stressful stimulation, a shift in hypothalamic signals for ACTH release in favour of AVP may ensue as it has been found in rats (De Goeij et al., 1992).

Experimental analysis in rats at the level of CRH and AVP responses in the PVN measured by primary transcript (heteronuclear) RNA and messenger RNA has confirmed that there is a desensitisation of CRH, but not AVP transcription responses to repeated restraint stress. It has also been demonstrated that animals adapted to a chronic homotypic stress show a greater response of CRH and AVP gene transcription in the parvocellular PVN after a novel, heterotypic stress. The hypothalamus clearly has the flexibility to adapt to homotypic stress while at the same time maintaining its ability to respond to novel stressors (Ma et al., 1999). These experiments show that, as to the responses of the HPA-axis, vasopressin is a mediator for the discrimination between chronic and acute, homotypic and heterotypic stressors, which, to some extent, can be controlled independently from CRH. In human depression not only an increase in CRH expressing neurones in the PVN was found, but also an increased co-expression of AVP and of AVP *per se* (Hoogendÿk et al., 2000). If PTSD is indeed the mirror image of depression it seems to be, the enhanced feedback of cortisol on the hypothalamus should be the result of parallel inhibition by another central mechanism.

Glucocorticoid Receptor Gene Polymorphism

A possibility that has not been considered by researchers in the field of the psychobiology of PTSD until now is the existence of a receptor polymorphism accounting for lower than expected circulating levels of cortisol and increased dexamethasone feedback sensitivity. In an epidemiological field study of an elderly population, a close relationship was found between basal cortisol levels and the feedback sensitivity of the HPA axis to a low dose of dexamethasone, lower cortisol corresponding with higher feedback effect which looks the same, so far, as in PTSD. This suggested a genetic influence on the set point of the HPA axis. Over a $2\frac{1}{2}$-year follow-up period, individual characteristics remained fairly constant, denying an effect of ageing on HPA activity or feedback sensitivity (Huizenga et al., 1998a). Among 216 elderly people, 13 heterozygotes for the N363S glucocorticoid receptor gene polymorphism (codon 363) were identified, showing increased cortisol suppression to 0.25 mg dexamethasone, but no differences in glucocorticoid receptor number or ligand binding affinity on peripheral mononuclear leukocytes (Huizenga et al., 1998b). In PTSD patients, increased receptor numbers on lymphocytes have been found and a correlation with specific symptomatology, which suggests that this is indeed a disease-specific phenomenon (Yehuda et al., 1991). Nevertheless, this finding calls for control of receptor polymorphism in studies on the HPA axis of PTSD patients.

Serotonin

Indirect evidence points to an important role of the serotonin system in the brain in patients with PTSD. Selective serotonin re-uptake inhibitors (SSRIs) are probably the most effective drugs to control a number of very disturbing symptoms in PTSD, especially impulsiveness and anger, and, to a substantial degree, also post-traumatic nightmares. They may be the first choice to be tried (Van der Kolk et al., 1994b). Impulsiveness can be an effective parameter for indication and follow-up (Ørner and De Loos, 1998). The way it is being expressed can vary largely but it is a potent cue in the recognition of socially disrupting symptoms, for both the patients and their families. Loss of temper is a very general phenomenon in PTSD but also panic can be understood as an impulse break-through. Many of these patients are "caged tigers" suffering from unexpressed irritability and anger. From an ethological point of view, rage and panic are closely related phenomena. They presumably have a common centre of organisation in the defence areas of the limbic system. The state of the central serotonergic system can be described at an overall level by decreased tonic activity resulting in increased sensitivity of the postsynaptic receptor systems. Phasic serotonin release would then result in strong responses corresponding with strong defence reactions, i.e. impulsiveness. The concept of receptor down-regulation by increasing the activity of serotonin with re-uptake inhibitors would both account for the initial increase of symptoms and the favourable effect of these agents in chronic application.

PSYCHOPHARMACOLOGIC CONNECTIONS

Useful pharmacological substances applied in the treatment of PTSD are the above-mentioned SSRIs, MAO inhibitors, the anti-kindling drugs carbamazepine and valproate, other serotonergic substances, clonidine, propranolol, anti-opioids and lithium.

REFERENCES

Adamec RE (1990) Does kindling model anything clinically relevant? *Biol Psychiatry* **27**: 249–279.

Aguilera G (1998) Corticotropin releasing hormone, receptor regulation and the stress response. *Trends Endocrinol Metab* **9**: 329–336.

Antoni FA (1993) Vasopressinergic control of pituitary adrenocorticotropin secretion comes of age. *Front Neuroendocrinol* **14**: 76–122.

Attias J, Bleich A, Furman V, Zinger Y (1996a) Event-related potentials in post-traumatic stress disorder of combat origin. *Biol Psychiatry* **40**: 373–381.

Attias J, Bleich A, Gilat S (1996b) Classification of veterans with post-traumatic stress disorder using visual brain evoked P3s to traumatic stimuli. *Br J Psychiatry* **168**: 110–115.

Baker DG, West SA, Nicholson WE, Ekhator NN, Kasckow JW, Hill KK, Bruce AB, Orth DN, Geracioti TD (1999) Serial CSF corticotropin-releasing hormone levels and adrenocortical activity in combat veterans with posttraumatic stress disorder. *Am J Psychiatry* **156**: 585–588.

Bhatnagar S and Meaney MJ (1995) Hypothalamic-pituitary-adrenal function in chronic intermittently cold-stressed neonatally handled and non-handled rats. *J Neuroendocrinol* **7**: 97–108.

Blanchard EB (1990) Elevated basal levels of cardiovascular responses in Vietnam veterans with PTSD: A health problem in the making? *J Anxiety Dis* **4**: 233–237.

Blanchard EB, Kolb LC, Gerardi RJ, Ryan D, Pallmeyer TP (1986) Cardiac response to relevant stimuli as an adjunctive tool for diagnosing posttraumatic stress disorder in Vietnam veterans. *Behav Ther* **17**: 592–606.

Blanchard EB, Kolb LC, Prins A (1991a) Psychophysiologic responses in the diagnosis of posttraumatic stress disorder in Vietnam veterans. *J Nerv Ment Dis* **179**: 97–101.

Blanchard EB, Kolb LC, Prins A, Gates S, McCoy GC (1991b) Changes in plasma norepinephrine to combat-related stimuli among Vietnam veterans with posttraumatic stress disorder. *J Nerv Ment Dis* **179**: 371–373.

Bleich A, Attias J, Furman V (1996) Effect of repeated visual traumatic stimuli on the event related P3 brain potential in post-traumatic stress disorder. *Int J Neurosci* **85**: 45–55.

Blomhoff S, Reinvang I, Malt UF (1998) Event-related potentials to stimuli with emotional impact in posttraumatic stress patients. *Biol Psychiatry* **44**: 1045–1053.

Bohus B, De Jong W, Hagan JJ, De Loos WS, Maas CM, Versteeg CAM (1983) Neuropeptides and steroid hormones in adaptive autonomic processes: implications for psychosomatic disorders. In Endröczi E, De Wied D, Angelucci L, Scapagnini U (eds) *Integrative Neurohumoral Mechanisms: Developments in Neuroscience*. Amsterdam: Elsevier Biomedical Press, **16**: 35–49.

Bohus B, Kovas GL, De Wied D (1978) Oxytocin, vasopressin and memory: Opposite effects on consolidation and retrieval processes. *Brain Res* **157**: 414–417.

Boscarino JA (1996) Posttraumatic stress disorder, exposure to combat, and lower plasma cortisol among Vietnam veterans: findings and implications. *J Consult Clin Psychol* **64**:

191–201.

Bremner JD (1999) Does stress damage the brain? *Biol Psychiatry* **45**: 797–805.

Bremner JD, Licinio J, Darnell A, Krystal JH, Owens MJ, Southwick SM, Nemeroff CB, Charney DS (1997b) Elevated CSF corticotropin-releasing factor concentrations in posttraumatic stress disorder. *Am J Psychiatry* **154**: 624–629.

Bremner JD, Randall P, Scott TM, Bronen RA, Seibyl JP, Southwick SM, Delaney RC, McCarthy G, Charney DS, Innis RB (1995) MRI-based measurement of hippocampal volume in patients with combat-related posttraumatic stress disorder. *Am J Psychiatry* **152**: 973–981.

Bremner JD, Randall P, Vermetten E, Staib L, Bronen RA, Mazure C, Capelli S, McCarthy G, Innis RB, Charney D (1997a) Magnetic resonance imaging-based measurement of hippocampal volume in posttraumatic stress disorder related to childhood physical and sexual abuse: A preliminary report. *Biol Psychiatry* **41**: 23–32.

Bremner JD, Staib LH, Kaloupek D, Southwick SM, Soufer R, Charney DS (1999) Neural correlates of exposure to traumatic pictures and sound in Vietnam combat veterans with and without posttraumatic stress disorder: A positron emission tomography study. *Biol Psychiatry* **45**: 806–816.

Brende JO (1992) Electrodermal responses in post-traumatic syndromes: A pilot study of cerebral hemisphere functioning in Vietnam veterans. *J Nerv Ment Dis* **170**: 352–361.

Butler RW, Braff DL, Rausch JL, Jenkins MA, Sprock J, Geyer MA (1990) Physiologic evidence of exaggerated startle response is a subgroup of Vietnam veterans with combat-related PTSD. *Am J Psychiatry* **147**: 1308–1312.

Cadenhead KS, Carasso BS, Swerlow NR, Geyer MA, Braff DL (1999) Prepulse inhibition and habituation of the startle response are stable neurobiological measures in a normal male population. *Biol Psychiatry* **45**: 360–364.

Casada JH, Amdur R, Larsen R, Liberzon I (1998) Psychophysiologic responsivity in posttraumatic stress disorder: Generalized hyperresponsiveness versus trauma specificity. *Biol Psychiatry* **44**: 1037–1044.

Chepkova AN, French P, De Wied D, Ontskul AH, Ramakers GMJ, Skrebitski VG, Gispen WH, Urban IJA (1995) Long-lasting enhancement of synaptic excitability of CA1/subiculum neurons of rat ventral hippocampus by vasopressin and vasopressin(4-8). *Brain Res* **701**: 255–266.

Cohen H, Kotler M, Matar MA, Kaplan Z, Miodownik H, Cassuto Y (1997) Power spectral analysis of heart rate variability in posttraumatic stress disorder patients. *Biol Psychiatry* **41**: 627–629.

Cohen H, Kotler M, Matar MA, Kaplan Z, Loewenthal U, Miodownik H, Cassuto Y (1998) Analysis of heart rate variability in posttraumatic stress disorder patients in response to a trauma-related reminder. *Biol Psychiatry* **44**: 1054–1059.

De Bellis MD, Baum AS, Birmaher B, Keshavan MS, Eccard CH, Boring AM, Jenkins FJ, Ryan ND (1999a) Developmental traumatology part I: Biological stress systems. *Biol Psychiatry* **45**: 1259–1270.

De Bellis MD, Chrousos GP, Dorn LH, Burke L, Helmers K, Kling MA, Trickett PK, Putnam FW (1994) Hypothalamic-pituitary-adrenal axis dysregulation in sexually abused girls. *J Clin Endocrinol Metab* **78**: 249–255.

De Bellis MD, Keshavan MS, Clark DB, Casey BJ, Giedd JN, Boring AM, Frustaci K, Ryan ND (1999b) Developmental traumatology part II: Brain development. *Biol Psychiatry* **45**: 1271–1284.

De Goeij DCE, Binnekade R, Tilders FJH (1992) Chronic stress enhances vasopressin but not corticotropin-releasing factor secretion during hypoglycaemia. *Am J Physiol* **263**: E394–399.

De Goeij DCE, Kvetnansky R, Whitnall MH, Jezova D, Berkenbosch F, Tilders FJH (1991) Repeated stress-induced activation of corticotropin-releasing factor neurons enhances vasopressin stores and co-colisation with corticotropin-releasing factor in the median eminence of rats. *Neuroendocrinology* **53**: 150–159.

Denenberg VH (1964) Critical periods, stimulus input, and emotional reactivity: A theory of infantile stimulation. *Psychol Rev* **71**: 335–351.

De Wied D (1999) Behavioural pharmacology of neuropeptides related to melanocortins and the neurohypophyseal hormones. *Eur J Pharmacol* **375**: 1–11.

Driver HS, Shapiro CM (1993) Parasomnias. *Br Med J* **306**: 921–924.

Fuller KH, Waters WF, Scott O (1994) An investigation of slow-wave sleep processes in chronic PTSD patients. *J Anxiety Disord* **8**: 227–236.

Garrick NA, Hill JL, Szele FG, Tomai TP, Gold PW, Murphy DL (1987) Corticotropin-releasing factor: A marked circadian rhythm in primate cerebrospinal fluid peaks in the evening and is inversely related to the cortisol circadian rhythm. *Endocrinology* **121**: 1329–1334.

Glover H (1992) Emotional numbing: A possible endorphin-mediated phenomenon associated with post-traumatic stress disorders and other allied psychopathological states. *J Trauma Stress* **5**: 643–675.

Glover H (1993) A preliminary trial of nalmefene for the treatment of emotional numbing in combat veterans with post-traumatic stress disorder. *Isr J Psychiatry Relat Sci* **30**: 255–263.

Goenjian AK, Yehuda R, Pynoos RS, Steinberg AM, Tashjian M, Yang RK, Najarian LM, Fairbanks LA (1996) Basal cortisol, dexamethasone suppression of cortisol, and MHPG in adolescents after the 1988 earthquake in Armenia. *Am J Psychiatry* **153**: 929–934.

Gold PW, Goodwin FK, Chrousos GP (1988) Clinical and biochemical manifestations of depression: Relation to the neurobiology of stress. Part II. *N Engl J Med* **319**: 413–420.

Goldfinger DA, Amdur RL, Liberzon I (1998) Psychophysiologic responses to the Rorschach in PTSD patients, non-combat and combat controls. *Depress Anx* **8**: 112–120.

Granovsky Y, Sprecher E, Hemli J, Yarnitsky D (1998) P300 and stress in mild head injury patients. *Electroencephalography Clin Neurophysiol* **108**: 554–559.

Grillon C, Morgan CA 3rd, Davis M, Southwick SM (1998a) Effects of experimental context and explicit threat cues on acoustic startle in Vietnam veterans with posttraumatic stress disorder. *Biol Psychiatry* **44**: 1027–1036.

Grillon C, Morgan CA 3rd, Davis M, Southwick SM (1998b) Effect of darkness on acoustic startle in Vietnam veterans with PTSD. *Am J Psychiatry* **155**: 812–817.

Heim C, Ehlert U, Hanker JP, Hellhammer DH (1998) Abuse-related posttraumatic stress disorder and alterations of the hypothalamic-pituitary-adrenal axis in women with chronic pelvic pain. *Psychosom Med* **60**: 309–318.

Hockings GI, Jackson RV, Grice JE, Ward WK, Jensen GR (1994) Cell-mediated immunity in combat veterans with post-traumatic stress disorder. *Med J Aust* **161**: 287–288.

Hoffman L, Burges Watson P, Wilson G, Montgomery, J (1989) Low plasma β-endorphin in posttraumatic stress disorder. *Aust N Z J Psychiatry* **23**: 269–273.

Hoogendyk WJG, Meynen G, Eikelenboom P, Swaab DF (2000) Brain alterations in depression. *Acta Neuropsychiatrica* **12**: 54–58.

Huizenga NATM, Koper JW, De Lange P, Pols HAP, Stolk RP, Grobbee DE, De Jong FH, Lamberts SWJ (1998a) Interperson variability but intraperson stability of baseline plasma cortisol concentrations, and its relation to feedback sensitivity of the hypothalamo-pituitary-adrenal axis to a low dose of dexamethasone in elderly individuals. *J Clin Endocrinol Metab* **83**: 47–54.

Huizenga NATM, Koper JW, De Lange P, Pols HAP, Stolk RP, Burger H, Grobbee DE, Brinkmann AO, De Jong FH, Lamberts SWJ (1998b) A polymorphism in the glucocorticoid receptor gene may be associated with an increased sensitivity to glucocorticoids in vivo. *J Clin Endocrinol Metab* **83**: 144–151.

Jacobson L, Sapolsky R (1991) The role of the hippocampus in feedback regulation of the hypothalamic-pituitary-adrenocortical axis. *Endocr Rev* **12**: 118–134.

Kaufman J, Birmaher B, Perel J, Dahl RE, Moreci P, Nelson B, Wells W, Ryan ND (1997) The corticotropin-releasing hormone challenge in depressed abused, depressed non-abused, and normal control children. *Biol Psychiatry* **42**: 669–679.

Keane TM, Kolb LC, Kaloupek DG, Orr SP, Blanchard EB, Thomas RG, Hsieh FY, Lavori PW (1998) Utility of psychophysiological measurement in the diagnosis of posttraumatic stress disorder: Results from a Department of Veterans Affairs Cooperative Study. *J Consult Clin Psychol* **66**: 914–923.

Kellner M, Baker DG, Yehuda R (1997) Salivary cortisol in operation desert storm returnees. *Biol Psychiatry* **42**: 849–850.

Kocijan-Hercigonja D, Sabioncello A, Rijavec M, Folnegovi-Šmalc V, Matijevi Lj, Dunevski I, Tomaši J, Rabati S, Dekaris D (1996) Psychological condition hormone levels in war trauma. *J Psychiatr Res* **30**: 391–399.

Kosten TR, Mason JW, Giller EL, Ostroff RB, Harkness L (1987) Sustained urinary norepinephrine and epinephrine elevation in post-traumatic stress disorder. *Psychoneuroendocrinology* **12**: 13–20.

Krystal H (1988) *Integration and Self-healing: Affect, Trauma, Alexithymia*. With a contribution from JH Krystal. Hillsdale, NJ: Lawrence Erlbaum Associates, Inc.

Kudler H, Davidson J, Mendor K, Lipper S, Ely T (1987) The DST and posttraumatic stress disorder. *Am J Psychiatry* **144**: 1068–1071.

LeDoux J (1998) Fear and the brain: Where have we been, and where are we going? *Biol Psychiatry* **44**: 1229–1238.

Lenz HJ, Raedler A, Greten H, Brown MR (1987) CRF initiates biological actions within the brain that are observed in response to stress. *Am J Physiol* **252**: R34–39.

Levine S (1957) Infantile experience and resistance to physiological stress. *Science* **126**: 405–406.

Liberzon I, Abelson JL, Flagel SB, Raz J, Young EA (1999b) Neuroendocrine and psychophysiologic responses in PTSD: A symptom provocation study. *Neuropsychopharmacology* **21**: 40–50.

Liberzon I, Taylor SF, Amdur R, Jung TD, Chamberlain KR, Minoshima S, Koeppe RA, Fig L (1999a) Brain activation in PTSD in response to trauma-related stimuli. *Biol Psychiatry* **45**: 817–826.

Liu D, Diorio J, Tannenbaum B, Caldji C, Francis D, Freedman A, Sharma S, Pearson D, Plotsky PM, Meaney MJ (1997) Maternal care, hippocampal glucocorticoid receptors, and hypothalamic-pituitary-adrenal responses to stress. *Science* **277**: 1659–1662.

Lynch G, Muller D, Seubert P, Larson L (1988) Long-term potentiation: Persisting problems and recent results. *Brain Res Bull* **21**: 363–372.

Ma XM, Lightman S, Aguilera G (1999) Vasopressin and corticotropin-releasing hormone gene responses to novel stress in rats adapted to repeated restraint. *Endocrinology* **140**: 3623–3632.

Maes M, Lin A, Bonaccorso S, van Hunsel F, van Gastwel, A, Delmeire L, Biondi M, Bosmans E, Kenis G, Scharpé S (1998) Increased 24-hour urinary cortisol excretion in patients with post-traumatic stress disorder and patients with major depression, but not in patients with fibromyalgia. *Acta Psychiatr Scand* **98**: 328–335.

Mason JW, Giller EL, Kosten TR, Ostroff RB, Podd L (1986) Urinary free-cortisol levels in posttraumatic stress disorder patients. *J Nerv Ment Dis* **174**: 145–149.

McCaffrey RJ, Lorig TS, Pendrey DL, McCutcheon NB, Garrett JC (1993) Odor-induced EEG changes in PTSD Vietnam veterans. *J Trauma Stress* **6**: 213–224.

McEwen BS, Gould EA, Sakai RR (1992) The vulnerabililty of the hippocampus to protective and destructive effects of glucocorticoids in relation to stress. *Br J Psychiatry* **160**: 18–24.

McEwen BS (1998) Protective and damaging effects of stress mediators. *N Engl J Med* **338**: 171–179.

McEwen BS, Magariños M (1997) Stress effects on morphology and function of the hippocampus. In Yehuda R, McFarlane AC (eds) *Psychobiology of Posttraumatic Stress Disorder. Ann N Y Acad Sci* **821**: 271–284.

Meaney MJ, Aitken DH, Viau V, Sharma S, Sarrieau A (1989) Neonatal handling alters adrenocortical negative feedback sensitivity and hippocampal type II glucocorticoid receptor binding in the rat. *Neuroendocrinology* 50: 597–604.

Mellman TA, Kulick-Bell R, Ashlock LE, Nolan B (1995) Sleep events among veterans with combat-related posttraumatic stress disorder. *Am J Psychiatry* 152: 110–115.

Morgan CA 3rd, Grillon C (1999) Abnormal mismatch negativity in women with sexual assault-related posttraumatic stress disorder. *Biol Psychiatry* 45: 827–832.

Morgan CA 3rd, Grillon C, Southwick SM, Davis M, Charney DS (1995) Fear-potentiated startle in posttraumatic stress disorder. *Biol Psychiatry* 38: 378–385.

Morgan CA 3rd, Grillon C, Southwick SM, Davis M, Carney DS (1996) Exaggerated acousic startle reflex in Gulf War veterans with posttraumatic stress disorder. *Am J Psychiatry* 153: 64–68.

Muraoka MY, Carlson JG, Chemtob CM (1998) Twenty-four-hour ambulatory blood pressure and heart rate monitoring in combat-related posttraumatic stress disorder. *J Trauma Stress* 11: 473–484.

Ørner RJ, De Loos WS (1998) Second World War veterans with chronic post-traumatic stress disorder. *Adv Psychiat Treatment* 4: 211–218.

Ornitz EM, Guthrie D (1989) Long-term habituation and sensitisation of the acoustic startle response in the normal adult human. *Psychophysiology* 26: 166–173.

Ornitz EM, Pynoos RS (1989) Startle modulation in children with posttraumatic stress disorder. *Am J Psychiatry* 146: 866–870.

Ornitz EM, Russell AT, Hanna GL, Gabikian P, Gehricke JG, Song D, Guthrie D (1999) Prepulse inhibition of startle and the neurobiology of primary nocturnal enuresis. *Biol Psychiatry* 45: 1455–1466.

Orr SP, Lasko NB, Metzger LJ, Berry NJ, Ahern CE, Pitman RK (1998b) Psychophysiologic assessment of women with posttraumatic stress disorder resulting from childhood sexual abuse. *J Consult Clin Psychol* 66: 906–913.

Orr SP, Lasko NB, Shalev AY, Pitman R (1995) Physiologic responses to loud tones in Vietnam veterans with posttraumatic stress disorder. *J Abnorm Psychol* 104: 75–82.

Orr SP, Meyerhoff JL, Edwards JV, Pitman RK (1998a) Heart rate and blood pressure resting levels and responses to generic stressors in Vietnam veterans with posttraumatic stress disorder. *J Trauma Stress* 11: 155–164.

Orr SP, Solomon Z, Peri T, Pitman RK, Shalev AY (1997) Physiologic responses to loud tones in Israeli veterans of the 1973 Yom Kippur War. *Biol Psychiatry* 41: 319–326.

Paige SR, Reid GM, Allen MG, Newton JEO (1990) Psychophysiological correlates of posttraumatic stress disorder in Vietnam veterans. *Biol Psychiatry* 27: 419–430.

Pallmeyer TP, Blanchard EB, Kolb LC (1986) The psychophysiology of combat-induced post-traumatic stress disorder in Vietnam veterans. *Behav Res Ther* 24: 645–652.

Perry BD, Giller EL, Southwick SM (1987) Altered platelet alpha$_2$-adrenergic binding sites in posttraumatic stress disorder. *Am J Psychiatry* 144: 1511–1512.

Pitman RK, Orr SP, Forgue DF, De Jong JB, Claiborn JM (1987) Psychophysiologic assessment of posttraumatic stress disorder imagery in Vietnam combat veterans. *Arch Gen Psychiatry* 44: 970–975.

Pitman RK, Orr SP, Lasko NB (1993) Effects of intranasal vasopressin and oxytocin on physiologic responding during personal combat imagery in Vietnam veterans with posttraumatic stress disorder. *Psychiatry Res* 48: 107–117.

Pitman RK, Orr SP, Steketee GS (1989) Psychophysiological investigations of posttraumatic stress disorder imagery. *Psychopharmacol Bull* 25: 426–431.

Pitman RK, Van der Kolk BA, Orr SP, Greenberg MS (1990) Naloxone-reversible analgesic response to combat related stimuli in posttraumatic stress disorder. *Arch Gen Psychiatry* 47: 541–544.

Post RM, Weiss SMB, Smith M (1995) Sensitisation and kindling: Implications for the evolving neural substrate of PTSD. In Friedman MJ, Charney DS, Deutsch AJ (eds) *Neurobiology and Clinical Consequences of Stress: From Normal Adaptation to PTSD.* Philadelphia: Lippincott-Raven Publishers, pp. 203–224.

Racine R (1978) Kindling: The first decade. *Neurosurgery* **3**: 234–252.

Reisine T, Pasternak G (1996) Opioid analgesics and antagonists. In Hardman JG, Limbird LE, Molinoff PB, Ruddon RW, Gilman AG (eds) *Goodman & Gilman's the Pharmacological Basis of Therapeutics.* 9th edition. New York: MacGraw-Hill, pp. 521–555.

Resnick HS, Yehuda R, Pitman RK, Foy DW (1995) Effect of previous trauma on acute plasma cortisol level following rape. *Am J Psychiatry* **152**: 1675–1677.

Ross RJ, Ball WA, Dinges DF, Kribbs MB, Morrison AR, Silver SM, Mulvaney FD (1994) Rapid eye movement sleep disturbance in posttraumatic stress disorder. *Biol Psychiatry* **35**: 195–202.

Sallinen J, Haapalinna A, Viitamaa T, Kobilka BK, Scheinin M (1998) Adrenergic α_{2C}-receptors modulate the acoustic startle reflex, prepulse inhibition, and aggression in mice. *J Neurosci* **18**: 3035–3042.

Sapolsky RM (1996) Why stress is bad for your brain. *Science* **273**: 749–750.

Sapolsky RM (1997) The importance of a well-groomed child. *Science* **277**: 1620–1621.

Sapolsky RM, Zola-Morgan S, Squire LR (1991) Inhibition of glucocorticoid secretion by the hippocampal formation in the primate. *J Neurosci* **11**: 3695–3704.

Schiffer F, Teicher MH, Papanicolaou AC (1995) Evoked potential evidence for right brain activity during the recall of traumatic memories. *J Neuropsychiatry* **7**: 169–175.

Schreuder JN (1996) Posttraumatic re-experiencing in older people: Working through or covering up? *Am J Psychother* **50**: 231–242.

Schulkin J, Gold PW, McEwen BS (1998) Induction of corticotropin-releasing hormone gene expression by glucocorticoids: Implications for understanding the states of fear and anxiety and allostatic load. *Psychoneuroendocrinology* **23**: 219–243.

Scott LV, Medbak S, Dinan TG (1999) Desmopressin augments pituitary-adrenal responsivity to corticotropin-releasing hormone in subjects with chronic fatigue syndrome and in healthy volunteers. *Biol Psychiatry* **45**: 1447–1454.

Seeman TE and Robbins RJ (1994) Ageing and hypothalamic-pituitary-adrenal response to challenge in humans. *Endocr Rev* **15**: 233–260.

Shalev AY, Bonne OB, Peri T (1996) Auditory startle response during exposure to war stress. *Compr Psychiatry* **37**: 134–138.

Shalev AY, Freedman S, Peri T, Brandes D, Sahar T, Orr SP, Pitman RK (1998) Prospective study of posttraumatic stress disorder and depression following trauma. *Am J Psychiatry* **155**: 630–637.

Shalev AY, Orr SP, Peri T, Schreiber S, Pitman RK (1992) Physiologic responses to loud tones in Israeli patients with posttraumatic stress disorder. *Arch Gen Psychiatry* **49**: 870–875.

Shalev AY, Orr SP, Pitman RK (1993) Psychophysiologic assessment of traumatic imagery in Israeli civilian patients with posttraumatic stress disorder. *Am J Psychiatry* **150**: 620–624.

Shalev AY, Peri T, Gelpin E, Orr SP, Pitman RK (1997) Psychophysiologic assessment of mental imagery of stressful events in Israeli civilian posttraumatic stress disorder patients. *Compr Psychiatry* **38**: 269–273.

Shalev AY, Rogel-Fuchs Y (1992) Auditory startle reflex in post-traumatic stress disorder patients treated with clonazepam. *Isr J Psychiatry Relat Sci* **29**: 1–6.

Shin LM, Kosslyn SM, McNally RJ, Alpert NM, Thompson WL, Rauch SL, Macklin ML, Pitman RK (1997) Visual imagery and perception in posttraumatic stress disorder: A positron emission tomographic investigation. *Arch Gen Psychiatry* **54**: 233–241.

Sifneos PE (1973) The prevalence of "alexithymia" characteristics in psychosomatic patients. *Psychother Psychosom* **22**: 255–262.

Smith MA, Davidson J, Ritchie JC, Kudler H, Lipper S, Chappell P, Nemeroff CB (1989) The corticotropin-releasing hormone test in patients with posttraumatic stress disorder. *Biol*

Psychiatry **26**: 349–355.

Southwick SM, Krystal JH, Morgan CA, Johnson D, Nagy LM, Nicolaou A, Heninger GR, Charney DS (1993a) Abnormal noradrenergic function in posttraumatic stress disorder. *Arch Gen Psychiatry* **50**: 266–274.

Southwick SM, Morgan CA 3rd, Charney DS, High JR (1999) Yohimbine use in a natural setting: Effects on posttraumatic stress disorder. *Biol Psychiatry* **46**: 442–444.

Southwick SM, Yehuda R, Giller EL (1993b) Personality disorders in treatment seeking combat veterans with postraumatic stress disorder. *Am J Psychiatry* **150**: 1020–1023.

Spivak B, Segal M, Mester R, Weizman A (1998) Lateral preference in post-traumatic stress disorder. *Psychol Med* **28**: 229–232.

Stein MB, Koverola C, Hanna C, Torchia MG, McClarty B (1997) Hippocampal volume in women victimised by childhood sexual abuse. *Psychol Med* **27**: 951–959.

Sterling P, and Eyer J (1988) Allostasis: a new paradigm to explain arousal pathology. In Fisher S, Reason J (eds) *Handbook of Life Stress, Cognition and Health.* Chichester: John Wiley & Sons, Ltd, pp. 629–649.

Teyler FJ, DiScenna P (1987) Long-term potentiation. *Ann Rev Neuroscience* **10**: 316–361.

Toni C, Cassano GB, Perugi G, Murri L, Mancino M, Petracca A, Akiskal H, Roth M (1996) Psychosensorial and related phenomena in panic disorder and in temporal lobe epilepsy. *Compr Psychiatry* **37**: 125–133.

Van der Kolk, Burbridge JA, Suzuki J (1995) Current status of the psychobiology of posttraumatic stress disorder. *Acta Neuropsychiatrica (Interdisciplin Soc Biol Psychiatry)* **7**(3S): S34–37.

Van der Kolk BA, Dreyfuss D, Michaels M, Shera D, Berkowitz R, Fisler R, Saxe G (1994b) Fluoxetine in posttraumatic stress disorder. *J Clin Psychiatry* **55**: 517–522.

Van der Kolk BA, Greenberg MS, Orr SP, Pitman RK (1989) Endogenous opioids and stress induced analgesia in post-traumatic stress disorder. *Psychopharmacol Bull* **25**: 108–112.

Van der Kolk BA, Hostetler A, Herron N, Fisler RE (1994a) Trauma and the development of borderline personality disorder. *Psychiatr Clin North Am* **17**: 715–729.

Van der Kolk BA, Saporta S (1991) The biological response to psychic trauma: mechanisms and treatment of intrusion and numbing. *Anxiety Res* **4**: 199–212.

Wan R, Diamant M, De Jong W, De Wied D (1992) Differential effects of $ACTH_{4–10}$, DG-AVP, and DG-OXT on heart rate and passive avoidance behaviour in rats. *Physiol Behav* **51**: 507–513.

Webster RA (1989) The catecholamines (noradrenaline and dopamine). In Webster RA, Jordan CC (eds) *Neurotransmitters, Drugs and Disease.* Oxford: Blackwell Scientific Publications, pp. 95–125.

Wolf M, Lipper S, Mosnaim A (1990) Carbamazepine and the kindling hypothesis of PTSD. *Biol Psychiatry* **27**: 165A–166A.

Yehuda R, Boisoneau D, Lowy MT, Giller EL (1995c) Dose response changes in plasma cortisol and lymphocyte glucocorticoid receptors following dexamethasone administration in combat veterans with and without posttraumatic stress disorder. *Arch Gen Psychiatry* **52**: 583–593.

Yehuda R, Kahana B, Binder-Brynes K, Southwick SM, Mason JW, Giller EL (1995b) Low urinary cortisol in holocaust survivors with posttraumatic stress disorder. *Am J Psychiatry* **152**: 982–986.

Yehuda R, Keefe RSE, Harvey PD, Levengood RA, Gerber DK, Geni J, Siever LJ (1995a) Learning and memory in combat veterans with posttraumatic stress disorder. *Am J Psychiatry* **152**: 137–139.

Yehuda R, Levengood RA, Schmeidler J, Wilson S, Ling Song Guo, Gerber D (1996b) Increased pituitary activation following metyrapone administration in post-traumatic stress disorder. *Psychoneuroendocrinology* **21**: 1–16.

Yehuda R, Lowy MT, Southwick SM, Shaffer D, Giller EL (1991) Lymfocyte glucocorticoid receptor number in posttraumatic stress disorder. *Am J Psychiatry* **148**: 499–504.

Yehuda R, Perry BD, Southwick SM, Giller EL (1990b) Platelet alpha$_2$-receptor binding in PTSD, generalized anxiety disorder, and major depressive disorder. *New Res Abstr* **143**: NR286.

Yehuda R, Resnick HS, Schmeidler J, Yang R-K, Pitman RK (1998b) Predictors of cortisol and 3-methoxy-4-hydroxyphenylglycol responses in the acute aftermath of rape. *Biol Psychiatry* **43**: 855–859.

Yehuda R, Siever LJ, Teicher MH, Levengood RA, Gerber DK, Schmeidler J, Yang R-K (1998a) Plasma norepinephrine and 3-methoxy-4-hydroxyphenylglycol concentrations and severity of depression in combat posttraumatic stress disorder and major depressive disorder. *Biol Psychiatry* **44**: 56–63.

Yehuda R, Southwick SM, Giller EL, Ma X, Mason JW (1992) Urinary catecholamine excretion and severity of PTSD symptoms in Vietnam combat veterans. *J Nerv Ment Dis* **180**: 321–325.

Yehuda R, Southwick SM, Krystal JH, Bremner D, Charney DS, Mason JW (1993) Enhanced suppression of cortisol following dexamethasone admission in posttraumatic stress disorder. *Am J Psychiatry* **150**: 83–86.

Yehuda R, Southwick SM, Nussbaum G, Wahby V, Giller EL, Mason JW (1990a) Low urinary cortisol excretion in patients with posttraumatic stress disorder. *J Nerv Ment Dis* **178**: 366–369.

Yehuda R, Teicher MH, Trestman RL, Levengood RA, Siever LJ (1996a) Cortisol regulation in posttraumatic stress disorder and major depression: a chronobiological analysis. *Biol Psychiatry* **40**: 79–88.

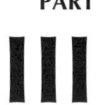

Research Methods

Methods of Experimental Psychology

Learning Perspectives on Anxiety Disorders

P. Eelen, D. Hermans and F. Baeyens

University of Leuven, Leuven, Belgium

INTRODUCTION

One of the intriguing themes within psychology (and philosophy) has always been the "nature–nurture" debate. The extreme standpoints within this discussion are well known, although seldom clearly articulated. The extreme nature-position defends a sort of biogenetically prepared hardware of behavioral output: favorite research themes within this tradition are topics such as typology (as old as Greek philosophical ideas), personality traits, and—more recently—the genetic basis of behavior. The extreme nurture-position assumes a "tabula rasa" idea: nothing is programmed and the behavior of the individual is shaped as a result of experiences. Although psychologists no longer adhere to one of these extreme positions, most current behavioral research tends to lean towards one end of this bipolar dimension. This bipolarity has not only its impact on psychology in general, but is also influential on conceptualizations and theories about the origin of so-called abnormal behavior or psychopathology. The present chapter is written from a nurture-position, because the psychology of learning has its roots in this position. Before illustrating this position with regard to the etiology and treatment of anxiety disorders, the phenomenon of learning is introduced.

THE PHENOMENON OF LEARNING

While most people have a sense of what is meant by the term *learning* (most often they associate it with the educational perspective of school learning), the precise meaning of how this concept has been used in psychology is difficult to specify. The following is the most commonly accepted definition:

Anxiety Disorders: An Introduction to Clinical Management and Research. Edited by E. J. L. Griez, C. Faravelli, D. Nutt and J. Zohar. © 2001 John Wiley & Sons, Ltd.

Learning refers to the change in a subject's behavior or behavior potential to a given situation brought about by the subject's repeated experiences in that situation, provided that the behavior change cannot be explained on the basis of the subject's native response tendencies, maturation, or temporary states (such as fatigue, drunkenness, drives, and so on).

(Bower and Hilgard, 1981, p. 12)

Basically, learning refers to the capacity of a living organism to alter its behavior as a result of experience. This idea can be reduced to a rather simple schema: there is evidence of learning if an organism (animal or human) has an experience at time 1, and as a result of this experience the behavior of the organism changes at time 2.

While this schema looks very simple and straightforward, it reflects the basic problems which have plagued the scientific study of a learning process. Reasons for these problems are mainly twofold. On the one hand, not every change in behavior is due to a learning process. Behavior potentials can change for reasons other than learning. For instance, becoming paralysed through an accident (experience) might seriously change a person's potential for behavior, but nobody wants to consider this change as due to learning. The same is true for all changes in behavior, due to natural maturation, brain damage, or any other organic cause of behavior change. If we deny or overlook this possibility, we are tempted to "psychologize" any behavioral change, and this is especially true in the domain of psychopathology. On the other hand, not every experience results in a behavioral change. Therefore in the above-mentioned definition, Bower and Hilgard (1981) refer to a change in behavioral *potential*. For this reason, psychologists have made a distinction between *learning* and *performance*, where the former refers to what exactly happens at t_1 and the latter at t_2. The basic problem, however, is that we have never direct access to t_1: we can only infer the consequences of t_1 through the behavioral change at t_2. This leads to the rather strange assertion that we can never be sure whether something was learned at t_1: all we can conclude is whether this eventual learning is manifested into overt behavior at t_2. Anderson (1995) has used Figure 13.1 to illustrate what is happening in a learning episode. The rectangle, representing the environment in Figure 13.1, is what can be observed: the situational experiences of the organism on the one hand (t_1) and the behavior (t_2) on the other hand. Within the oval are theoretical processes within the organism, introduced to explain the link between experience and behavior. This general schema will guide us in the further discussion about the application of this learning perspective on anxiety disorders.

LEARNING PARADIGMS

Learning paradigms have been distinguished, on the basis of the sort of experiences an organism is exposed to.

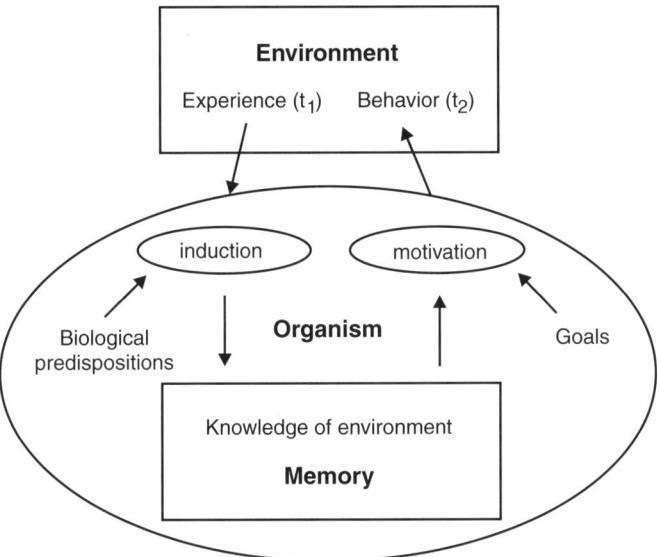

FIGURE 13.1 Learning episode and theoretical processes involved
Source: Reproduced by permission of Anderson, 1995, p. 154.

First Paradigm: Exposure to a Stimulus

The *first paradigm* is related to what happens when an organism is merely exposed to a repeated confrontation with a stimulus. It is called a non-associative paradigm. Repeated exposure to a stimulus results most often in habituation which means that the original reaction towards the stimulus diminishes in intensity or even disappears. Even while this form of learning refers to very basic mechanisms (it can be demonstrated in almost all animals), there is some evidence that it requires some primitive form of memorial representation, and that is not merely due to adaptation of the sensorial or motor system (Sokolov, 1975; Öhman, 1979). In this sense, it is a form of learning, conforming to the definition of learning as the capacity to change behavior as a consequence of experience.

Second Paradigm: Relationship between Stimuli

The *second learning* paradigm is known as classical or Pavlovian conditioning (Pavlov, 1927). In its bare essence, the Pavlovian paradigm offers a way to investigate the conditions through which an organism learns a relation between event A and event B. Thus, conditioning can be defined as the process whereby an organism, through the exposure to spatio-temporal relations between events, establishes associations between the representations of these events. In Pavlov's seminal studies, a dog started to salivate (conditioned reaction, CR) upon the presentation of a neutral stimulus (the conditioned stimulus, CS) when this stimulus was paired with the delivery of food substances (the unconditioned stimulus, US, or reinforcer), evoking an unconditioned reaction (UR). Pavlov defined the US as an innate trigger of a specific reaction (UR). We prefer to call the US a reinforcer to avoid the rather reflexological viewpoint of Pavlov. A reinforcer is any event, the occurrence of which in relation to other events (it can be either a neutral stimulus or some behavior of the organism, see the third paradigm) supports some change in behavior (Mackintosh, 1983). This change can either be an increase or a decrease in the occurrence of a response. It is tempting to describe these reinforcers also as having some motivational significance within the pleasure-pain or approach-avoidance dimensions.

Indeed, everyone seems to agree that for a particular organism some stimuli are rather intrinsically evoking either an approach behavior (appetitive reinforcers) or avoidance or escape behavior (aversive reinforcers). As prototypes of both classes of reinforcers, animal studies have used food as an example of an appetitive reinforcer and shock as an example of an aversive reinforcer. Even while the final criterion for the classification of appetitive and aversive stimuli has to be based on their behavioral effects, it might be a good heuristic to look at classical conditioning as a learning process whereby rather neutral stimuli acquire a new meaning (expressed in behavior) as a consequence of their relation to what happens with an "appetitive" or "aversive" reinforcer, either through an experimental manipulation, or through what happens in "real life". It should be clear that classical conditioning is, in principle, not restricted to the learning of an association between a neutral stimulus and a "reinforcing" stimulus. Therefore, we defined it as a paradigm to investigate learning of relations between two events, whatever their nature. However, by using a reinforcing stimulus as one of these events, the learning of the association will be expressed (and can be measured) in a behavioral change. This leads us to the following classification (see Table 13.1).

In Pavlovian terminology, the presentation of a reinforcer with a CS will produce *excitatory* conditioning; the disappearance or omission of the reinforcer produces *inhibitory* conditioning, a process opposed to excitatory conditioning. The distinction between disappearance and omission is, at least at the procedural level, obvious: in the first case, an appetitive or aversive reinforcer is present and its disappearance evokes some behavioral change; in the second case, an appetitive or aversive reinforcer is omitted: omission can only be psychologically relevant when it is preceded by learning that either an appetitive or aversive reinforcer will be delivered. Whereas Pavlov considered excitatory and inhibitory conditioning as equally important, there has been a tendency to identify classical conditioning with the behavioral change due

TABLE 13.1 Classification of classical conditioning procedures as a function of what happens with reinforcing stimuli contingent upon the presentation of a CS

	Appetitive reinforcer	Aversive reinforcer
Delivery	(1) excitatory conditioning	(2) excitatory conditioning
Disappearance	(3) inhibitory conditioning	(4) inhibitory conditioning
Omission	(5) inhibitory conditioning	(6) inhibitory conditioning

to the presentation of a reinforcer (excitatory conditioning), whereas the phenomenon of inhibitory conditioning has been largely neglected.

A closer look at Table 13.1 makes it clear that each of the six cases will produce a particular emotional state within the organism. Neutral stimuli (CSs) associated with one of these six events will acquire an emotional significance. Table 13.2 gives a label to these different emotional states. Three cases within this configuration will give rise to rather positive emotional states (cases 1, 4, 6) whereas the other three cases (2, 3, 5) will produce rather negative emotions.

Another advantage of this classification is that it offers a model for understanding the conflicting meaning of a stimulus. We have to remember that one of the students of Pavlov introduced the first paradigm of experimental neurosis without using any aversive reinforcer. It was the well-known circle–oval experiment: each time when a circle (CS +) was presented, food was given to the dog (case 1 in Table 13.1) whereas an oval figure (CS −) was not followed by food. One can imagine that the dog did not differentiate at the beginning of the experiment between the circle and the oval, so that he expected food after the presentation of both figures. After some trials, a clear differentiation was established: the circle evoked salivation (case 1 in Table 13.1) and the oval figure not (case 5 in Table 13.1). Making the oval figure gradually more circular, the dogs started to manifest "neurotic behavior": according to Pavlov, it was due to a clash between excitatory and inhibitory conditioning. In other words: losing predictability within the environment might be a major cause for the development of "neurotic symptoms".

TABLE 13.2 Emotional change towards a neutral stimulus (CS) when it is associated with what happens to reinforcing stimuli

	Appetitive reinforcer	Aversive reinforcer
Delivery	(1) hope	(2) fear
Disappearance	(3) sadness	(4) relief
Omission	(5) frustration	(6) safety

Third Learning Paradigm: Relationship between Behavior and Consequences

The third learning paradigm is called operant or instrumental learning, introduced by Thorndike but further developed by Skinner. In his prototypical studies of instrumental conditioning, Thorndike placed a hungry cat in a box and the animal had to perform some arbitrary response, such as pressing a panel, in order to get access to the food outside the box. Skinner refined this procedure by letting an animal freely move in a closed environment whereby a particular response, pressing a lever (for rats) or pecking a key (for pigeons) delivered food. Notice that, in this learning paradigm, a contingency is introduced between a subject's behavior and a reinforcer, whereas in classical or Pavlovian conditioning, there is a relationship between a CS and a reinforcer regardless of the subject's behavior. These different rules for the delivery of reinforcers are the defining criteria of classical and instrumental or operant learning.

Because of this procedural difference, classical conditioning may be considered as the study of how organisms learn the *predictability* of their environment whereas the instrumental or operant paradigm reflects the learning of *controllability*.

The different contingencies between a CS and a reinforcer were illustrated in Table 13.1. The same schema can now be used to illustrate the contingencies between some behavior and reinforcing stimuli (see Table 13.3).

It should be clear that the three cases in Table 13.2 which were associated with positive emotions (cases 1, 4, 6) will lead to a reinforcement of the behavior (manifested for instance in an increase of frequency or probability), whereas the other three cases (2, 3, 5) will lead to punishment (decrease in frequency or probability of the behavior). The terms "positive" and "negative" to differentiate two forms of reinforcement and two forms of punishment might be misleading if one identifies them with an affective connotation: how can, for instance, the delivery of an aversive reinforced upon a response be positive? However, the terms are referring to a positive or negative contingency between some behavior and appetitive or aversive reinforcers.

As was made clear from Table 13.1 for classical conditioning, stimuli may acquire a conflicting meaning. The same is true with regard to the conflict between some behavioral consequences (Table 13.3): the same behavior may lead either to a form of reinforcement or to a form of punishment. The classical demonstration of how such a conflict may lead to "neurotic" behavior was offered by Masserman: the same instrumental behavior for cats was either followed by food or by an aversive air-puff (Masserman, 1943). After a while, the cats showed signs of neurotic behavior. So we have to remember that a major source for the origin of neurotic disorders, including anxiety, may exist in the *loss* of predictability and *loss of* controllability, a hypothesis which was convincingly defended by Mineka and Kihlstrom (1978) and Mineka and Henderson (1985).

TABLE 13.3 Classification of operant learning procedures as a function of what happens with reinforcing stimuli contingent upon some behavior of the organism

	Appetitive reinforcer	Aversive reinforcer
Delivery	(1) positive reinforcement	(2) positive punishment
Disappearance	(3) negative punishment	(4) negative reinforcement
Omission	(5) negative punishment	(6) negative reinforcement

Interaction between Classical and Instrumental Conditioning

It is important to underline the close interaction between the classical and instrumental learning paradigm, especially in the context of this chapter on anxiety. One of the first to notice this interaction was Mowrer, introducing the two-factor theory on the basis of an avoidance learning paradigm (Mowrer, 1947; Mowrer, 1960). The basic setting is illustrated in Figure 13.2.

The animal subject is placed in a box with two compartments. A signal (light or tone) announces the delivery of shock. As soon as the shock is experienced, the animal tries to escape it and eventually runs to the other side of the box. After a few trials, the animal will run to the other side upon the presentation of the signal without experiencing the shock. This simple experimental paradigm, which has been used in several variants, illustrates the interaction of classical and instrumental learning: first, the animal has to learn the relation between the signal and the shock (classical conditioning) and second, it must learn the relation between running to the other side and the omission of shock (instrumental learning). Whereas there have been several theoretical discussions about the mechanisms underlying this avoidance behavior, the phenomenon itself illustrates the role of both learning paradigms: through a process of classical conditioning, stimuli in the environment acquire a new meaning (the signal for shock becomes aversive) and through a process of instrumental conditioning, the organism learns to react appropriately towards this stimulus.

From Two-term towards Three-term Contingencies

Thus far, we have described classical and operant learning in a two-term contingency. In classical conditioning a relation is learned between a CS and a reinforcing event, whereas in operant learning a relation is learned between some behavior and a reinforcing event. However, right from the beginning, Skinner introduced a third term into an operant learning episode: the discriminative stimulus, or S^D. Indeed, the

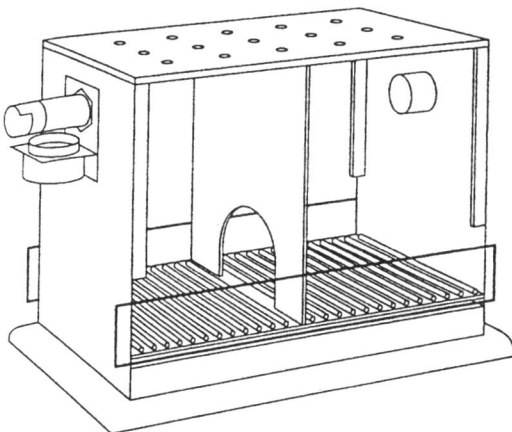

FIGURE 13.2   An illustration of a two-way shuttle-box. Several variants have been used. In a one-way box, shock is only delivered on one side. Also the escape- or avoidance behavior can be different

relation between a response and a reinforcing stimulus is most often dependent upon the presence either of a discrete stimulus (for instance, a rat can learn that pressing a lever produces food only if a light is illuminated) or of some general contextual stimuli. It is only in more recent years, that an analogue has been studied with regard to classical conditioning: the relation between a CS and a reinforcing event might also be dependent upon the presence of a third discrete stimulus or a particular context: this phenomenon is called *occasion-setting* which might be especially relevant to understand anxiety disorders and their treatment.

LEARNING PARADIGMS AND ANXIETY DISORDERS

Given the conceptual and empirical richness of the research on learning, it is sometimes frustrating to realize that a behavioral approach towards the origin of fears, phobias and anxiety states is often only identified with the famous case study of Watson and Rayner (1920). They induced a phobic reaction in a 11-month-old baby, Albert, through the pairing of a neutral stimulus (a white rat) with a strong aversive reinforcer (an intense aversive noise). On the other hand, this study has fulfilled a pioneering role: considering phobic reactions as a result of Pavlovian conditioning, it opened straightforward options for therapy. Pavlov had demonstrated that conditioned reactions disappear through extinction (repeated exposure towards the CS) or through counterconditioning (pairing a CS, which has been associated with an aversive reinforcer, with an appetitive reinforcer). These ideas were formulated in another seminal study by Mary-Cover Jones for the treatment of a young child, Peter, who was afraid of rabbits (Jones, 1924a; Jones 1924b).

It was only in the 1960s that this learning approach became more influential in clinical psychology. A major step for understanding some of the anxiety disorders was the two-factor theory of Mowrer (1960) wherein avoidance behavior was considered to be a crucial factor in the maintenance of fear and anxiety. The animal experimental paradigm of avoidance learning has already been described (see Figure 13.2): avoidance responses are considered as motivated by classically conditioned fear (cell 2 in Table 13.1) and negatively reinforced by fear or anxiety reduction (cell 4 and 6 in Table 13.3). It was, however, also Rachman who formulated the major critical comments on this conditioning approach (Rachman, 1977; Rachman, 1991). Similar critical comments were formulated by Merckelbach et al. (1996), with regard to the etiology of specific phobias.

Classical conditioning, which is at the heart of avoidance behavior, seemed to be inappropriate as a model for the following reasons:

1. Many clients with fears and phobias have not experienced a traumatic conditioning episode in the past.
2. On the other hand, many persons who are victims of traumatic experiences, do not develop anxiety disorders.
3. Fears and phobias do not develop towards any stimulus or situation associated

with traumatic experiences. There seems to exist a selective basis whereby some objects or situations are more easily associated with aversive events.

4. Finally, why are fears and phobias—if they are based on Pavlovian conditioning—so resistant to extinction, and why do we observe often a return of fear after successful treatment?

Most of these critiques against a conditioning model have been challenged in an important study by Mineka and Zinbarg (1996). They argue, based on solid experimental evidence, that most of these critiques are reflecting the rather old-fashioned Watsonian view on conditioning, not taking into account more recent conceptual and empirical developments within this domain. For instance, they refer to (a) the experimental evidence on the role of vicarious conditioning; (b) the demonstrated influence of temperament and a multitude of experiential variables occurring before, during or following a traumatic or an observational conditioning experience on the amount of acquired fear and anxiety; (c) the experimental evidence demonstrating the selectivity in development of fear; and finally (d) the more recent insights in the phenomenon of extinction. Mineka and Zinbarg (1996) conclude that clinical theorists interested in anxiety disorders have to abandon their critiques of outmoded conditioning models and to explore the many hypotheses for further understanding of the anxiety disorders that stem from these new developments.

We fully agree with this conclusion. An associative account of anxiety disorders—which is, by the way, very close to a Freudian perspective—remains very valuable. The experimental basis of the conditioning literature still has a strong heuristic value to understanding not only the etiology but also the ways of treatment of anxiety disorders.

However, in the meantime, these critical comments on a conditioning approach were rather uncritically accepted, especially by cognitive therapists. They subscribed eagerly to the arguments that the model of conditioning was inappropriate. Since then, a false dichotomy has been created between a conditioning and a cognitive approach within behavior therapy. The falsity of this dichotomy is already clear from Figure 13.1. Nobody can deny that even in the "simple" Pavlovian conditioning paradigm, some cognitive processes are involved: it is up to the dog to make an inference that there is a link between the neutral and the reinforcing stimulus. Some biological predispositions may facilitate this inference process which may explain the selectivity of this associative learning (Seligman, 1971; Mineka, 1987). The animal has to keep this link "in mind" through some memorial representation and it will manifest this knowledge through salivation when it is hungry. So, there are hardly any arguments to dismiss a conditioning approach as non-cognitive. As was mentioned before, the chapter by Mineka and Zinbarg (1996) offers convincing evidence for a conditioning approach. One extra-argument is the following: in the critical comments on a conditioning viewpoint, one has a tendency to identify the etiology of anxiety disorders only with cell 2 of Table 13.1. This is reflected in the research, trying to discover through retrospective reports whether clients of phobic disorders can still remember some discrete traumatic experience, associated with the object or the situation of their phobia (e.g. Öst and Hugdahl, 1981; Merckelbach et al., 1989). It seems that quite often the clients do not explicitly remember a traumatic experience. Even while this research might be worthwhile at some level, it cannot be used as an argument against a conditioning approach. First, because there is now ample evidence—even outside the clinical domain—of the phenomenon of *implicit* memory. Framing it within Figure 13.1, this means that behavioral changes can be due to some previous experiences, without any awareness of the subject (client) of these experiences. Second, this kind of research does not sufficiently take into account the different sources for the development of anxiety disorders. Experiences of unpredictability and uncontrollability (see above) can hardly be detected in these retrospective clinical studies, whereas they might play a major role in the development of anxiety disorders.

We end up with the conclusion that an associative account can hardly be falsified. Therefore, we understand why Rachman claims that the new approach to conditioning (for instance, as advocated by Mineka and Zinbarg in 1996) is "still too liberal. It lacks limits and there is little that it disallows" (Rachman, 1991: 169). But do we have to disallow this approach?

The alternative is that we take a "nature"-standpoint: fears and phobias are genetically determined. However, as psychologists, we have to test the limits of a nurture-standpoint and start from the assumption that at least some anxiety disorders are (partly) based on associative learning, even while the learning episode(s) can no longer be reconstructed by the client. The advantage of making this assumption is that it may offer some better theoretical insights in the effects of the treatment. Some authors (e.g. Menzies and Clarke, 1995) have argued that the disappearance of anxiety responses towards some stimuli or situations through repeated confrontation can be considered as habituation (first learning paradigm). Implicitly, they defend a non-associative account for the existence of anxiety responses (Merckelbach et al., 1996). However, an extinction perspective, referring to an original associative learning process, offers a more fruitful therapeutic framework. Next, we will illustrate this perspective.

NEW PERSPECTIVES ON EXTINCTION

As was mentioned before, Mary-Cover Jones was the first to apply the conditioning hypothesis of Watson, with regard to the etiology of phobias, in the treatment of a specific phobia for rabbits in a young boy, Peter (Jones, 1924b). The Pavlovian principle of extinction offered one of the main sources of inspiration for the treatment. It is interesting to note that Mary-Cover Jones (1924a) describes practically all the basic methods which would only become popular years later, like cognitive therapy, modelling, contra-conditioning, desensitization, etc. Formally, an extinction procedure refers to the fact that a CS is no longer followed by the reinforcing stimulus (US), and the result is that the conditioned reaction disappears. In Peter's case, by confronting the child repeatedly with a rabbit, the fear reaction disappeared. So, the procedure and the usual results of an extinction procedure are well documented. However, with regard to the theoretical explanation of this phenomenon, the picture is less clear. Some traditional associative accounts of Pavlovian conditioning consider extinction as a weakening or even disappearance of the associative strength between the CS and the reinforcing event (see Donegan et al., 1989). However, there are some new (and some old!) intriguing findings, contradicting the idea that an extinction procedure results in simple unlearning or forgetting of the previously acquired association between a CS and the reinforcing event. It appears that only the behavioral expression of the learned association is inhibited. The Watsonian identification of learning with behavior changes (the disappearance of behavior change means therefore unlearning) has plagued our view on classical conditioning. Especially, because Pavlov himself, the founder of the paradigm, was convinced that through a procedure of extinction the excitatory link between the CS and the reinforcer (see cell 1 and 2 in Table 13.1) was not abolished, but inhibited (see cell 5 and 6). Two lines of recent empirical observations subscribe to this position, and they are especially relevant to the return of fear after successful treatment.

Evidence from the Animal Literature

The first line of evidence that convincingly argues against the "extinction-implies-unlearning" position has recently been reviewed by Bouton (Bouton, 1988; Bouton, 1994; Bouton and Bolles, 1985; Bouton and Swartzentruber, 1991). Four well-established phenomena from the animal laboratory demonstrate that an extinction procedure may leave an acquired CS–US association intact, while simultaneously affecting performance as apparent from a complete disappearance of conditioned responding. These phenomena are (1) renewal; (2) spontaneous recovery; (3) reinstatement; and (4) rapid reacquisition.

1. Renewal of extinguished CRs refers to the observation that when a CS that was completely extinguished in a context (B) different from the acquisition context (A) is reintroduced in the acquisition context (A), a strong recovery or renewal of conditioned responding towards the CS can be observed (Bouton and Swartzentruber, 1996). The findings on the renewal phenomenon further suggest the hypothesis that extinction may be specific to the context in which it occurred. Rather than forgetting that the CS co-occurred with the US, the subject may learn that "in this particular context, the CS-US relation does not hold".

2. Spontaneous recovery was described as early as in Pavlov's *Conditioned Reflexes*: when conditioned responding has been abolished completely through an extinction procedure, the mere passage of time may cause CRs to recover spontaneously (Pavlov, 1927). Again, this argues against the hypothesis that extinction would be based on forgetting or unlearning of the original CS–US relation.

3. In a reinstatement procedure, a previously conditioned stimulus is first extinguished until conditioned responding disappears. Next, a few USs are administered without any contiguous CS presentations. When the previously

extinguished CS is finally represented, conditioned responding to the CS (partially) reappears (e.g. Bouton and Bolles, 1979; Rescorla and Heth, 1975).
4. A final demonstration that the originally acquired CS–US association survives an extinction procedure is provided by studies on reacquisition. In a typical reacquisition experiment, subjects are first exposed to a CS–US acquisition contingency. Next, in an extinction phase, CS only presentations are scheduled until any sign of conditioned responding disappears. In the crucial third phase, CS–US acquisition pairings are resumed. It has been demonstrated repeatedly that conditioned responding reappears more rapidly than during the original learning phase (within-subject comparison) or than in a control group, not subjected to the original CS–US pairings (between-subject comparison).

Based on these findings, Bouton argues for an interpretation of extinction that stresses that the original CS–US relation is never unlearned, but is rather supplemented by new, additional knowledge implying that in some contexts or at some moments in time, the CS–US relation does not hold. Hence, it is proposed that the subject has learned both a dominant rule, namely that the CS predicts the US, and exceptions to the rule, namely, that in certain contexts or at certain moments the CS does not predict the US. As a result, an extinguished CS becomes an ambiguous stimulus, the meaning of which may be controlled by contextual stimuli.

In general, these findings on the effects of an extinction procedure with regard to the disappearance of conditioned (fear) reactions, offer a rather pessimistic perspective towards the effects of exposure therapy modelled upon an extinction procedure. It is no wonder that Bouton and Swartzentruber gave the article, wherein they documented these findings, the title: "Sources of relapse after extinction in Pavlovian and instrumental learning" (Bouton and Swartzentruber, 1991). Indeed, the general lesson from these findings is that contextual-bound processes might play a major role in the extinction of learned responses, whereas the acquisition of these responses seems to be less restricted to one particular context or stimulus and is easily generalized towards other contexts or stimuli.

There is additional evidence from the animal literature that a process of inhibitory conditioning may suppress excitatory conditioning. This process may play a major role in avoidance behavior. If an individual learns that (s)he can do something to avoid an aversive event, this avoidance behavior may function as an inhibitory or safety stimulus, suppressing the behavioral expression of anxiety evoked by a danger stimulus. At the phenomenal level, fear reactions are no longer observed. But, as soon as the avoidance behavior is no longer successful, the original excitatory fear conditioning will reappear (Mineka, 1979).

Evidence from Human Evaluative Learning

A second line of evidence has been a central research topic in our laboratory. As was illustrated in Tables 13.1 and 13.2, a Pavlovian procedure may not only lead to a change in the predictive characteristics of a CS (behaviorally expressed as excitatory or inhibitory conditioning) but also in the emotional or affective meaning of the CS. This *evaluative conditioning*, as it was first called by Martin and Levey (1987), has been extensively studied by Baeyens (e.g. Baeyens et al., 1995). There is now ample evidence that the *acquired predictive function* of a CS shows other characteristics than the *acquired valence* of the CS, especially in the procedure of extinction. Whereas the predictive value of a CS seems to diminish through a procedure of extinction, the acquired evaluative change seems to be resistant to extinction.

The evidence was originally only based on overt verbal ratings of the CSs by human experimental subjects. However, it has recently been corroborated by using a more unobtrusive non-verbal measure of stimulus valence. This procedure is derived from the standard sequential semantic priming procedure (e.g. Neely, 1991) and is better known as the affective priming paradigm (Hermans et al., 1994). In a standard affective priming study (e.g. Hermans et al., 1994), a series of positive or negative target stimuli is presented, which have to be evaluated as quickly as possible as either "positive" or "negative". Each target is immediately preceded by a prime stimulus, which can be positive, negative, or neutral, and which has to be ignored by the participant. Nevertheless, results show that the time to evaluate the target stimuli is mediated by the valence of the primes. If targets are preceded by an evaluatively congruent prime, response latencies are significantly smaller than on evaluatively incongruent trials. This effect is based on the automatic processing of the valence of the prime, and is not dependent upon controlled response strategies (Hermans et al., 1998). Hence, the affective priming paradigm is an excellent method to assess the (newly acquired) valence of the conditioned stimuli in a way that is unobtrusive and—in contrast to standard evaluative ratings—cannot be biased by demand effects. In fact, recently we were able to replicate these priming effects for initially neutral, nonsense words, which had acquired their positive or negative valence in a preceding evaluative conditioning procedure (De Houwer et al., 1998). This priming effect remained even after an extinction procedure. Once again, these findings offer a rather pessimistic viewpoint on the possibilities of successful treatment. Eventually, we might change the predictive value of stimuli or situations but not their acquired valence. As far as documented from the same line of research, this acquired valence can only be changed through a procedure which conceptually comes down to a contra-conditioning procedure (Baeyens et al., 1989). Of course, this experimental research on human subjects can never simulate exactly the processes involved of what happens when subjects are confronted with strong emotional traumatic events. But these findings corroborate the idea that a procedure of exposure cannot be identified with unlearning.

Relevance for Treatment

Because nowadays in the clinical literature the more neutral concept of *exposure* is preferred, instead of *extinction*, to describe treatment procedures for anxiety disorders, the danger exists that we are losing track with the rich empirical research, inspired by an associative account of anxiety disorders. This account stems from a long philosophical tradition. In his famous book *An Essay Concerning Human Understanding*, Locke, the founder of empiricism, reflected on the origin of some phobic fears:

> *Wrong connexion of ideas: a great cause of errors*—This wrong connexion in our minds of ideas in themselves loose and independent of one another, has such an influence, and is of so great force to set us awry in our actions, as well moral as natural, passions, reasonings, and notions themselves, that perhaps there is not any one thing that deserves more to be looked after.
>
> *An instance*—The ideas of goblins and spirits have really no more to do with darkness than light: yet let but a foolish maid inculcate these often on the mind of a child, and raise them there together, possibly he shall never be able to separate them again so long as he lives, but darkness shall ever afterwards bring with it those frightful ideas, and they shall be joined, that he can no more bear to one than the other.
>
> (Locke, 1894)

The great merit of the Pavlovian contribution has been to translate this "connexion of ideas" into behavioral indices. Pavlov himself noted the resemblance: "Are there any grounds for differentiation, for distinguishing between that which the physiologist calls the temporary connection and that which the psychologist terms association? They are fully identical, they merge and absorb each other" (Pavlov, 1955: 251).

It would be unwise to abandon this learning approach as old-fashioned. It still offers the clinical psychologist a strong heuristic framework for conceptualizing his therapeutic endeavours. And it is still an ideal meeting ground between theory and practice.

REFERENCES

Anderson JR (1995) *Learning and Memory: An Integrated Approach*. New York: John Wiley & Sons.

Baeyens F, Eelen P, Crombez G (1995) Pavlovian associations are forever: On classical conditioning and extinction. *J Psychophysiology* **9**: 127–141.

Baeyens F, Eelen P, Van den Bergh O, Crombez G (1989) Acquired affective-evaluative value: Conservative but not unchangeable. *Behav Res Ther* **27**: 279–287.

Bouton ME (1988) Context and ambiguity in the extinction of emotional learning: Implications for exposure therapy. *Behav Res Ther* **26**: 137–149.

Bouton ME (1994) Conditioning, remembering, and forgetting. *J Experimental Psychology: Animal Behavior Processes* **20**: 219–231.

Bouton ME, Bolles RC (1979) Role of conditioned contextual stimuli in reinstatement of conditioned fear. *J Experimental Psychology: Animal Behavior Processes* **5**: 368–378.

Bouton ME, Bolles RC (1985) Contexts, event-memories and extinction. In Balsam PD, Tomie A (eds) *Context and Learning*. Hillsdale, NJ: Erlbaum.

Bouton ME, Swartzentruber D (1991) Sources of relapse after extinction in Pavlovian and instrumental learning. *Clin Psychology Review* **11**: 123–140.

Bouton ME, Swartzentruber D (1996) Analysis of the associative and occasion-setting properties of contexts participating in a Pavlovian discrimination. *J Experimental Psychology: Animal Behavior Processes* **12**: 333–350.

Bower GH, Hilgard ER (1981) *Theories of Learning*, 5th edition. Englewood Cliffs, NJ: Prentice-Hall.

De Houwer J, Hermans D, Eelen P (1998) Affective and identity priming with episodically associated stimuli. *Cognition and Emotion* **12**: 145–169.

Donegan NH, Gluck MA, Thompson RF (1989) Integrating behavioral and biological models of classical conditioning. *The Psychology of Learning and Motivation* **23**: 109–156.

Hermans D, Baeyens F, Eelen P (1998) Odours as affective processing context for word evaluation: A case of cross-modal affective priming. *Cognition and Emotion* **12**: 601–613.

Hermans D, De Houwer J, Eelen P (1994) The affective priming affect: Automatic activation of evaluative information in memory. *Cognition and Emotion* **8**: 515-533.

Jones MC (1924a) The elimination of children's fears. *J Experimental Psychology* **7**: 383–390.

Jones MC (1924b) A laboratory study of fear: the case of Peter. *Pedalogical Seminary* **31**: 308–315.

Locke J (1894) *An Essay Concerning Human Understanding* (2 vols). Fraser AC (ed.). London: Oxford University Press, 1690; 1700.

Mackintosh NJ (1983) *Conditioning and Associative Learning*. Oxford: Clarendon Press.

Martin I, Levey AB (1987) Learning what will happen next: Conditioning, evaluation and cognitive processes. In Davey G (ed.) *Cognitive Processes and Pavlovian Conditioning in Humans*. New York, Wiley & Sons, pp. 57–82.

Masserman JH (1943) *Behavior and Neurosis*. Chicago: University of Chicago Press.

Menzies RG, Clarke JC (1995) The etiology of phobias: A non-associative account. *Clinical Psychology Review* **15**: 23–48.

Merckelbach H, De Jong P, Muris P, Van den Hout M (1996) The etiology of specific phobias: A review. *Clinical Psychology Review* **16**: 337–361.

Merckelbach H, De Ruiter C, Van den Hout MA, Hoekstra R (1989) Conditioning experiences and phobias. *Behav Res Ther* **27**: 657–662.

Mineka S (1979) The role of fear in theories of avoidance learning, flooding and extinction. *Psychological Bull* **86**: 985–1010.

Mineka S (1987) A primate model of phobic fears. In Eysenck H, Martin I (eds) *Theoretical Foundations of Behavior Therapy*. New York: Plenum Press.

Mineka S, Henderson RW (1985) Controllability and predictability in acquired motivation. *Annual Review of Psychology*, vol. 36. Palo Alto, CA: Annual Reviews Inc.

Mineka S, Kihlstrom J (1978) Unpredictable and uncontrollable aversive events. *J Abnorm Psychol* **87**: 256–271.

Mineka S, Zinbarg R (1996) Conditioning and ethological models of anxiety disorders: Stress-in-dynamic context anxiety models. In Hope DA (ed.) *Perspectives on Anxiety, Panic and Fear*. Vol. 43 of the Nebraska Symposium on Motivation, Lincoln, University of Nebraska Press.

Mowrer OH (1947) On the dual nature of learning. A reinterpretation of "conditioning" and "problem solving". *Harvard Educational Review* **17**: 102–148.

Mowrer OH (1960) *Learning Theory and Behavior*. New York: Wiley.

Neely JH (1991) Semantic priming effects in visual word recognition: A selective review of current findings and theories. In Besner D, Humphreys GW, Glyn W (eds) *Basic Processes in Reading: Visual Word Recognition*. Hillsdale, NJ: Lawrence Erlbaum Associates, pp. 264–336.

Öhman A (1979) The orienting response, attention and learning: An information-processing perspective. In Kimmel HD, Van Holst EH, Orlebeke JF (eds) *The Orienting Reflex in Humans*. Hillsdale, NJ: Erlbaum.

Öst LG, Hugdahl K (1981) Acquisition of phobias and anxiety response patterns in clinical patients. *Behav Res Ther* **16**: 439–447.

Pavlov IP (1927) *Conditioned Reflexes*. London: Oxford University Press.

Pavlov IP (1955) *Selected Works*. J. Gibbons (ed). Moscow: Foreign Languages Publishing House.

Rachman SJ (1977) The conditioning theory of fear acquisition: A critical examination. *Behav Res Ther* **15**: 375–388.

Rachman SJ (1991) Neoconditioning and the classical theory of fear acquisition. *Clin Psychology Review* **11**: 155–173.

Rachman S, Eysenck HJ (1966) Reply to a "critique and reformulation" of behaviour therapy.

Psychological Bull **65**(3): 165–169.

Rescorla RA, Heth C (1975) Reinstatement of fear to an extinguished conditioned stimulus. *J Experimental Psychology: Animal Behavior Processes* **1**: 88–96.

Seligman MEP (1971) Phobias and preparedness. *Behav Ther* **2**: 307–320.

Sokolov EN (1960) Neuronal models and the orienting reflex. In Brazier MA (ed.) *The Central Nervous System and Behavior*. New York: Macy.

Sokolov EN (1975) The neuronal mechanisms of the orienting reflex. In Sokolov EN, Vinogradova OS (eds) *Neuronal Mechanisms of the Orienting Reflex*. Hillsdale, NJ: Erlbaum.

Watson JB, Rayner R (1920) Conditioned emotional reactions. *J Experimental Psychology* **3**: 1–14.

Current Trends in Cognitive Behaviour Therapy for Anxiety Disorders

Ph. Fontaine, E. Mollard, S.N. Yao and J. Cottraux

Hôpital Neurologique et Neuro-Chirurgical, Lyons, France

INTRODUCTION

For a number of years, clinicians have been making a case for more integration between behaviourism and cognitivism. In the 1970s, a major stream of research clearly demonstrated the mutually beneficial effects of a symbiosis between behaviourism and cognitivism.

Historically, behaviour therapy was defined as the application of learning theory and conditioning principles, that is classical and operant conditioning. Classical conditioning refers to the ways people come to associate events that are contiguous in time, operant conditioning stipulates that behaviours are conditioned by their consequences (reinforcers). In that way, Mowrer's two factor-theory encompassed components of both classical and operant conditioning, suggesting fear stimuli are acquired through classical conditioning, and that the subject learns how to reduce this fear when avoiding the conditioned stimuli (negative reinforcement). This prevents the fear from being extinguished through habituation. At this stage, behaviour therapy focused mainly on developing specific conditioning techniques to modify particular problems (e.g. systematic desensitisation for phobias, aversion conditioning for alcoholism). The main focus was on conditioning procedures.

The first formal concern with social variables in behaviour therapy was introduced in 1969 by Bandura with his social learning theory and his research on vicarious learning. His self-efficacy theory (1977) is based on self-attribution of behaviour change. In carrying out exposure and response prevention methods, the aim is to help patients to attribute success experiences to their own mastery. The success of the therapy is guided by its effects on the patient's perceived mastery.

It then appeared important to counteract the patient's dysfunctional cognitive bias by attributing successful performances to sources other than himself. Beck (1976) has emphasised this type of dysfunctional cognition in his conceptualisation and treatment of depression, also suggesting that dysfunctional and negative thinking play a

Anxiety Disorders: An Introduction to Clinical Management and Research. Edited by E. J. L. Griez, C. Faravelli, D. Nutt and J. Zohar. © 2001 John Wiley & Sons, Ltd.

central role in triggering and maintaining negative emotions. According to Beck, this negative view emerges from unconscious negative schemas representing oneself, the world and the future, which have to be discussed "socratically" in order to help the patient to modify his or her beliefs and consequently his or her behaviour. "Behavioural experiments" are then given to the patient in order to test the change in his or her beliefs. Beck's theory and therapy for depression have been extended to many dimensions of psychopathology, especially anxiety disorders, eating disorders, and personality disorders. This chapter deals with cognitive behaviour therapy (CBT) trends and results in anxiety disorders.

PANIC DISORDER AND AGORAPHOBIA

Methods

Although infrequent or single panic attacks are seen in approximately 30% of the general population (Norton et al., 1986), panic disorder occurs in up to 4% of the general population. This rather frequent and distressing condition has been the centre of great interest since the pioneering work of Wolpe on systematic desensitization. To date, a wide range of behavioural procedures have been carried out to manage the disorder, with special focus on avoidance (i.e. agoraphobia) and symptoms control (i.e. breathing retraining, using Valsalva reflex to control tachycardia).

More recently, the cognitive model has been applied to this condition, with special emphasis on the panic component. Cognitive therapy of phobias aims at modifying erroneous assumptions concerning danger (Beck et al., 1985). Clark (1986) proposed a cognitive explanation of the interaction and the negative feed-back loop between cognitions, hyperventilation and external or internal triggering events. These authors established a treatment plan with two main strategies: cognitive restructuring on misinterpretations of bodily sensations and breathing retraining in order to control the physiological effects of hyperventilation. This model also involves exposure with emphasis on behavioural experiments aimed at testing the restructured assumptions of danger. To date, the case of panic disorder represents a good illustration of the merging of cognitive and behaviour therapies (CBT) that becomes more and more a frame of reference for the doctors. Treatment typically includes about 15–20 sessions and can be summarised as follows:

1. Modifying panic attacks (PA):
   (a) Breathing retraining to control the hyperventilatory sensations frequently involved in PA.
   (b) Valsalva technique to control tachycardia.
   (c) Cognitive restructuring to modify misinterpretations of bodily sensations and postulates concerning danger.
2. Modifying avoidance behaviours through graded exposure. Generally the therapy starts with imaginal exposure confronting the patient step by step with the

feared situations until habituation occurs. Then graded *in vivo* exposure is carried out. Exposure *in vivo* represents the final common pathway of all the techniques. Each session of exposure *in vivo* or in imagination may last up to 45 minutes which is, in general, the maximum length of time required to habituate the anxiety responses.

3. Adjunctive techniques could be used as relaxation, social skills training, problem solving, family therapy, etc.

Results

Results of Exposure Treatments

Barlow's review (1984) showed a significant improvement for 70% of the patients with a total symptom elimination for only 18%. The drop-out rate was 12% but reached 25–40% when anti-depressants were added. Relapse was as high as 50% but in general was easily treated with booster sessions. No symptom substitution was found. The clinical significance of exposure treatment also appeared also in the meta-analysis by Jacobson et al. (1988). Using stringent criteria, they found that out of 11 studies there was an average improvement of 58% with only 27% of patients free of symptoms at the end of therapy. A review of 10 long-term follow-ups (up to 9 years) was conducted by O'Sullivan and Marks (1990). Some 474 patients out of 553 were followed up in controlled studies for a mean duration of four years. They found a 76% improvement in the cumulated samples with residual symptoms as a rule; 15–25% of the patients continued to have depressive episodes after treatment. In the longer follow-ups, up to 50% consulted practitioners for their psychological problems and 25% saw psychiatrists for depression and/or agoraphobia. However, the consultation rate decreased.

Cognitive Therapy as an Adjunct to Exposure

The majority of the studies tended to show that cognitive therapy was a clear adjunct to exposure with positive results up to 80% (Cottraux, 1993). The most complete study was conducted by Clark et al. (1994). They found that CBT (84%) was superior to relaxation (40%), imipramine up to 300 mg/day (42%) and a waiting list at a one year follow-up where all intent-to-treat groups received self-exposure instructions. This study confirms the superiority of CBT over the non-specific relaxation and that imipramine, the drug of reference, is neither the only effective treatment, nor the most efficient.

Relaxation

In two studies, cognitive therapy appeared to be superior to Jacobson's relaxation (Barlow, 1988; Öst, 1988). In their two-year follow-up study, Craske et al. (1991) suggested that Jacobson's relaxation could even alter the result of behaviour therapy. In contrast, the Applied Relaxation of Öst (Öst et al., 1993; Öst and Westling, 1995) has been found as effective as CBT. But it contains cognitive coping strategies as well as exposure assignments. Accordingly, the Applied Relaxation is more a form of CBT than a pure relaxation technique.

Psychotropic Drugs and CBT: Antidepressants

Some of them are known to have specific effects on panic, although side effects result in frequent non-compliance by patients and relapse after discontinuation is common: 25% to 100% (Noyes et al., 1986). Reviews of CBT-antidepressant combination suggest a better outcome in the short term, but the gain seems to vanish after withdrawal (Zitrin et al., 1980). However, antidepressants are useful in case of depression or in panic attacks continuing to be frequent and intense after six weeks of exposure (Marks, 1987; Wolfe and Maser, 1994).

Benzodiazepines

High potency benzodiazepines have an intrinsic therapeutic activity alone or combined with CBT, but only on a short-term basis (Wardle et al., 1994; Marks et al., 1993). A negative interaction is found after withdrawal, although CBT can facilitate discontinuation (Otto et al., 1993; Spiegel et al., 1994). Only buspirone demonstrated a positive interaction on agoraphobia in the short term without negative effect at follow-up (Cottraux et al., 1995).

Meta-analyses

The first four meta-analyses on panic disorder (Mattick et al., 1990; Cox et al., 1992; Clum et al., 1993; Van Balkom, 1994) found *in vivo* exposure as a critical component of treatment but disagreed on its results in combination with antidepressants, anxiolytics and cognitive intervention. A more recent meta-analysis by Gould et al. (1995) found a higher effect for CBT compared with pharmacotherapy and combination of medication with therapy, with the lowest drop-out rate and the best cost-efficacy ratio.

GENERALISED ANXIETY DISORDER (GAD)
Methods

GAD is four times as frequent as panic disorder. Since the first operationalised definition of the disorder in the DSM-III (APA, 1980), the pathogenesis has been clearly centred on the concept of excessive worry (DSM-III-R, APA, 1987). This cognitive view tended to consider the somatic symptoms as secondary manifestations. Moreover, the DSM-IV (APA, 1994) paid allegiance to the cognitive model with another criterion: the difficulty to control the worry. This new trend was supported by numerous studies assessing normal and abnormal thoughts. The distress seemed to relate to the frequency, the intensity of the thoughts, and the difficulty of ignoring them (Clark, 1986; England and Dickerson, 1988; Kent and Janbunather, 1989). Worry correlated more with anxiety and the uncontrolabillity of the thought than with the sense of internal tension (Borkovec and Inz, 1990; Clark, 1986).

A central key feature appeared to be the sense of uncertainty that prevented the patient from using existing coping strategies (Blais et al., 1993). Worries are viewed as cognitive distortions, resulting from maladaptive schemas of danger, triggered by trivial situations, preventing normal coping. In that way, Krohne's model (Krohne, 1989; Krohne, 1993) postulates that patients are perpetually switching between intolerance of uncertainty leading to an approach behaviour and intolerance to emotional arousal leading to avoidance. This prevents the patient from dealing correctly with any coping strategy despite the belief that worry has a preventive value. With respect to the treatment, the patient is taught to consider his or her catastrophic view up to its ultimate consequences (downward arrow technique) This allows him/her, through socratic questioning, to substitute a more probabilistic view instead and to establish coping strategies for the worst case. He or she can also be exposed in their imagination to the catastrophic scenes to reach habituation. Finally, basic schemas of danger are questioned in a tactful and socratic way.

Ladouceur et al. (1995) proposed a typology of worries with specific guidelines. Ladouceur's model classifies worries into three types and offers treatment guidelines for each of these three types:

1. Realistic and modifiable (e.g., a conflict at work which may be solved by assertion training and problem-solving techniques).
2. Realistic but not modifiable (e.g., having real physical illness): teaching coping skills, problem solving and flooding in imagination would be the treatment.
3. Remote events that are not realistic, unpredictable, improbable and consequently not modifiable: the treatment could be flooding in imagination, cognitive modification and problem solving.

The main aims of the treatment are to help the patient to recognise worries as approach-avoidance behaviour, to discriminate between different types of worries, and to apply the correct strategy to each type of worry. Evaluation of this treatment package is underway.

As in other cognitive behaviour therapies, cognitive interventions are combined with other techniques such as relaxation and exposure.The treatment classically involves about 15 sessions. We can describe three main levels of intervention:

1. Cue-controlled relaxation.
2. Cognitive therapy: several techniques are used:
   (a) considering the worst possibility
   (b) evaluation of probability for the worry
   (c) problem solving
   (d) discussing basic schemas (e.g., usefulness and efficacy of worry)
   (e) exposure in imagination in order to obtain habituation to highly improbable situation
3. Avoidance modification: this is useful as avoidance prevents the patient from using his/her own coping strategies.

Results

To date, numerous controlled studies permit a first evaluation of the non-pharmacological procedures to treat the condition. The meta-analysis by Chambless and Gillis (1993) demonstrates the effectiveness of CBT on worry and anxiety compared with a waiting list and placebo. Furthermore, the results were maintained at 6 to 12 months follow-up. Borkovec and Whisman (1996) found similar results, but failed to find any superiority of CBT over non-specific treatment like non-directive therapy or between cognitive, behavioural and cognitive behaviour therapy. A more recent meta-analysis by Gould et al. (1997) found CBT and pharmacotherapy equally effective, but the drug samples had a higher drop-out rates and showed a loss of efficacy at withdrawal, while the effects of CBT were maintained. However, studies assessing the CBT–drug combination are lacking.

Moreover, psychotherapy could facilitate withdrawal. Within the field of psychotherapy, CBT appeared superior to cognitive or behaviour therapy alone. CBT for GAD also appeared to be more effective in reducing comorbid depressive symptomatology. One should also notice the very cost-effective method called "Stresspac" (White, 1995), which consists of a self-management book that has been found superior to counselling and a waiting list.

POST-TRAUMATIC STRESS DISORDER

Methods

Prevalence of PTSD is evaluated at 1–14% in the general population, reaching 3–58% in a risk population. Treatment of PTSD is the centre of a growing interest in the literature. PTSD could be viewed as the lack of schema for treating unexpected and inconceivable information concerning danger. Therapeutic programmes involve relaxation, beneficial in the case of high emotional arousal, exposure to avoided situations or images related to the trauma, and cognitive therapy. Six methods have been proposed:

1. Systematic desensitisation means presenting the feared stimuli under relaxation in a graded way before *in vivo* exposure.
2. Exposure in imagination and *in vivo* aim at habituating the patient to the aversive stimulus, by reducing abnormal reactivity and avoidance.
3. Stress management emphasises coping strategies when confronted to feared stimulus (relaxation, social skills training, modification of anxious verbalisation, thought stopping).
4. Cognitive therapy also proposes imaginal exposure and representation of coping strategies but puts a greater emphasis on tackling automatic thoughts and dysfunctional attitudes (personalisation, culpability, illusion of a safe world, necessity of vengeance).
5. Eye Movement Desensitisation and Reprocessing (EMDR) consists in inducing eye movements when concentrated on feared imagery, bodily sensations and negative statements associated with the trauma, in order to reduce anxiety, then to modify the cognitions and the flashbacks (Shapiro, 1989). This method is hypothesised to work on neuropsychological functions.
6. Debriefing is early intervention (no more than 48 hours after the trauma) that aims at preventing the development of PTSD. Emphasis is put on the expression of the emotions. Normalisation of the fear response and the deculpabilisation are stressed. In some cases, it is also necessary to provide psychosocial rehabilitation and alcohol/drug withdrawal.

Results

Most of the studies showed positive results but they are still few (see Table 14.1). Follow-up studies never exceed six months. Thus, the interpretation of the results must be cautious and further research is needed, especially with longer follow-up. Stress management appears to reduce vegetative symptoms, while exposure tackles avoidance. One must be aware of the fact that exposure can cause depression, panic disorder or alcohol relapse in some population (like veterans). In the same way, early intervention could not always be beneficial.

OBSESSIVE-COMPULSIVE DISORDER

Methods

Epidemiological studies emphasised the prevalence of the illness as high as 2% of the general population with a duration before consultation up to 13 years. High comor-

TABLE 14.1 Controlled studies on PTSD

Technique	Result	Researcher
Systematic desensitisation	Positive	Peniston (1986) DS > WL
		Brom et al. (1989)
		DS = ANA = HYP > WL
Exposure	Positive:	Boudewyns et al. (1990)
		Cooper and Clum (1989)
		Keane et al. (1989)
		Foa et al. (1991)
Cognitive therapy	Positive:	Resick (1992)
		Echeburua et al. (1996)
Stress management	Positive:	Resick and Schnicke (1992)
		Foa et al. (1991)
Eye movement	Positive:	Wilson et al. (1995) EMDR > WL
desensitisation		(follow-up: 3 months)
and reprocessing	Negative:	Jensen (1994) EMDR = WL
		Vaughan et al. (1994)
		EMDR = Relaxation = Flooding
Early intervention	Positive:	André et al. (1997)
		Chemtob et al. (1997)
	Negative:	Bisson et al. (1997)

Notes: WL = waiting list, HYP = hypnosis, ANA = Psychoanalysis, DS = Systematic Desensitisation.

bidity is common, especially with depression (30–50%). Obsessional symptomatology could be divided into two main dimensions: overt compulsions (ritualisers), for whom a greater emphasis is put on behavioural techniques, and covert compulsions (obsessional ruminators), for whom greater emphasis is put on cognitive techniques. The therapeutic tools encompass behavioural, cognitive and pharmacological (serotonergic) interventions, mostly combined.

The main behavioural strategy is *in vivo* exposure with response prevention (Marks, 1987), which means exposure is carried out while compulsions are not allowed and prevented to occur. The aim is to reach habituation to the triggering stimuli. Nonetheless, it is just as effective, less time-consuming and very cost-effective to give homework assignments which are agreed on with the patient (Emmelkamp and Kraanen, 1977; Marks et al., 1988). It is also helpful to involve the patient's partner as co-therapist (Hand et al., 1979). For patients for whom the trigger is more internal, e.g. fear of internal representation rather than environmental cues or having covert rituals, prolonged exposure in imagination is the recommended procedure (Foa et al., 1980). Although the effectiveness of behaviour therapy for OCD is well established, the limitations (especially for obsessional ruminations) justify testing adjunctive procedures like cognitive interventions (Rachman, 1996; Rachman, 1997).

Since RET (Rationale Emotive Therapy) and self-instructional training have been the main cognitive strategies for the past 10 years, a cognitive behavioural model for OCD has been proposed by Salkovskis (1985). First, the intrusive thought, unacceptable, egodystonic is viewed as a "normal" process failing to habituate for biological and/or psychological reasons. Four surveys showed that more than 80% of normal subjects have intrusive thoughts with content similar to those found in OCD (Rachman and De Silva, 1978; Salkovskis and Harrison, 1984; Niler and Beck, 1989; Freeston et al., 1991).

Second, the obsessive thought (automatic thought) is an evaluation of the intrusive ideas through over-responsibility schemas (Ladouceur et al., 1995; Lopatka and Rachman, 1995) deep-seated in the long-term memory. This leads to rituals (covert behaviour) and to neutralising thoughts (covert behaviour) which represent an attempt to control and suppress intrusive thoughts. Such an "undoing process" prevents habituation to intrusive thoughts occurring. Hence, Salkovskis proposed a triple intervention: cognitive exposure to intrusive thoughts with neutralisation prevention, socratic questioning of the automatic thoughts and over-responsibility schemas, followed by behavioural experiments (*in vivo* exposure) to disconfirm the schemas. Treatment classically involves 20–25 sessions with several components.

1. Cognitive components
    (a) Dedramation of the worst consequence of automatic thoughts.
    (b) Reattribution of guilt.
    (c) Questioning automatic thoughts or irrational postulates.
    (d) Reassurance behaviours is discouraged.
2. Behavioural components
    (a) Exposure with response prevention to modify the rituals.
3. Specific treatment of ruminations
    (a) Exposure in imagination to the automatic thought without cognitive neutralisation (e.g., loop tape, writing down repeatedly, deliberate thought evocation).
    (b) Exposure in imagination (flooding) to the worst consequence of the thoughts.

Results

Results of Behaviour Therapy

Behaviour therapy demonstrates a clear superiority over placebo and relaxation. The outcome of behaviour therapy is close to that of serotonergic antidepressants which have detrimental side-effects and a high relapse rate after withdrawal (Marks, 1987). The limitations of behaviour therapy could be summed up as follows: drop-out or refusals 25%, no or poor effect 25%, relapse 20% (three months to three years) (Salkovskis and Warwick, 1988).

The controlled studies combining behaviour therapy with antidepressants show a better outcome on rituals and depression in the short term, vanishing after time, especially after withdrawal (see Table 14.2). In particular, Cottraux et al. (1993) showed fluvoxamine plus behaviour therapy compared with placebo plus behaviour

TABLE 14.2 Obsessions-compulsions: exposure + response prevention and antidepressants study

Study	N		Hamilton DEPRESSION (17 items)
Solyom, 1977	27		SHORT TERM: (6 weeks) Ruminations: CMI = imagal flooding CMI > thought stopping Rituals: CMI < E
Marks, 1980	40	17	SHORT TERM (7 weeks) CMI + E > CMI + R
	37		LONG TERM (2 years): CMI + E > PBO + E in weeks 7–18, waning at week 36
Marks, 1988	49	10	SHORT TERM (17 weeks) CMI + E > CMI + A
	39		LONG TERM (2 years): CMI + E > PBO + E at week 8, waning at week 17
Cottraux, 1990	60	19	SHORT TERM (8 weeks): FLV + E and FLV > PBO + E on rituals
	44		MID-TERM (24 weeks): FLV + E and FLV > PBO + E on depression
	37		LONG TERM (1 year): FLV + E = PBO + E = FLV
Cottraux, 1993	33		LONG TERM (18 months) FLV + E = PBO + E = FLV still under antidepressants: PBO + E and FLV + E = 18% versus FLV = 60% (P < 0.05)
Foa, 1990	19	20	SHORT TERM (6 weeks): IMI > PBO on depression LONG TERM (2 years):
	19	11	IMI + E = PBO + E
	19	20	IMI + E = PBO + E
Baxter, 1992	18	9	SHORT TERM (10 weeks): FLUOX = E on OC symptoms and reduction of right caudate hypermetabolism (PET)
Van Balkom, 1994	104		SHORT TERM: FLV = TCC > LA (rituals) TCC > FLV > LA (anxiety)

CMI = Clomipramine;   FLV = Fluvoxamine;   Fluox = Fluoxetine;   IMI = Imipramine; PBO = Placebo; E = Exposure; R = Relaxation; A = Anti-exposure; PET = Positron Emission Tomography.

therapy gave better results at three months for rituals and at six months for depression with equivalent results at 12 and 18 months.

It has to be noted that the results by Van Balkom are part of a larger multicentre study assessing cognitive and behaviour therapy, alone or combined with fluvoxamine (De Haan et al., 1997; Van Balkom, 1998; Van Oppen et al., 1995).

When addressing long-term follow-up, O'Sullivan and Marks (1990) reviewed nine cohorts of patients over one to six years (mean of three years). They found 9% drop-out and 78% improvement with a 60% mean reduction in rituals. Nonetheless, residual symptoms were a rule and liability for depression remained unchanged.

Results of Cognitive Therapy

To date, the usefulness of cognitive therapy for OCD has been assessed in five controlled studies. Emmelkamp et al. (1980) did not find a superior effect when adding cognitive modifications to *in vivo* exposure. Nevertheless, the design of the experiment aimed at teaching the patient to replace negative thoughts by positive ones. This could have been used as neutralising thoughts.

Emmelkamp et al. (1988) compared cognitive therapy without exposure to self-managed exposure. Six months after the end of the treatment, both group showed equivalent reduction in rituals, generalised anxiety and social anxiety. Only the cognitive group showed change on the measures of depression. In a study with a more impaired population, Emmelkamp and Beens (1991) found similar results at a six-month follow-up.

Van Oppen et al. (1995) randomised 71 patients in either Beckian cognitive therapy or exposure. They found after 16 sessions a superiority of cognitive interventions over exposure. Danger schemas were better modified by cognitive therapy than by exposure. Unfortunately, this study had no long-term follow-up.

Freeston et al. (1997) presented a study comparing a waiting list to a group treated with the Salkovskis' model of CBT. They found, with a group of obsessional with exclusively covert rituals a superiority over the waiting list maintained at six months follow-up. Although there is a clear need for more controlled studies, there are elements arguing for a positive effect of cognitive approach for OCD.

SOCIAL PHOBIA

Methods

According to Kessler et al. (1994), social phobics represent more than 13% of the general population. However, there are more subjects who suffer from deficient social competence and situational anxiety, causing many difficulties or even handicaps in their family or socio-professional lives. This view leads to the conception of a continuum from shyness to restricted and generalised social phobia and avoidance personality disorder as an extreme form (Rapee and Heimberg, 1997). Several effective psychological treatments for social phobia have been developed over the past two decades, especially the behavioural and cognitive approach and their merging into CBT.

Behavioural intervention is based on the notion of lacking or unadaptive skills. Social skills training through role play with rehearsal, shaping and modelling by the therapist is effective in treating social phobics. The therapy can be practised in individual or group settings, although the group formula is generally considered more effective. The rationale of such a treatment refers to both exposure and social learning principles. First, the therapy specifies the anxiogenic situation: for instance, making a request or a refusal, expressing or receiving a critic, expressing or giving a compliment, conversational skills. The situation is role-played by the patient and the therapist or another patient. Positive feedback is given by the therapist. Then, the patient is taught to observe others playing the situation and to discriminate what is positive in each scene (modelling). After this modelling phase the patient has to elicit more appropriate behaviours during the group sessions. At the end of each group session the patients agrees on a task to be carried out in real-life situations (homework). According to the cognitive model of social phobia (Beck et al., 1985), cognitive factors may be particularly important in the development and maintenance of the negative emotion and the avoidant behaviour in social phobia. The patients assume that other people are inherently critical and attach particular importance to being positively appraised by others (Rapee and Heimberg, 1997). This could be related to a basic schema in terms of inferiority (Yao et al., 1998). When in a social situation, patients form a mental representation of themselves as presumably seen by the audience and simultaneously focus their attentional resources onto both this representation and onto any perceived threat in the environment. The representation relies on internal cues (proprioception, physical symptoms) and external cues (audience feedback). In addition to the allocation of attentional resource to these perceived threats and representation, the subjects formulate a prediction of a perceived performance standard or norm. A discrepancy between norm and representation is seen as the likelihood of a negative evaluation. The anxiety elicited has physiological, cognitive and behavioural components that are prone to influence self-representation, thus renewing the cycle (Rapee and Heimberg, 1997). Cognitive therapy consists in identifying negative automatic thoughts and schemas, and then modifying them by more realistic interpretations. Current models tend to mix cognitive and behavioural methods. The patient's evidence for his/her negative belief is cognitively questioned but a greater emphasis is placed on behavioural experiments to test the irrational assumptions (e.g. dropping safety behaviours, video and audio feedback, intentional performance of the fears). Emphasis is also placed on replacing internal by external focus. As we can see, the behavioural model is based more on the notion of lack in social skills, while the cognitive one is based on skills impeded by misinterpretation of social situations.

Treatment classically involves about 15–20 sessions and has several phases. Cognitive phase with assessment and discussion of automatic thoughts in social situations, replacement of negative thoughts by positive ones isolating and challenging the schemas. Behavioural experiments are proposed to disconfirm the schemas. The behavioural phase consists generally of the implementation of social skills training in a group format.

Results

Results of Behaviour Therapy

Systematic desensitisation and role play have been found to be more effective than the waiting list (Marzillier et al., 1976). However, Butler et al. (1984) found *in vivo* exposure to be superior to the waiting list. Long-term gains of exposure techniques seemed to be maintained (O'Sullivan and Marks, 1990). Shaw (1979) demonstrated that imagination exposure was similar to role play. Nonetheless, the gains seemed to be limited for some patients and it appeared that cognitive factors prevented patients from full recovery of anxiety even with exposure.

Result of Cognitive Behaviour Therapy

The first studies assessing the effectiveness of cognitive therapy in social phobia shared positive results compared with a waiting list or other therapies (Kanter and Goldfried, 1979; Emmelkamp et al., 1985; Jerremalm et al., 1986). Stravinsky et al. (1982), at six-month follow-up, found no advantage of cognitive restructuring over behaviour therapy. Two other studies (Butler et al., 1984; Mattick et al., 1989) found a superiority of the merging in CBT over exposure alone. Heimberg et al. (1990, 1993) demonstrated the efficacy of CBT in group settings over supportive therapy on a six-year follow-up. Nonetheless, a comparison of CBT in the Heimberg's setting with graded *in vivo* exposure reported a slight advantage to exposure.

Emmelkamp and Scholing (1993) showed, for limited phobias, no difference when comparing cognitive therapy before or after behaviour therapy or the merging in CBT. Scholing and Emmelkamp (1993) suggested, for generalised phobias, that cognitive therapy before behaviour therapy was preferable to the contrary or a mixed CBT.

A French multicentric study (Cottraux et al., 2000) compared an individual cognitive therapy followed by group therapy (social skill training) with supportive therapy. They found a clear advantage over supportive therapy presented as usual. Significant gains were made with cognitive therapy but the main effects were seen after social skills training in group. However, the individual cognitive approach seemed to diminish the high drop-out rate seen when patients were directly engaged in group therapy.

All these results clearly suggest that exposure whenever alone or in CBT represents a critical part of the treatment of social phobia. In the same vein, a meta-analysis by

Freske and Chambless (1995) concluded that CBT had no clear advantage over exposure on cognitive measures. These results also suggest that exposure has cognitive effect. Nevertheless, cognitive therapy is necessary at least for those who cannot enter directly into group therapy.

Drug Therapy versus CBT

Gelernter et al. (1991) compared four groups: CBT, phenelzine, alprazolam and placebo. All four groups received instruction in self-exposure. All groups improved significantly at two months with few differences between them. However, this equal improvement could have resulted in exposure that is therapeutic by itself.

Liebowitz (1993, 1996) compared phenelzine, placebo, CBT and support. Phenelzine showed a superiority over the other groups at six weeks. At post-test, CBT and phenelzine were both superior to the other groups. Phenelzine appeared superior to CBT until withdrawal.

Recently, moclobemide was also studied in four controlled studies (Versiani et al., 1996; Noyes et al., 1997; The International Multicenter Clinical Trial Group, 1997; Schneier et al., 1998), but only Versiani's first study found really robust effects.

These few studies tended to demonstrate the effectiveness of certain drugs on social phobia compared with CBT but at the cost of an indefinite maintenance. More studies are needed to assess the usefulness of combining drug therapy with CBT in treating social phobia.

SPECIFIC PHOBIA

Methods

Specific phobia is often considered a normal fear like the fear of animals or of blood, nevertheless, it affects 7% of the general population. In some cases, anxiety and avoidance behaviours become a handicap severe enough to lead to consultation. The general principle of the treatment for phobias is *in vivo* exposure in order to obtain habituation. We can describe about five varieties. In systematic desensitisation, the subject is relaxed and presented a hierarchy of graded stimuli, first in imagination and after, *in vivo*. In *in vivo* desensitisation, the patient is relaxed and gradually exposed to real situations. During *in vivo* graded exposure, he or she is confronted step by step with feared situations. One can also use modelling by the therapist to guide and precede the patient into the situation. Through flooding therapy, the subject is exposed in their imagination to the most fearful image until habituation occurs. During exposure (or flooding) *in vivo*, the patient is confronted with the most feared situation until habituation occurs. The cognitive model is also proposed, to correct irrational postulates and schemas of danger. Treatment classically involves about 10 sessions.

Results

There is a lack of controlled studies. In many controlled trials simple phobias are often part of mixed samples of phobic patients. Follow-up studies showed a 54% improvement from baseline which is maintained at follow-up ranging from one to five years with behaviour therapy (O'Sullivan and Marks, 1990). Two early controlled studies of cognitive therapy showed negative results (Biran and Wilson, 1981; Ladouceur, 1983). A more recent study by Getka and Glass (1992) compared four groups for dentist phobia: systematic desensitisation, cognitive therapy and stress management, interview with a warmth practitioner prior to intervention and waiting list. At a one-year follow-up, behaviour and cognitive therapy showed equivalent results superior to the two other conditions, but this needs more investigation.

Considering pharmacology, Zitrin et al. (1978) showed in a controlled study that imipramine was ineffective and may have detrimental effects. Recently, virtual reality was introduced as a means of treating height and plane phobias with positive results in a controlled study (Rothbaum et al., 1995). To summarise, despite a scarce literature, *in vivo* exposure seems to be the treatment of choice for specific phobia.

WHERE ARE WE NOW AND WHERE SHOULD WE GO?

Behavioural and cognitive approaches have merged into CBT, and CBT tends now to dominate clinical research and practice. A case in point is the panic model by Clark (1986). Results of CBT in the other anxious disorders are actually promising. One should note the influence of panic theory on the development of theories for other anxiety disorders: the special focus on misinterpretation of internal or external cues as danger signs leading to anxiety. Along with Rachman (1996), we want to point out some important issues in the future of CBT.

In the future, CBT will be shaped by external forces, like the cost-containment issues (Rachman, 1996). This will lead our procedures to become increasingly refined and cost-effective. In the long term, we will have to transform many techniques into self-help procedures (Marks et al., 1983), computer-assisted therapy (Gosh et al., 1988), non-specialist therapy (e.g., nurses or social workers, Welkowitz et al., 1991), or group therapy (Marks, 1987).

There is a growing amount of treatment manuals that provide empirically validated therapies to non-specialised or even lay therapists. This has a central role to play in the dissemination and availability of health care (Persons, 1997). Yet, therapy offered in a manual has limitations, especially when the therapists are facing patients with multiple problems. In the same way, research uses problem-focused manuals, as opposed to diagnostic-focused manuals in order to find a balance between controlled procedures and flexibility (Eiffert et al., 1997).

Another challenge is the current development in biological psychiatry. Although there is not necessarily a conflict between biological and psychological explanations, in practice, the theories and procedures are in competition. For a variety of reasons, including the cost, the availability, and the dominant influence of medicine, drug therapy for psychological problems tends to be the norm despite the demonstrated efficacy and effectiveness of CBT. This leads us to think about the future of the relationship between physicians and other health care practitioners.

Since the fundamental decision to adopt empiricism in the study of normal and abnormal psychology and the pioneering works in learning theory, one should notice that the interest for fundamental psychology has tended to fade away. The first behaviourists relied heavily on fundamental research work, but the gap between practice and basic sciences has grown larger and larger (Foa and Kozak, 1997). Three related issues might be of relevance here. First, experimental psychology is still too theoretical to offer much guidance on clinical problems. Second, experimental psychopathology has not made relevant use of the knowledge for their clinical application. Finally, therapy researchers have made limited use of the existing knowledge of basic research. Only the refreshing cognitive model gave rise to a renewed enthusiasm in theory building. However, the fact remains that our efficacy is better than our theoretical knowledge: hence we tend to shift from science to technology.

The merging into CBT, for example, is more driven by empirical clinical considerations than by fundamental research. In that way, we need to determine, for instance, the extent to which the cognitive explanation can account for the therapeutic effects of exposure and pharmacological treatment.

Moreover, contemporary attempts to advance the field of CBT have been eclectic or integrationist, involving various therapies or components, in an effort to surpass the efficacy of the individual parts. This led more to incremental improvements than to efficacy breakthroughs. Although a better enrichment is to wait from fundamental psychology, biological factors could also account for the relative slowing in progress. Learning has undoubtedly biological boundaries and there is growing evidence for the involvement of biological factors such as genetics in psychopathology. CBT has largely ignored this body of knowledge. Maybe we are still haunted by the mind–body dualism which suggests that so-called "biological" disorders should be dealt with biological means and so-called "psychological" disorders with psychological treatments. Some results suggest that many disorders involve both biological and psychological processes. In the long term, the trend could be to move towards a bio-psychosocial model accounting for many variables implied in human behaviours and cognitions.

REFERENCES

American Psychiatric Association (1980) *Diagnostic and Statistical Manual of Mental Disorders* 3rd edition. Washington, DC: American Psychiatric Association.

American Psychiatric Association (1987) *Diagnostic and Statistical Manual of Mental Disorders* 3rd revised edition. Washington, DC. French transl. P Pichot, JD Guelfi (1988) *Manuel diagnostique et statistique des troubles mentaux.* Paris: Masson.

American Psychiatric Association (1994) *Diagnostic and Statistical Manual of Mental Disorders* 4th edition. Washington, DC: American Psychiatric Association.

André C, Lelord F, Légeron P, Reigner A, Delattre A (1997) Etude contrôlée de l'efficacité à six mois d'une prise en charge précoce de 132 conducteurs d'autobus victimes d'une agression. *L'Encéphale* **23**: 65–71.

Bandura A (1977) *Social Learning Theory*. Englewoods Cliffs, NJ: Prentice Hall.

Barlow D (1984) The psychosocial treatment of anxiety disorders: current status future directions. In Williams JB, Spitzer RL, *Psychotherapy Research*. New York: Guilford Press, pp. 89–105.

Barlow D (1988) *Anxiety and its Disorder: The Nature and Treatment of Anxiety and Panic*. New York: Guilford Press.

Baxter L, Schwartz J, Bergman K, Szuba M, Guze B, Mazziota J, Alazraki A, Selin C, Huan-Kwang F, Munford P, Phelps M (1992) Caudate glucose metabolic rate changes with both drug and behavior therapy for obsessive-compulsive disorder. *Arch Gen Psychiatry* **49**: 681–689.

Beck AT (1976) *Cognitive Therapy and the Emotional Disorders*. New York: International Universities Press.

Beck AT, Emery G, Greenberg R (1985) *Anxiety Disorders and Phobias: A Cognitive Perspective*. New York: Basic Books.

Biran M, Wilson GT (1981) Treatment of phobic disorders using cognitive and exposure methods: A self-efficacy analysis. *J Consult Clin Psychology* **49**(6): 886–899.

Bisson JI, Jenkins PL, Alexander J, Bannister C (1997) Randomised controlled trial of psychological debriefing for victims of acute burn trauma. *Br J Psychiatry* **167**: 171.

Blais F, Ladouceur R, Dugas MJ, Freeston MH (1993) Résolution de problème et inquiétude: distinction clinique (Problem solving and worry: clinical distinction). Paper presented at the annual meeting of the Société Québécoise pour la recherche en psychologie, Québec, Canada, November.

Borkovec TD, Inz J (1990) The nature of worry in generalized anxiety disorders: A predominance of thought activity. *Behav Res Ther* **28**: 153–158.

Borkovec TD, Whisman MA (1996) Psychosocial treatments for generalized anxiety disorders. In Mavissakalian M, Prienar R (eds) *Long-term Treatment of Anxiety Disorders*. Washington, DC: American Psychiatric Association.

Boudewyns P, Hyser L, Woods M, Harrison W, Mc Cranie E (1990) PTSD among Vietnam veterans: An early look at treatment outcome using direct treatment exposure. *J Traum Stress* **3**: 359–365.

Brom D, Kleber RJ, Defares PB (1989) Brief psychotherapy for post-traumatic stress disorders. *J Consult Clin Psychology* **57**: 607–612.

Butler G, Cullington A, Monby M (1984) Exposure and anxiety management in the treatment of social phobia. *J Clin Psychology* **52**: 642–650.

Chambless DL, Gillis MM (1993) Cognitive therapy of anxiety disorders. *J Consult Clin Psychology* **61**: 248–260.

Chemtob CM, Tomas S, Law W, Cremniter D (1997) Post-disaster psychological interventions: A field study of the impact of debriefing on psychological disasters. *Am J Psychiatry* **154**(3): 415–417.

Clark DA (1986) A cognitive approach to panic. *Behav Res Ther* **4**(24): 461–470.

Clark D, Salkovskis P, Hackmann A, Middleton H, Anastasiades P, Gelder M (1994) A comparison of cognitive therapy, applied relaxation and imipramine in the treatment of panic disorder. *Br J Psychiatry* **164**: 759–769.

Clum GA, Clum G, Surls R (1993) A meta-analysis of treatments for panic disorder. *J Consult Clin Psychology* **61**: 317–326.

Cooper N, Clum B (1989) Imaginal flooding as a supplementary treatment for PTSD in combat veterans: A controlled study. *Behav Ther* **20**: 381–391.

Cottraux J (1991) *Cognitive-behavior Therapy*. Report to the WHO scientific group on treatment of psychiatric disorders. Geneva, November 20–24, 1989, Revised December 31, 1991.

Cottraux J (1993) Behavior therapy. In Sartorius N, De Girolamo G, Andrews G, German A, Eisenberg L (eds) *Treatment of Mental Disorders: A Review of Effectiveness*. WHO, Washington: American Psychiatric Press, pp. 199–232.

Cottraux J (1994) Alternatives thérapeutiques non-médicamenteuses dans le traitement des troubles anxieux et des troubles du sommeil. Utilisation pratique courante. Paper presented at Conférence de consensus: anxiolytiques, hypnotiques, optimiser la prescription, Euro-médecine 94, Montpellier, 11 November.

Cottraux J (1998) *Les thérapies comportementales et cognitives* 3rd edition. Editions Masson, pp. 303–304.

Cottraux J, Mollard E, Bouvard M, Marks I (1993) Exposure therapy, Fluvoxamine or combination treatment in obsessive-compulsive disorder: one year follow-up. *Psychiatry Research* 49: 63–75.

Cottraux J, Mollard E, Bouvard M, Marks I, Sluys M, Nury AM, Douge R, Cialdella Ph (1990) A controlled study of fluvoxamine and exposure in obsessive-compulsive disorder. *Inter Clin Psychopharmacology* 5: 17–30.

Cottraux J, Note ID, Cungi C et al. (1995) A controlled study of cognitive-behavior therapy with buspirone or placebo in panic disorder with agoraphobia: a one year follow-up. *Br J Psychiatry* 167: 635–641.

Cox BJ, Endler NS, Lee PS, Swinson RP (1992) A meta-analysis of treatments for panic disorder with agoraphobia: Imipramine, alprazolam and in vivo exposure. *J Behav Ther Experimental Psychiatry* 23: 175–182.

Craske MG, Brown TA, Barlow DH (1991) Behavioural treatment of panic disorders: a two year follow-up. *Behav Ther* 22(3): 289–304.

De Haan F, Van Oppen P, Van Balkon AJLM, Spinhoven P, Hoogduin KAL, Van Dyck R (1997) Prediction of outcome and early vs late improvement in OCD patients treated with cognitive behavior therapy and pharmacotherapy. *Acta Psychiatr Scand* 96: 354–361.

Echeburua E, De Corral P, Sarasua B, Zubizarreta I (1996) Treatment of acute postraumatic stress disorder in rape victims: An experimental study. *J Anx Dis* 10(3): 185–199.

Eifferts GH, Schulk D, Zvolensky MJ, Lejucz CW, Lan AW (1997) Manualized behavior therapy: Merits and challenges. *Behav Ther* 28: 499–509.

Emmelkamp P, Beens H (1991) Cognitive therapy with obsessive-compulsive disorder: A comparative evaluation. *Behav Res Ther* 29(3): 293–300.

Emmelkamp P, Kraanen J (1977) Therapist controlled exposure versus self-controlled exposure in vivo: A comparison with obsessive-compulsive patients. *Behav Res Ther* 15: 341–346.

Emmelkamp P, Mersch PP, Vissia E, Van der Helm M (1985) Social phobia: A comparative evaluation of cognitive and behavioral interventions. *Behav Res Ther* 23: 365–369.

Emmelkamp PMG, Scholing A (1993) Cognitive and behavioral treatments of fear of blushing, sweating or trembling. *Behav Res Ther* 31(2): 155–170.

Emmelkamp P, Van der Helm M, Van Zanten B, Plochg I (1980) Contribution of self-instructional training to the effectiveness of exposure in vivo: a comparison with obsessive-compulsive patients. *Behav Res Ther* 18: 61–66.

Emmelkamp P, Visser S, Hoekstra RJ (1988) Cognitive therapy versus in vivo exposure in the treatment of obsessive-compulsive patients. *Cognitive Therapy and Research* 12(1): 103–114.

England SL, Dickerson M (1988) Intrusive thoughts: Unpleasantness not the major cause of uncontrollability. *Behav Res Ther* 26: 279–282.

Freske U, Chambless DL (1995) Cognitive behavioral versus exposure only treatment for social phobia. *Behav Ther* 26: 695–720.

Foa EB, Kozak MJ (1997) Beyond the efficacy ceiling? Cognitive behavior therapy in search of theory. *Behav Ther* 28: 601–611.

Foa EB, Kozak M, Steketee G, McCarthy PR (1992) Treatment of depressive and obsessive-compulsive symptoms in obsessive-compulsive disorder by imipramine and behavior therapy. *Br J Clin Psychology* **31**: 279–292.

Foa EB, Rothbaum BO, Riggs DS, Murdock TB (1991) Treatment of posttraumatic stress disorder in rape victims: A comparison between cognitive-behavioral procedures and counseling. *J Consult Clinical Psychology* **59**: 715–723.

Foa EB, Steketee G, Turner RM, Fischer S (1980) Effects of imaginable exposure to feared disasters in obsessive compulsive checkers. *Behav Res Ther* **18**: 449–455.

Freeston M, Ladouceur R, Gagnon F, Thibodeau N, Rhéaume J, Letarte H, Bujold A (1997) Cognitive-behavioral treatment of obsessive-thoughts: A controlled study. *J Consult Clin Psychology* **65**(3): 405–413.

Freeston MH, Ladouceur R, Thibodeau H et al. (1991) Cognitive intrusions in non clinical population. I: Response style subjective experience and appraisal. *Behav Res Ther* **25**: 585–597.

Gerlernter C, Uhde T, Cimbolic P, Arnkoff D, Vittone B, Tancer M, Bartko J (1991) Cognitive-behavioral and pharmacological treatments of social phobia: A controlled study. *Arch Gen Psychiatry* **48**: 938–945.

Getka EJ, Glass CR (1992) Behavioral and cognitive-behavioral approaches to the reduction of dental anxiety. *Behav Ther* **23**: 433–448.

Gould RA, Otto MW, Pollack MH (1995) A meta-analysis of treatment outcome for panic disorder. *Clinical Psychology Review* **8**: 819–844.

Gould RA, Otto MW, Pollack MH, Yay L (1997) Cognitive behavioral and pharmacological treatment of generalized anxiety disorder: A preliminary meta-analysis. *Behav Ther* **28**: 285–305.

Gosh A, Marks IM, Carr AC (1988) Therapist contact and outcome of self-exposure treatment to phobias: A controlled study. *Br J Psychiatry* **152**: 234–238.

Hand I, Tichazky M (1979) Behavioral group therapy for obsessions and compulsions: First results of a pilot study. In *Trends in Behavior Therapy*. London: Academic Press.

Heimberg R, Dodge C, Hope D, Kennedy C, Zollo L (1990) Cognitive behavioral group treatment for social phobia: Comparison with a credible placebo control. *Cognitive Therapy and Research* **14**(1): 1–23.

Heimberg R, Salzman D, Holt C, Blendell K (1993) Cognitive behavioral group treatment for social phobia: Effectiveness a five year follow-up. *Cognitive Therapy and Research* **17**(4): 325–339.

Jacobson N, Wilson L, Tupper C (1988) The clinical significance of treatment gains resulting from exposure-based intervention for agoraphobia: A reanalysis of outcome data. *Behav Ther* **19**: 539–554.

Jensen J (1994) An investigation of eye movement desensitization and reprocessing (EMDR/R) as a treatment for post-traumatic stress disorder (PTSD) symptoms in Vietnam combat veterans. *Behav Ther* **25**: 311–325.

Jerremalm A, Jansson L, Ost LG (1986) Cognitive and physiological reactivity and the effects of different behavioral methods in the treatment of social phobias. *Behav Res Ther* **24**: 171–180.

Kanter NJ, Goldfried MR (1979) Relative effectiveness of rational restructuring and self-control desensitization in the reduction of interpersonal anxiety. *Behav Ther* **10**: 472–490.

Keane T, Fairbank J, Cadel J, Zimering R (1989) Implosive (flooding) therapy reduces symptoms of PTSD in vietnam combat veterans. *Behav Ther*: 245–260.

Kent G, Janbunather P (1989) A longitudinal study of the intrusiveness of cognitions in test anxiety. *Behav Res Ther* **27**: 43–50.

Kessler RC, McGonagle KA, Zhao S, Nelson CB, Hughes M, Eshleman S, Wittchen HU, Kendler KS (1994) Lifetime and 12-month prevalence of DSM–3-R psychiatric disorder in the United States: Results from the national comorbidity survey. *Arch Gen Psychiatry* **51**: 8–19.

Krohne HW (1989) The concept of coping modes: Relating cognitive person variable to actual coping behavior. *Advances in Behavior Research and Therapy* **11**: 235–247.

Krohne HW (1993) Vigilance and cognitive avoidance as concept in coping research. In Krohne HW (ed.) *Attention and Avoidance*. Seattle: Hogrefe and Huber Publishers, pp. 19–50.

Ladouceur R (1983) Participant modeling with or without cognitive treatment for phobias. *J Consult Clin Psychology* **51**(6): 942–944.

Ladouceur R (1996) Obsessions, ruminations obsédantes, et responsabilité, trouble anxieux généralisé. Diplôme Universitaire de Thérapie Comportementale et Cognitive, Université de Lyon, 30 March.

Ladouceur R, Rhéaume J, Freeston MH, Aublet F, Jean K, Lachance S, Langlois F, De Pokomandy-Motin K (1995) Experimental manipulations of responsabilité: An analogue test for models of obsessive compulsive disorder. *Behav Res Ther* **33**: 937–946.

Liebowitz MR (1993) Pharmacological treatment of social phobia: Traditional MAOI and moclobemide. *European Neuropsychopharmacology* **3**(3): 193–194.

Liebowitz MR (1996) *Mixed Anxiety, Depression, and Personality Disorders*. New York: American Psychiatric Association.

Lopatka C, Rachman S (1995) Perceived responsibility and compulsive checking: An experimental analysis. *Behav Res Ther* **33**: 673–684.

Marks I (1987) *Fears, Phobias, and Rituals: Panic, Anxiety, and their Disorders*. New York: Oxford University Press.

Marks I, Gray S, Cohen D, Hill R, Mawson D, Ramm L, Stern R (1983) Imipramine and brief therapist aided exposure in agoraphobics having self-exposure homeworks. *Arch Gen Psychiatry* **40**: 153–161.

Marks I, Lelliott P, Basoglu M, Noshirvani H, Monteiro W, Kasvikis Y (1988) Clomipramine, self-exposure and therapist aided exposure in obsessive-compulsive ritualisers. *Br J Psychiatry* **152**: 522–534.

Marks I, Stern RS, Mawson D, Cobb J, Mc Donald R (1980) Clomipramine and exposure for obsessive-compulsive rituals. *Br J Psychiatry* **136**: 1–25.

Marks I, Swison R, Basoglu M et al. (1993) Alprazolam and exposure alone or combined in panic disorder with agoraphobia: A controlled study in London and Toronto. *Br J Psychiatry* **162**: 776–787.

Marzillier J, Lambert C, Kellett J (1976) A controlled evaluation of systematic desensitization and social skills training for socially inadequate psychiatric patients. *Behav Res Ther* **14**: 225–238.

Mattick R, Peters L, Clarke C (1989) Exposure and cognitive restructuring for social phobia: A controlled study. *Behav Ther* **20**: 3–23.

Mattick R, Andrews G, Hadzi-Pavlovic D et al. (1990) Treatment of panic and agoraphobia: An integrative view. *J Nervous and Mental Disease* **178**: 567–576.

Niler ER, Beck SJ (1989) The relationship among guilt, dysphoria, anxiety and obsessions in a normal population. *Behav Res Ther* **27**: 213–220.

Norton GR, Dorward J, Cox BJ (1986) Factors associated with panic attacks in non-clinical subjects. *Behav Ther* **17**: 239–252.

Noyes R, Chaudry R, Domingo D (1986) Pharmacologic treatment of phobic disorders. *J Clin Psychiatry* **47**(9): 445–452.

Noyes R, Moroz G, Davidson JRT (1997) Moclobemide in social phobia: A controlled dose-response trial. *J Clinical Psychopharmacology* **17**: 247–254

O'Sullivan G, Marks I (1990) Long-term follow-up of agoraphobia, panic, and obsessive-compulsive disorders. In Noyes R, Roth M, Burrows GD (eds) *Handbook of Anxiety* Vol. 4. Amsterdam: Elsevier.

Öst LG (1988) Applied relaxation versus progressive relaxation in the treatment of panic disorder. *Behav Res Ther* **26**(1): 13–22.

Öst LG, Westling B (1995) Applied relaxation vs cognitive behavior therapy in the treatment of panic disorder. *Behav Res Ther* **33**(2): 145–158.

Öst LG, Westling B, Hellström K (1993) Applied relaxation, exposure in vivo and cognitive methods in the treatment of panic disorder with agoraphobia. *Behav Res Ther* **31**(4): 383–394.

Otto M, Pollack MH, Sachs G, Reiter S, Meltzer-Brody S, Rosenbaum J (1993) Discontinuation of benzodiazepine treatment: Efficacy of cognitive-behavioral therapy for patients with panic disorder. *Am J Psychiatry* **150**(10): 1485–1490.

Peniston EG (1986) EMG biofeedback-assisted desensitization treatment for Vietnam combat veterans post-traumatic stress disorder. *Clinical Biofeedback and Health* **9**: 35–41.

Persons JB (1997) Dissemination of effective methods: Behavior therapy's next challenge. *Behav Ther* **28**: 465–471.

Rachman SJ (1996) *Trends in Cognitive and Behavioral Therapy* (ed.) PM Salkovskis. Chichester: John Wiley & Sons Ltd.

Rachman S (1997) A cognitive theory of obsessions. *Behav Res Ther* **35**(9): 793–802.

Rachman S, De Silva P (1978) Abnormal and normal obsessions. *Behav Res Ther* **16**: 233–248.

Rapee RM, Heimberg RG (1997) A cognitive behavioral model of anxiety in social phobia. *Behav Res Ther* **35**(7): 741–756.

Resick PA, Jordan CG, Girelli SA, Hutter CK, Marhoefer-Dvorak S (1988) A comparative outcome study of behavioral group therapy for sexual assault victims. *Behav Ther* **19**: 385–401.

Resick PA, Schnicke MK (1992) Cognitive processing therapy for sexual assault victims. *J Consult Clin Psychology* **60**(5): 748–756.

Rothbaum BO, Hodges LF, Kooper R, Opdyke D, Williford JS, North M (1995) Effectiveness of computer-generated (virtual reality) graded exposure in the treatment of acrophobia. *Am J Psychiatry* **152**: 626–628.

Salkovskis PM (1985) Obsessional-compulsive problems: A cognitive behavioral analysis. *Behav Res Ther* **23**(5): 571–583.

Salkovskis PM, Harrison J (1984) Abnormal and normal obsessions: A replication. *Behav Res Ther* **22**: 549–552.

Salkovskis PM, Warwick H (1988) Cognitive therapy for obsessive compulsive disorder. In Perris C, Blackburn I, Perris H (eds) *Cognitive Therapy: The Theory and Practice*. Berlin: Springer Verlag.

Schneier FR, Goetz D, Camplas R, Fallon B, Marshall R, Liebowitz MR (1998) Placebo controlled trial of moclobemide in social phobia. *Br J Psychiatry* **172**: 70–77.

Scholing A, Emmelkamp PMG (1993) Exposure with and without cognitive therapy for generalized social phobia: Effects of individual and group treatment. *Behav Res Ther* **31**(7): 667–681.

Shapiro F (1989) Eye movement desensitization: A new treatment for post-traumatic stress disorder. *J Behavior Therapy and Experimental Psychiatry* **20**: 211–217.

Shaw P (1979) A comparison of three behavior therapies in the treatment of social phobia. *Br J Psychiatry* **134**: 620–623.

Solyom L, Sookman D (1977) A comparison of clomipramine hydrochloride (Anafranil) and behavior therapy in the treatment of obsessive-compulsive neurosis. *Journal of Internal Medicine Research* **5** Suppl. 5: 49–61.

Spiegel D, Bruce T, Gregg B et al. (1994) Does cognitive behavior therapy assist slow-taper alprazolam discontinuation in panic disorder? *Am J Psychiatry* **151**(6): 876–881.

Stravinsky A, Marks I, Yule W (1982) Social skills problems in neurotic out-patients. *Arch Gen Psychiatry* **39**: 1378–1385.

The International Multicenter Clinical Trial Group (1997) Moclobemide in social phobia. *Eur Arch Clin Neurosci* **247**: 71–80.

Van Balkom AJL, De Haan E, Van Oppen P, Spinhoven P, Hoogduin KA, Van Dyck R (1998) Cognitive and behavioral therapies alone versus in combination with fluvoxamine in the treatment of obsessive-compulsive disorder. *J Nervous Mental Dis* **186**(8).

Van Oppen P, De Haan E, Van Balkom AJ, Spinhoven P, Hogduin K, Van Dyck R (1995) Cognitive therapy and exposure in vivo in the treatment of obsessive-compulsive disorder. *Behav Res Ther* **33**(4): 379–390.

Vaughan K, Armstrong MS, Gold R, O'Connor N, Jenneke W, Tarrier N (1994) A trial of eye movement desensitization compared to image habituation training and applied muscle relaxation in post-traumatic stress disorder. *J Behavior Therapy and Experimental Psychiatry* **25**(4): 283–291.

Versiani M, Nardi AP, Mundim FD, Pinto S, Saboya E, Kovacs R (1996) The long-term treatment of social phobia with moclobemide. *Clinical Psychopharmacology* **11** Suppl. 3: 83–88.

Wardle J, Hayward P, Higgit A et al. (1994) Effects of concurrent diazepam treatment on the outcome of exposure therapy in agoraphobia. *Behav Res Ther* **32**: 203–215.

Welkowitz L, Laszlo A, Cloitre M, Liebowitz M, Martin L, Gorman J (1991) Cognitive-behavior therapy for panic disorder delivered by psychopharmacologically oriented clinicians. *J Nervous and Mental Disease* **179**(8): 473–477.

White J (1995) Stresspac: A controlled trial of a self-help package for anxiety disorder. *Behavioral Psychotherapy* **23**: 89–107.

Wilson SA, Becker LA, Tinker RH (1995) Eye movement desensitization and reprocessing (EMDR) treatment for psychologically traumatized individuals. *J Consult Clin Psychology* **63**(6): 928–937.

Wolfe BE, Maser JD (1994) *Treatment of Panic Disorder: A Consensus Development Conference.* Washington, DC: American Psychiatric Press.

Wolpe J (1975) *La pratique de la thérapie comportementale.* Transl. J. Rognant, Masson, Paris.

Yao SN, Cottraux J, Martin R, Mollard E, Bouvard M, Guérin J, Hanauer MT (1998) Inferiority in social phobics, obsessive-compulsive and non-clinical controls: A controlled study with the inferiority scale. In Sanavio E (ed.) *Behaviour and Cognitive Therapy Today: Essays in Honour of Hans J Eysenck.* London: Elsevier.

Zitrin C, Klein D, Woerner M (1978) Behavior therapy, supportive psychotherapy, imipramine and phobias. *Arch Gen Psychiatry* **35**: 307–316.

Zitrin C, Klein D, Woerner M (1980) Treatment of agoraphobia with group in vivo exposure and imipramine. *Arch Gen Psychiatry* **37**: 63–72.

Methods of Environmental Research

15

The Experience Sampling Method in Stress and Anxiety Research

M.W. deVries, C.I.M. Caes and P.A.E.G. Delespaul

Maastricht University, Maastricht, The Netherlands

NEW WAYS OF ASSESSING STRESS AND ANXIETY

Over the past twenty years, a new research trend has emerged that has shifted the focus from categories of disorders to time and context. This shift has blossomed into an increase in daily life and time-based studies in the psychological and psychiatric literature (Tennen et al., 1991; deVries and Kaplan, 1993; Delespaul, 1995; Fahrenberg and Myrtek, 1996; deVries, 1997; Stone et al., 2000; Reis and Gable, 2000).

However, most studies on stress and anxiety have been carried out in a laboratory setting or rely on retrospective recall. In order to obtain true-to-life descriptions, research has to be carried out in the natural environment and should involve situations and activities from daily life. Clinical assessment should focus on the extent to which situations and social processes co-determine the appearance of stress and anxiety.

Studies carried out in the natural environment provide a fresh picture of the physiological, psychological and behavioural processes involved in stress and anxiety disorders: a picture that often differs from that derived from experiments, questionnaires and interviews. The power of daily life studies lies in the ability to assess time and context effects and their ecological validity without retrospective distortions.

Time and Context

Psychopathology is not randomly or evenly distributed across a population nor is it constantly present in the lives of individuals. At both the population and the person level, psychopathology varies with time and context. By condensing observations over a time period, moment to moment variability is lost. Prospective studies carried out in the natural environment highlight the variability in experiences between and within subjects. Time-based studies may further uncover diurnal variations in the

Anxiety Disorders: An Introduction to Clinical Management and Research. Edited by E. J. L. Griez, C. Faravelli, D. Nutt and J. Zohar. © 2001 John Wiley & Sons, Ltd.

patterning of stress and the onset of anxiety. Moreover, profiles of the experience of symptoms in context over time allow treatment and rehabilitation to be tailored to the real needs of the patient (Massimini et al., 1987; Dijkman-Caes and deVries, 1987; Delespaul, 1995).

In daily life studies, a majority of panic attacks was found to be associated with external or internal cues and precipitating events (Freedman et al., 1985; Margraf et al., 1987; Street et al., 1989; Basoglu et al., 1992). In one study, panic attacks which were expected and associated with external cues occurred with more stressful life events at the time of the attack than panic attacks which were unexpected and not associated with external cues (Street et al., 1989). In another study, spontaneous attacks were found to occur more often at home than situational panic attacks (Margraf et al., 1987). Situational attacks were registered most frequently in a car, and often while driving on a motorway. When a spontaneous attack occurred at home, little information was gathered about the circumstances. Nevertheless, in the few cases that a description of the circumstances was provided, patients were alone or just had a fight with their spouses. In this study, a rather large number of the panic attacks which were labelled by the patients as "spontaneous" appeared to occur in the same situations as situational attacks, for instance, while eating in a restaurant, leaving home or driving a car.

Ecological Validity

Ecological validity refers to the occurrence and distribution of stimulus variables in the natural or customary habitat of an individual (Brunswick, 1949). Based on this definition, a study is considered to be ecologically valid if it is carried out in the natural environment and involves situations and activities from daily life. This definition is, however, too narrow. The ecological validity of a study should not merely depend on the setting in which it is carried out, but also to what extent the research method measures what it is supposed to measure. As Bronfenbrenner has pointed out: "Ecological validity refers to the extent to which the environment experienced by the subject in a scientific investigation has the properties it is supposed or assumed to have by the investigator" (1979: 29). This definition urges that the research setting is evaluated in terms of its psychological meaning to the subject. Characteristics of the research setting may influence the processes that take place within that situation and may affect the interpretation and generalisability of the findings. In a study by Barlow et al. (1984b), for instance, some subjects were able to complete a standardised behavioural avoidance test in a naturalistic setting though they reported they would not have been able to do so if it were not a test.

If it is our goal to provide true-to-life descriptions of stress and anxiety, research has to be carried out in the natural environment or in carefully selected settings, having similar connotations as daily life situations. The reciprocity of perceiver and environment is a central notion in ecological psychology (Gibson, 1979). We would argue that the reciprocity between perceiver and environment is central to our relationship to the world. Environmental cues are not objective entities, but are perceived differently by each individual and at each moment. A "stimulus" is always a "stimulus-for-the-subject".

Retrospective Distortions

Another important advantage of prospective daily life studies is that they minimise retrospective distortions. Looking back upon events provides a totally different view on momentary experiences. Individuals are often unable to recall variability in mood and the occurrence of events. Variance in the subject's retrospective reports of agoraphobic avoidance, for instance, has been identified as a major source of bias in diagnostic interviews (Mannuzza et al., 1989). Problems such as difficulty in remembering specific situations in which mental states occurred and the selectivity of memory in relation to current motivation and psychophysiological state have all been shown to have an impact on the information retrieved (Wheeler and Reis, 1991). From an extensive overview of studies about the relationship between mood and memory, Blaney concluded that mood-congruent events are more easily recalled (Blaney, 1986). Martin et al. (1983) further demonstrated that selective recall of negative information about the self is associated with neuroticism. Subjects with high scores on a neuroticism scale were found to be more likely to attend selectively to negative information.

Retrospective measures and time-based assessments provide different results. Diary studies on the relationship between anxiety and the menstrual cycle challenged the findings from retrospective studies, showing a retrospective exaggeration of pre-menstrual anxiety symptoms (Cameron et al., 1988; Stein et al., 1989). Moreover, there is evidence that the frequency and severity of panic attacks are over-reported in retrospective reports. A sample of patients who retrospectively reported having more than 4–6 panic attacks per week (often an inclusion criterion in pharmaceutical trials) was measured prospectively using time and event sampling methods. They reported a lower number of weekly panic attacks (Beurs et al., 1992; deVries, 1992; Margraf et al., 1987; Rapee et al, 1990). Margraf et al. (1987) also found important differences between retrospective and prospective reports of panic symptoms. Event sampling of panic symptoms indicated that palpitations, dizziness, dyspnea, nausea, sweating and chest pain or discomfort were noted most frequently. Fear of going crazy, faintness, trembling or shaking and fear of dying were reported more often in retrospect than in the panic diaries.

METHODS OF DAILY LIFE RESEARCH

Methods of research in daily life can be classified into three main categories: event sampling, time sampling and continuous recordings. In event sampling studies, subjects are instructed to collect information about the occurrence of specific events.

Subjects are asked to complete a self-report each time a specific event (e.g., a panic attack) occurs. In time sampling studies, subjects record information about their actual experience at different time points. Continuous recordings are mainly used to monitor psychophysiological responses.

Event Sampling Techniques

Event sampling techniques have been used in a number of studies to estimate the frequency and distribution of panic attacks and anxiety episodes in daily life (Uhde et al., 1985; Gurguis et al., 1988; Basoglu et al., 1992). Other studies compared daily panic diaries of panic patients with and without agoraphobia (Street et al., 1989; Ganellen et al., 1986). Different types of instructions were given to the subjects. In the study by Street et al. (1989), for instance, subjects filled out questionnaires during or immediately after the occurrence of each of three consecutive panic attacks. The questionnaires included questions about the extent to which the panic attack was expected, whether the attack was associated with external cues, whether they expected to panic again in similar circumstances in the future, whether they expected to have a good or bad day. Subjects also rated items about mood, stressful life events, maladaptive thoughts, fear and severity of bodily sensations at the time of the attack. Ganellen et al. (1986), on the other hand, instructed subjects to classify panic attacks as spontaneous major panic (no apparent cause, at least three symptoms), spontaneous minor attacks (one or two symptoms) or situational attacks (in a phobic situation or during anticipation of a phobic situation, three or more symptoms). As a consequence, the results of different studies are difficult to compare.

Time Sampling Techniques

In time sampling studies, subjects are asked to describe several times a day how they feel, where and with whom they are, what they do and so on. Subjects are instructed to fill out a self-report form either at fixed or at randomised time points during the day. An example of random time sampling is the Experience Sampling Method (ESM), which will be described in further detail later.

The combination of time sampling of psychological and psychophysiological responses at fixed time points is found in prospective studies on circadian rhythms in the severity of symptoms in patients with panic disorder (Cameron et al., 1986). Panic patients and normal subjects rated their level of anxiety five times a day at fixed time points. Time of sleep and waking was recorded. Pulse rates and oral temperature were measured at each time point. The results of this study were compared with a retrospective study on fluctuations in anxiety levels.

Recently, increasingly sophisticated devices combining time and event sampling techniques have been developed. Taylor et al. (1990) for instance, used a programmable hand-held computer to collect time and event sampling data. The device produced a signal and administered a set of questions at every hour between 7.00 a.m. and 11.00 p.m. Subjects were further instructed to answer the same set of questions when they were having a panic attack. The computer also recorded the time when the questions were completed.

Continuous Recordings

Several types of psychophysiological responses have been registered in daily life by means of ambulatory monitoring equipment (for an overview of monitoring techniques, see Fahrenberg and Myrtek, 1996). Ambulatory monitoring of psychophysiological responses has been combined with event and time sampling recordings of psychological and behavioural responses. Hibbert and Pilsbury (1988, 1989), for instance, investigated the role of hyperventilation during panic attacks by combining ambulatory transcutaneous carbon dioxide monitoring with event sampling in diaries. At the end of the monitoring period, subjects underwent a hyperventilation provocation test. Several studies combined either event samplings (Taylor et al., 1986; Margraf et al., 1987) or time sampling techniques with ambulatory monitored ECGs, heart rates and physical activity levels (Taylor et al., 1983; Shear et al., 1987; Gaffney et al., 1988). Some studies combined both event and time sampling techniques with continuous recordings of various psychophysiological responses (Freedman et al., 1985; Kenardy et al., 1989; Anastasiades et al., 1990).

The Choice of Method

A large number of innovative and increasingly sophisticated techniques have been developed to study stress and anxiety in daily life. Different methods may provide different kinds of information. The choice of the method is of paramount importance if we want to quantify specific aspects of stress and anxiety. The diversity in techniques should allow the researcher to select a method, which is optimally suited to address specific questions about daily life experiences.

In event sampling studies, one could expect that reliance on retrospective recall is kept to a minimum, at least when the reports are filled out immediately after the occurrence of the event. However, this is not always true. Event sampling techniques ask the subject to reflect on an event in the past. Even when it is in the very near past, they ask the subjects to look back at an event. Moreover, events like panic attacks may last several minutes to half an hour and it is not clear at what moment the reports are filled out. Was it while recovering from the attack when the subject was still shivering a bit or only after all symptoms of anxiety and distress disappeared? Unfortunately, several studies did not include information about the time the event sampling reports were filled out. Therefore, we recommend that data about compliance should be included in research reports. In one study, a majority of patients (77%) completed the self-report within one hour after the panic attack, but only 31% completed the form immediately after the attack (Rapee et al., 1990). There is some evidence that event sampling reports of the time of onset of panic attacks are not always accurate. Margraf et al. (1987) noted that a large number of panic attacks were reported to occur on the full or half hour. An advantage of time sampling techniques is that the number of missing responses is also registered. In event sampling studies, it is difficult to find out whether and when the subjects failed to record an event.

Time sampling techniques often require that information is gathered about momentary experiences. In comparison to diaries and event sampling approaches, the distortion due to retrospective recall is kept to a minimum. Even when this type of distortion is of less importance in diaries than in retrospective information over long periods of time, diaries also may suffer from selective recall. A comparison of ESM data with diary records from time budget studies revealed that "idling" (thinking about nothing in particular) is reported with ESM and not with diary approaches (Csikszentmihalyi and Larson, 1987). It seems that people do not find this type of behaviour important enough to mention it in their diaries.

Furthermore, with time sampling techniques it is easier to compare patients with normal controls. The relatively low incidence of psychopathology in normal subjects may hamper the comparison of event sampling data in different groups. In an event sampling study by Taylor et al. (1986), for instance, normal controls reported no panic attacks and only four episodes of anticipatory anxiety, with no more than one symptom.

An advantage of event sampling techniques, on the other hand, is that they reduce the risk of failing to catch an event with a short duration or a low frequency, such as a panic attack or an agoraphobic subject going to a public place. Yet, there is evidence that events with high frequencies are underestimated with event sampling techniques. A comparison of ESM with an event sampling technique to measure social interactions, for instance, demonstrated that the event sampling technique seriously underestimated the time subjects spent in interaction (Delespaul, 1995). Estimates of the frequency of symptoms and problem behaviour may also suffer from the reactive nature of monitoring techniques (Nelson, 1977; Barlow et al., 1984a). Reactivity can be minimised by using random time sampling procedures (Delespaul, 1992; Delespaul, 1995). Sampling with random intervals minimises the continuous self-awareness of individuals. The monitoring is not triggered by the occurrence of an event. It is only contingent on a time schedule and the target of the assessment is not so well defined. The target behaviours, cognitions and emotions are defocused. Therefore, time sampling approaches cover more than symptoms and illness. ESM, for instance, was found to be a useful method in evaluating treatment outcome at the level of the individual, not only by quantifying a decrease in symptoms, but also by adding a description of optimal experiences (Delle Fave and Massimini, 1992). Event sampling studies usually lack descriptions of positive experiences. And event sampling data cannot be compared with what happens when the event did not happen.

Event and time sampling techniques can both be supplemented by psychophysiological measures, although this type of assessment may also disrupt daily activities. An important disadvantage of the study by Cameron et al. (1986), for instance, is that the sampling method largely interferes with normal daily routine. Subjects were instructed to sit or lie down for at least 10 minutes and to avoid intense exercise for at least 30 minutes before the measurement of pulse rates and oral temperature, and these measurements were repeated five times a day.

Our choice of ESM was mainly based on the following considerations. We sought to enhance ecological validity by minimising the reactivity of the method. We wanted to minimise retrospective distortions and to gather detailed information about compliance. And last but not least, we wished to provide a general picture of stress and anxiety in daily life without narrowing our vision to symptoms and illness.

THE EXPERIENCE SAMPLING METHOD (ESM)

ESM has been applied in case studies to evaluate treatment outcome (Delle Fave and Massimini, 1992) and to explore the relationship between experiences of anxiety and the situational context (Dijkman-Caes and deVries, 1987). Dijkman-Caes and de-Vries (1991) have reported differences in experiences of anxiety in panic patients with and without agoraphobia. A comparison between panic patients and patients with other disorders has been offered by deVries et al. (1988). ESM has also been combined with time samplings of psychophysiological measures of stress, e.g. salivary cortisol (Nicolson, 1992; Nicolson et al., 1992; Van Eck and Nicolson, 1994; Van Eck et al., 1996a; Van Eck et al., 1996b).

Instruments and Procedures

ESM is designed to obtain self-reports about experiences at randomly chosen moments in daily life (deVries, 1987; Delespaul, 1995). To accomplish this, the subjects carry a digital watch (see Figure 15.1) that signals them several times a day. At each signal the subject completes a self-report form.

The self-report forms (see Figure 15.2) request a range of information about the subjects' objective and subjective state, usually 10 times per day for one week though the daily frequency can range between 6 and 20 times. Detailed aspects of the subjects' social, environmental, and emotional experience are assessed. This includes information about where subjects are, what they are doing, and who they are with, as well as information about their thoughts, moods, motivation, and both somatic and psychological symptoms. Items that assess experiences and symptoms are derived from the mental status examination, psychometric tests and DSM criteria as well as patients' descriptions of the illness experience gathered in focus groups. Responses are noted in small booklets of self-report forms.

Statistical packages and software are now available to manage the complex multi-level structure of the data sets. A guidebook for doing simple statistical analysis on the complex data set obtained with ESM is given by Larson and Delespaul (1992). New instruments for ambulatory monitoring, including improvements in the ease

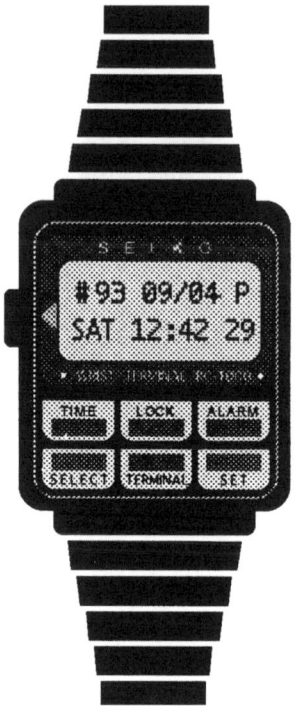

Figure 15.1   SEIKO RC-100 used as the ESM sampling device

with which the data may be logged in, downloaded and analysed are being developed (Delespaul, 1992).

Compliance and Reactivity Issues

Early research focused on such aspects of ESM as reactivity to being monitored on answers reported, reasons for drop-out or poor compliance, validity of self-reports with concurrent observation and time use comparisons as well as the feasibility of sampling individuals with various disorders (Hormuth, 1986; Csiksentmihalyi and Larson, 1987; Delespaul, 1995). Compliance to signals has consistently remained at the 75% level across all disorders except active psychosis, severe dementia, melancholia and obsessive-compulsive disorders (deVries, 1992). Studying these populations is not impossible, but definitely more demanding. Dijkman-Caes (1993) gives detailed information on compliance and reactivity issues in panic patients. Since compliance is the key element which can make or break a study of this kind, procedures that assure a research alliance have been of paramount importance, such as practice periods, briefings and debriefings (deVries, 1997).

ESM Research on Panic Disorder and Agoraphobia

Agoraphobic patients differed from panic patients without agoraphobia and normal controls in the amount of time spent in different social contexts and places in daily life (Dijkman-Caes et al., 1993a; Dijkman-Caes et al., 1993b). Agoraphobic patients spent more time at home and were more often with family than panic patients without agoraphobia and normal controls. Furthermore, they reported less often being alone or in public places than normal subjects. However, agoraphobic patients also differed from the other groups on demographic variables. The group of agoraphobic patients included more women and more unemployed subjects. Similar differences in demographic data, more specifically the preponderance of housewives among agoraphobic patients have been reported in other studies (Thorpe and Burns, 1983). This time allocation pattern, then, may largely depend on demographic features, such as living with family and being unemployed. On the other hand, there may be a cause–effect relationship: illness may cause demographic characteristics in the long run (Delespaul, 1995). Agoraphobic patients, for instance, may continue an unhappy marriage because they feel not able to live alone.

Panic patients in general were not found at home more than their counterparts with depression or pain (deVries et al., 1988). In this case, it seemed that the crucial variable in agoraphobia is not the avoidance of places nor the retreat to a safe home, but rather that these individuals tend to be found more often in the presence of family members than individuals without this diagnosis. This is further substantiated by the fact that anxiety patients in general reported being in public places no less often than subjects with other disorders. This finding challenges theories of agoraphobia, based on avoidance of public places, and instead supports social and attachment theories of anxiety. Moreover, behavioural treatment, e.g. desensitisation may be inappropriate if avoidance of public places plays no or only a limited role (deVries, 1989).

What people actually do should be considered the background on which the ongoing dynamics of cognitions and mood play. Time budgets help us broaden our understanding of behavioural aspects of individuals within diagnostic groups. At the same time, they provide insight into individual responses to treatment. Indeed, modest changes in mental state over time or in the experience of comorbidity, e.g. anxiety with varying subtle levels of comorbid depression, may have a significant limiting impact on behavioural time budgets (deVries et al., 1987; deVries et al., 1990). Differences were found not only in the number of social situations such as places frequented, but also in the length of time they remained in them.

ESM Stress Research

Recent research has alerted us to the fact that it is not only a massive disruption in personal and social life that affects individuals, but minor daily events, hassles and family problems do so as well. These studies represent a shift in research design and methods away from the clarification of a single event to an attempt at understanding

What do I think?

....

....

....

This thought is

	not		a little		rather		very
pleasant	1	2	3	4	5	6	7
clear	1	2	3	4	5	6	7
agitated	1	2	3	4	5	6	7
normal	1	2	3	4	5	6	7

I feel

cheerful	1	2	3	4	5	6	7
uncertain	1	2	3	4	5	6	7
lonely	1	2	3	4	5	6	7
relaxed	1	2	3	4	5	6	7
anxious	1	2	3	4	5	6	7
angry	1	2	3	4	5	6	7
complaint 1 troubles me	1	2	3	4	5	6	7
complaint 2 troubles me	1	2	3	4	5	6	7
I feel short of breath, choking	1	2	3	4	5	6	7
I have palpitations, pain on the chest	1	2	3	4	5	6	7
I feel weak, dizzy, unsteady	1	2	3	4	5	6	7
I feel unreal	1	2	3	4	5	6	7
I am afraid to die, to go crazy or to lose control	1	2	3	4	5	6	7

Where am I now?

....

....

....

How far from home is this?   ....km

With whom am I?

....

....

....

How many men?.........women?.........children?.........

What am I doing?

....

....

....

FIGURE 15.3   The ESM anxiety booklet

the ongoing social and personal context of the individual as he or she adapts to environmental circumstances (deVries, 1987). Stone et al. (1999) summarise the results of ESM studies measuring stress and coping with palmtop computers. Subjects experiencing high levels of work stress or marital stress described every 40 minutes

	not		a little		rather		very
I'd like to do something else	1	2	3	4	5	6	7
I'm active	1	2	3	4	5	6	7
I'm in control	1	2	3	4	5	6	7
I can't concentrate	1	2	3	4	5	6	7
I'm hungry	1	2	3	4	5	6	7
I'm tired	1	2	3	4	5	6	7
I don't feel well	1	2	3	4	5	6	7

I'm standing / lying down / sitting / walking around (circle your choice)
I used nothing / alcohol / medication / coffee / ....

This beep was disturbing	1	2	3	4	5	6	7

It is now .... h ....min

Notes:
....
....
....
....
....
....

FIGURE 15.3 (*cont.*)

how they were coping with stressors. Answers on a retrospective questionnaire asking the same questions about the most stressful problem during the ESM research period ($2\frac{1}{2}$ days) were compared with the momentary ESM responses about the same event. Only modest correspondence between momentary and retrospective responses was found. And no strong person factors predicted discrepancies between responses.

ESM results indicate that minor events do contribute to mood fluctuations within as well as between days (Marco and Suls, 1993). Others demonstrated that minor events are generally followed by increases in negative affect and agitation (Van Eck et al., 1998). They also found that changes in mood depended on the type of events, with agitation being more sensitive to events that involved task demands. Future events had even greater effects on mood than prior events, possibly pointing at the anticipation of future events. The finding that the effect of future events was greater when the events were more predictable supports this assumption. Another body of data demonstrates that optimal, positive and supportive daily experiences (Csikszentmihalyi, 1991), in particular positively evaluated social contexts (deVries and Delespaul, 1989) may improve or correct the negative effects of stressful events.

Furthermore, psychosocial stressors, daily life events and activities were found to be capable of activating neuroendocrine and immunological responses (Nicolson, 1992; Stone et al., 1993; Van Eck et al., 1996a). The complex picture of daily life stress, therefore, may be best understood by studying both physical and psychological responses in the actual social contexts. ESM research focused on the relationship between stressful events, distress and cortisol dynamics in daily life contexts. In one study, white-collar workers with high versus low levels of perceived stress were sampled on routine work and weekend days (Van Eck and Nicolson, 1994; Van Eck et al., 1996a; Van Eck et al., 1996b). As soon as possible after each signal, subjects completed ESM forms and simultaneously collected their own saliva samples, by sucking on a normal dental wad while filling out the ESM form. Saliva samples were collected for determination of free cortisol levels. The central focus of this study was to determine whether common sources of stress in daily life, often referred to as hassles, contributed to increases in cortisol levels. In addition, the effect of individual differences in chronic perceived stress, anxiety and depressive symptoms on cortisol levels and reactivity to events was examined and the effects of different types of events (e.g. work, negative social interactions) and different event appraisals (e.g. controllability, predictability, importance) on cortisol reactivity was studied. To summarise the results, they found that minor daily stressors have small but significant effects on salivary cortisol levels. These neuroendocrine effects are mediated by negative mood states. Positive mood states have little or no effect on cortisol levels. And individuals scoring higher on anxiety or depression measures report more frequent daily stressors, more negative mood states in general and in response to stressors, have higher cortisol secretion throughout the day. In contrast, less neurotic individuals fail to show habituation of cortisol responses to recurrent daily stressors. These biological applications of ESM provide an innovative example of the types of studies that may be carried out using ESM in natural experimental settings

ESM in Clinical Practice

Clinically, time budget data provide a powerful tool for behavioural and directive therapies. They provide data such as the frequency, duration, and dynamic processes of disorders that are generally not obtained through traditional clinical evaluations. They elucidate specific areas for intervention, such as the preventive avoidance of situations associated with pathology or the active seeking of healthy contexts and situations. Time budget data also illuminate the effect of therapeutic intervention such as an increase in background socialising or the choice of active versus passive activities. ESM data have been found to provide sensitive measures of change in outcome assessment. Evidence of changes in real time use and in the appraisal of activities after pharmacological treatment has been demonstrated in depressed patients (Barge-Schaapveld et al., 1995). Quality of life improvements in response to drug treatment, not directly measured in interviews and questionnaires, also have been assessed (Barge-Schaapveld et al., 1997). Moreover, the application of ESM in treatment may focus on rearrangements in the social network so as to optimise patients' functioning by means of a more supporting social milieu (Delle Fave and Massimini, 1992). Changes in time budgets serve as a potential area for early detection in high-risk groups by providing the doctor with a window on the often under-reported world of deterioration or improvement in daily life.

What do these data add to improve clinical understanding? Psychopathology appears to be relatively variable, episodic and short-lived, as do moments of well-being. Periods of both well-being and symptoms fluctuate, challenging diagnostic descriptions which imply a static picture. A consequence of this variability is that the influence of immediate and specific situations may be assessed during, before, or after moments of illness or well-being, thus providing insight in dynamic and setting effects. The therapist may use this variability constructively and optimise the patient's daily coping.

Dijkman-Caes and deVries (1987), for instance, describe a case study of a 38-year-old woman, suffering from agoraphobia. After six months of treatment, she participated in ESM research. Although no panic attacks occurred during the ESM week, feelings of anxiety could be related to specific social contexts and activities. The ESM data revealed that she had very little social contacts in general and none in the neighbourhood she lived in. She was often alone at home and then kept cleaning the house. When she was alone in the house with nothing to do, feelings of anxiety and discomfort arose that she almost literally cleaned away. Subsequently, a treatment strategy was implemented in which she was instructed to practise specific interactions living nearby her house, such as with a neighbour or a storekeeper in the village. ESM allowed the application of a remedial developmental and behavioural strategy that allowed the patient to develop alternative coping skills that could support her sense of identity in a larger number of social contexts.

Finally, feedback on ESM data within the context of clinical care involves an interpersonal process in which the patient and the therapist construct and integrate a shared view of a patient's life. In the therapeutic process, the information gathered with ESM can be seen as a film of the daily life of the patient, that the patient and therapist project and view together. Viewing the week together fosters mutual respect and partnership. ESM can be very valuable in bridging the gap between the doctor "who knows" and the patient "who does not know". In ESM the patient is the specialist of his or her own life and becomes a partner in negotiating his or her treatment plan. As a consequence ESM offers a base for a true "negotiated medical care" (Delespaul, 1995).

CONCLUSION

With ESM, we sought to challenge psychiatric thinking with a new data set anchored more solidly in the experience of the person. We wished to place the person more central than he or she currently stands in diagnostic formulations by emphasising the actual daily life reality of individual illness experience and treatments tailored to the subject's own needs. We began to develop models not only to describe stress and anxiety, but also optimal experiences and well-being. The data thus far revealed new dimensions of stress and anxiety and opened up new avenues for treatment.

Bio-psychosocial research by means of simultaneously collecting physiological measures such as cortisol and blood pressure along with the moment-to-moment measures of mental state remains promising. Naturalistic studies that measure physiological parameters accurately and repeatedly outside the laboratory can facilitate the exchange of information with experimental studies within the laboratory. By systematically comparing the results of multiple assessments, the relative contribution of response types, sampling methods and characteristics of subjects and settings can be estimated. The best strategy, therefore, is not to select a single sampling technique measuring an isolated response, but to develop multi-method approaches including measurements of different responses under different conditions.

Daily life studies, then, may provide a more sophisticated description with a high level of individual, situational and temporal detail and supplement the general picture of stress and anxiety disorders that has been derived from cross-sectional research. These studies also provide a different picture than the pure types described in DSM-IV (APA, 1994). DSM-IV classifications of individual cases are of limited descriptive, clinical and prognostic value. New classification systems should be developed, in which subjects are not assigned to a single diagnostic category according to "all or none" criteria. A classification system in which the "resemblance" between the subject and the "pure types" of diagnostic categories are evaluated, would provide a more precise description of health and illness as it occurs in the natural context (Van Meter et al., 1987). Once we are able to gather quantitative and replicable data about individual variations in the experience of symptoms and in the quality of life, daily life measures could be added to the diagnostic procedures. They can provide valid descriptions of the severity of symptoms and the amount of psychosocial impairment experienced in everyday life. Diagnoses then can be further defined based on the processing of the environment, e.g. the occurrence of anxious reactions to intimate versus non-intimate (public and anonymous) social situations.

Time sampling data are especially suited to establish therapeutic approaches that are tailored to the needs of the individual patient. Time sampling data not only provide information on the frequency and severity of panic experiences (as many other self-monitoring approaches do), but also highlight sources of positive experiences. If the goal of the therapeutic strategies goes beyond the reduction of symptoms and problem behaviour, knowledge about sources of positive experiences can be used to develop strategies to increase the number of these experiences. Beside fear and phobia reduction, the therapeutic intervention then creates possibilities to improve the general quality of life.

ACKNOWLEDGEMENTS

This paper could not have been written without the collaboration of N. Nicolson, M. van Eck, the RIAGG/Vijverdal-combinatie and the Vijverdal Ambulatory Anxiety Clinic doctors and their patients. Manuscript support was provided by M.J. Duchateau. Funding is provided by the Letten F. Saugstad Foundation, the Solvay-Duphar Company, the Netherlands Science Foundation (NWO), the Nationaal Fonds voor Volksgezondheid (NcGv), Maastricht University, and the IPSER Institute.

REFERENCES

American Psychiatric Association (1994) DSM-IV *Diagnostic and Statistical Manual of Mental Disorders*. Washington, DC: American Psychiatric Association.

Anastasiades P, Clark DM, Salkovskis PM, Middleton H, Hackman A, Gelder M, Johnston DW (1990) Psychophysiological responses in panic and stress. *J Psychophysiology* **4**: 331–338.

Barge-Schaapveld DQCM, Nicolson NA, Van der Hoop RG, deVries MW (1995) Changes in daily life experience associated with clinical improvement in depression. *J Aff Dis* **34**: 139–154.

Barge-Schaapveld DQCM, Nicolson NA, Delespaul PAEG, deVries MW (1997) Assessing quality of life with the experience sampling method. In Katschnig H, Freeman H, Sartorius N (eds) *Quality of Life in Mental Disorders*. Chichester: John Wiley & Sons Ltd.

Barlow DJ, Hayes SC, Nelson RO (1984a) *The Scientist Practitioner: Research and Accountability in Clinical and Educational Settings*. New York: Pergamon Press.

Barlow DJ, O'Brien GT, Last CG (1984b) Couples treatment of agoraphobia. *Behav Ther* **15**: 41–58.

Basoglu M, Marks IM, Sengün S (1992) A prospective study of panic and anxiety in agoraphobia with panic disorder. *Br J Psychiatry* **160**: 57–64.

Beurs E, Lang A, Van Dijck R (1992) Self-monitoring of panic attacks and retrospective estimates of panic: Discordant findings. *Behav Res Ther* **30**: 411–413.

Blaney PH (1986) Affect and memory: A review. *Psychological Bull* **99**: 229–246.

Bronfenbrenner U (1979) *The Ecology of Human Development*. Cambridge, MA: Harvard University Press.

Brunswick E (1949) *Systematic and Representative Design of Psychological Experiments*. Berkeley, CA: University of California Press.

Cameron OG, Kuttesch D, McPhee K, Curtis GC (1988) Menstrual fluctuations in the symptoms of panic anxiety. *J Aff Dis* **15**: 169–174.

Cameron OG, Lee MA, Kotun J, McPhee KM (1986) Circadian symptom fluctuations in people with anxiety disorders. *J Aff Dis* **11**: 213–218.

Csikszentmihalyi M (1991) Flow. In *The Psychology of Optimal Experience: Steps towards Optimizing Quality of Life*. New York: Harper.

Csikszentmihalyi M, Larson R (1987) Validity and reliability of the Experience Sampling Method. *J Nervous and Mental Disease* **175**: 526–536.

Delespaul PAEG (1992) Technical note: Devices and time sampling procedures. In deVries MW (ed) *The Experience of Psychopathology: Investigating Mental Disorders in their Natural Settings*. Cambridge: Cambridge University Press, pp. 363–373.

Delespaul PAEG (1995) *Assessing Schizophrenia in Daily Life: The Experience Sampling Method*. IPSER Series in Ecological Psychiatry, Maastricht: Maastricht University.

Delle Fave A, Massimini F (1992) The ESM and the measurement of clinical change: A case of anxiety disorder. In deVries MW (ed) *The Experience of Psychopathology: Investigating Mental Disorders in their Natural Settings*. Cambridge: Cambridge University Press.

deVries MW (1987) Investigating mental disorders in their natural settings. *J Nervous and Mental Disease* **175**: 509–513.

deVries MW (1989) Angst: Altijd bij de hand. *Psychologie* **1**: 26–31.

deVries MW (ed.) (1992) *The Experience of Psychopathology: Investigating Mental Disorders in their Natural Settings*. Cambridge: Cambridge University Press.

deVries MW (1997) Recontextualizing psychiatry: Toward ecologically valid mental health research. *Transcultural Psychiatry* **34**: 185–218.

deVries MW, Delespaul PAEG (1989) Time, context and subjective experiences in schizophrenia. *Schizophrenia Bulletin* **15**: 233–244.

deVries MW, Delespaul PAEG, Dijkman-Caes CIM (1987) Anxiety and affect in daily life. In Racagni C, Smeraldi H (eds) *Anxious Depression.* New York: Raven Press.

deVries MW, Dijkman-Caes CIM, Delespaul PAEG (1988) De ontbrekende schakel: Diagnostiek in de natuurlijke omgeving. *Tijdschrift voor Psychiatrie* **2**: 94–114.

deVries MW, Dijkman-Caes CIM, Delespaul PAEG (1990) The sampling of experience: A method of measuring the co-occurrence of anxiety and depression in daily life. In Maser JD, Cloninger CR (eds) *Comorbidity of Mood and Anxiety Disorders.* Washington, DC: American Psychiatric Press, Inc.

deVries MW, Kaplan CD (1993) Missing links in mental health research. *Proceedings World Federation for Mental Health* 1993, 356–359.

Dijkman-Caes CIM (1993) Panic disorder and agoraphobia in daily life. PhD dissertation, Rijksuniversiteit Limburg Maastricht.

Dijkman-Caes CIM, deVries MW (1987) The social ecology of anxiety: Theoretical and quantitative perspectives. *J Nervous and Mental Disease* **175**: 550–557.

Dijkman-Caes CIM, DeVries MW (1991) Daily life situations and anxiety in panic disorder and agoraphobia. *J Anx Dis* **5**: 343–357.

Dijkman-Caes CIM, deVries MW, Kraan HF, Volovics A (1993a) Agoraphobic behavior in daily life: Effects of social roles and demographic characteristics. *Psychological Reports* **72**: 1283–1293.

Dijkman-Caes CIM, Kraan HF, deVries MW (1993b) Research on panic disorder and agoraphobia in daily life: A review of current studies. *J Anx Dis* **7**: 235–247.

Fahrenberg J, Myrtek M (eds) (1996) *Ambulatory Assessment: Computer-Assisted Psychological and Psychophysiological Methods in Monitoring and Field Studies.* Seattle: Hogrefe & Huber Publishers.

Freedman R, Ianni P, Ettedgui E, Puthezhath N (1985) Ambulatory monitoring of panic disorder. *Arch Gen Psychiatry* **42**: 244–248.

Gaffney FA, Fenton BJ, Lane LD, Lake CR (1988) Hemodynamic, ventilatory, and biochemical responses of panic patients and normal controls with sodium lactate infusion and spontaneous panic attacks. *Arch Gen Psychiatry* **45**: 53–60.

Ganellen RJ, Matuzas W, Uhlenhuth EH, Glass R, Easton CR (1986) Panic disorder, agoraphobia and anxiety relevant cognitive style. *J Aff Dis* **11**: 219–225.

Gibson JJ (1979) *The Ecological Approach to Visual Perception.* Boston: Houghton-Miffin.

Gurguis GNM, Cameron OG, Ericson WA, Curtis GC (1988) The daily distribution of panic attacks. *Comprehensive Psychiatry* **29**: 1–3.

Hibbert G, Pilsbury D (1988) Hyperventilation in panic attacks: Ambulant monitoring of transcutaneous carbon dioxide. *Br J Psychiatry* **153**: 76–80.

Hibbert G, Pilsbury D (1989) Hyperventilation: Is it a cause of panic attacks? *Br J Psychiatry* **155**: 805–809.

Hormuth SE (1986) The sampling of experiences in situ. *J Personality* **54**: 262–293.

Kenardy J, Evans L, Oei TPS (1989) Cognitions and heart rate in panic disorders during everyday activity. *J Anx Dis* **3**: 33–43.

Larson R, Delespaul PAEG (1992) Analyzing experience sampling data: A guidebook for the perplexed. In deVries MW (ed) *The Experience of Psychopathology: Investigating Mental Disorders in their Natural Settings.* Cambridge: Cambridge University Press, pp. 58–78.

Mannuzza S, Fyer AJ, Martin LY et al. (1989) Reliability of anxiety assessment. I. Diagnostic agreement. *Arch Gen Psychiatry* **46**: 1093–1101.

Marco CA, Suls J (1993) Daily stress and the trajectory of mood: Spillover, response assimilation, contrast and chronic negative affectivity. *J Personality and Social Psychology* **64**: 1053–1063.

Margraf J, Taylor CB, Ehlers A, Roth WT, Agras WS (1987) Panic attacks in the natural environment. *J Nervous and Mental Disease* **175**: 558–565.

Martin M, Ward JC, Clark DM (1983) Neuroticism and the recall of positive and negative personality information. *Behav Res Ther* **21**: 495–503.

Massimini F, Csikszentmihalyi M, Carli M (1987) The monitoring of optimal experience: A tool for psychiatric rehabilitation. *J Nervous and Mental Disease* **175**: 545–550.

Nelson RO (1977) Assessments and therapeutic functions of self-monitoring. In Hersen M, Eisler RM, Miller P (eds) *Progress in Behavior Modification* Vol 5. New York: Academic Press.

Nicolson NA (1992) Stress, coping and cortisol dynamics in daily life. In deVries MW (ed) *The Experience of Psychopathology: Investigating Mental Disorders in their Natural Settings.* Cambridge: Cambridge University Press, pp. 219–232.

Nicolson NA, Van Poll R, deVries MW (1992) Ambulatory monitoring of salivary cortisol and stress in daily life. In Kirschbaum C, Read GF, Hellhammer D (eds) *Assessment of Hormones and Drugs in Saliva in Biobehavioral Research.* Seattle: Hagrefe & Huber, pp. 163–173.

Rapee RM, Craske MG, Barlow DH (1990) Subject-described features of panic attacks using self-monitoring. *J Anx Dis* **4**: 171–181.

Reis HT, Gable SL (2000). Event-sampling and other methods for studying everyday experience. In Reis HT, Judd C (eds) *Handbook of Research Methods in Social and Personality Psychology.* New York: Cambridge University Press, pp. 190–222.

Schwartz JE, Neale J, Marco C, Shiffman SS, Stone AA (1999) Does trait coping exist? A momentary assessment approach to the evaluation of traits. *J Personality and Social Psychology* **77**: 360–369.

Shear MK, Kligfield P, Harshfield G, Devereux RB, Polan JJ, Mann JJ, Pickering T, Frances AJ (1987) Cardiac rate and rhythm in panic patients. *Am J Psychiatry* **144**: 633–637.

Stein MB, Schmidt PJ, Rubinow DR, Uhde TW (1989) Panic disorder and the menstrual cycle: Panic disorder patients, healthy control subjects, and patients with premenstrual syndrome. *Am J Psychiatry* **146**: 1299–1303.

Stone AA, Neale JM, Shiffman S (1993) Daily assessments of stress and coping and their association with mood. *Annals of Behavioral Medicine* **15**: 8–16.

Stone AA, Schwartz JE, Neale JM, Shiffman S, Marco CA, Hickcox M, Paty J, Porter LS, Cruise LJ (1998) How accurate are current coping assessments? A comparison of momentary versus end of day reports of coping efforts. *J Personality and Social Psychology* **74**: 670–680.

Stone AA, Shiffman SS, De Vries MW (1999) Ecological momentary assessment. In Kahneman D, Diener E, Schwarz N (eds) *Well-being: The Foundations of Hedonic Psychology.* New York: Russell Sage Foundation, pp. 26–39.

Stone AA, Turkkan JS, Bachrach CA, Jobe JB, Kurtzman HS, Cain VS (eds) (2000) *The Science of Self-Report: Implications for Research and Practice.* Mahwah, NJ: Lawrence Erlbaum Associates Publishers.

Street LL, Craske MG, Barlow DH (1989) Sensations, cognitions and the perception of cues associated with expected and unexpected panic attacks. *Behav Res Ther* **27**: 189–198.

Taylor CB, Fried L, Kenardy J (1990) The use of a real-time computer diary for data acquisition and processing. *Behav Res Ther* **28**: 93–97.

Taylor CB, Sheikh J, Agras WS, Roth WT, Margraf J, Ehlers A, Maddock RJ, Gossard D (1986) Ambulatory heart rate changes in patients with panic attacks. *Am J Psychiatry* **143**: 478–482.

Taylor CB, Telch MJ, Havvik D (1983) Ambulatory heart rate changes during panic attacks. *J Psychiatric Research* **17**: 261–266

Tennen H, Suls J, Affleck G (1991) Personality and daily experience: The promise and the challenge. *J Personality* **59**: 313–335.

Thorpe GL, Burns LE (1983) *The Agoraphobic Syndrome: Behavioral Approaches to Evaluation and Treatment.* New York: John Wiley & Sons.

Uhde TW, Boulenger JPh, Roy-Byrne PP, Geraci MF, Vittone BJ, Post RM (1985) Longitudinal course of panic disorder: Clinical and biological considerations. *Progress in Neuro-Psychopharmacology and Biological Psychiatry* **9**: 39–51.

Van Eck MM, Berkhof H, Nicolson N, Sulon J (1996a) The effects of perceived stress, mood state and stressful daily events on salivary cortisol in daily life. *Psychosomatic Medicine* **58**: 447–458.

Van Eck MM, Nicolson NA (1994) Perceived stress and salivary cortisol in daily life. *Annals of Behavioral Medicine* **16**(3): 221–227.

Van Eck MM, Nicolson NA, Berkhof H (1998) Effects of stressful daily events on mood states: Relationship to global perceived stress. *J Personality and Social Psychology* **75**(6): 1572–1585.

Van Eck MM, Nicolson N, Berkhof H, Sulon J (1996b) Individual differences in cortisol responses to a laboratory speech task and their relationship to responses to stressful daily events. *Biological Psychology* **43**: 69–84.

Van Meter KM, De Vries MW, Kaplan CD, Dijkman CIM (1987) States, syndromes and polythetic classes: The operationalization of cross-classification analysis in behavioral science research. *Bulletin de Méthodologie Sociologique* **15**: 22–38.

Wheeler L, Reis HT (1991) Self-recording of everyday life events: Origins, types and uses. *J Personality* **59**: 339–354.

Methods of Pharmacology

16

The Pharmacology of Human Anxiety

D.J. Nutt

Medical School, University of Bristol, Bristol, UK

INTRODUCTION

The study of anxiety disorders is of interest from both evolutionary/developmental as well as medical perspectives. Anxiety is a motivational state which promotes appropriate behaviour and achievement. However, when excessive, it impairs performance, narrows behavioural repertoire and leads to an inner sense of suffering. Excessive anxiety has been called either morbid or pathological anxiety. It is common, affecting up to 15% of the population at some time in their lives and can also be very disabling. Anxiety disorders themselves cause profound individual distress, suffering and reduced work and social achievement. There is also a major risk factor for other types of psychiatric disorders, particularly depression and alcohol/drug abuse. For these reasons, understanding the neural bases of anxiety, particularly the role of neuro-transmitters in the generation and treatment of anxiety is a key aspect of biological psychiatry.

The issue of the chemical bases of anxiety has been researched for nearly a century. Initial observations of individuals such as Canon and James suggested a role for autonomic modulators (later identified as adrenaline and noradrenaline) in anxiety. More recently there has been growing interest in the role of brain neuro-transmitters in anxiety. A synopsis of the various pharmacological theories is given in Figure 16.1. In very general terms these theories suggest that an increase in either amine or excitatory aminoacid (EAA) function leads to anxiety. There are conflicting theories about serotonin which suggest either an increase or a decrease in the brain is anxiogenic and there is about equal amount of evidence for each position (Bell and Nutt, 1998). Now, there is growing evidence that a down-regulation of the gamma amino butyric acid (GABA-A) function may underlie some forms of anxiety.

At least three peptide neuromodulators have also been implicated in anxiety. As these will not be described elsewhere they are briefly mentioned here. Cholecystokinin is a gut peptide which is involved with satiety and appetite. However, there are a large number of CCK receptors in the brain which fall into two classes CCK A and B. CCK A receptors are involved in eating behaviour and CCK B receptors,

Anxiety Disorders: An Introduction to Clinical Management and Research. Edited by E.J.L. Griez, C. Faravelli, D. Nutt and J. Zohar. © 2001 John Wiley & Sons, Ltd.

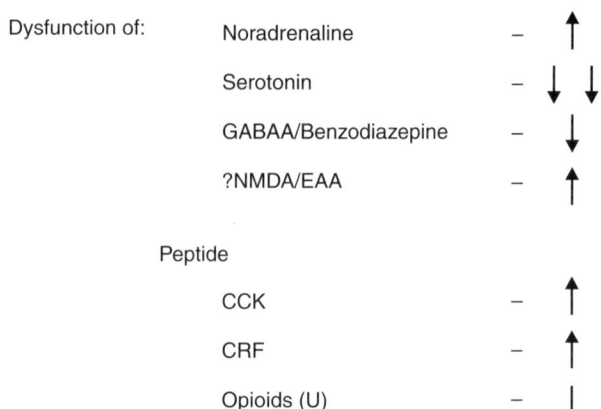

FIGURE 16.1   Human anxiety: pharmacological theories

among other things, are involved in anxiety (Montigney, 1989). It is not clear if the effect of administering CCK peptides is truly centrally mediated; it may be due to peripheral activation of the vagus or other peripheral nerves. A number of centrally active CCK antagonists have recently become available and a couple of clinical trials in humans with panic disorder have been conducted. The present results are equivocal perhaps due to poor brain penetration of drugs when administered orally. Nevertheless, it may yet turn out that CCK is an important neuro-transmitter in anxiety.

CRF (corticotrophin-releasing factor) is a hypothalamic peptide that causes ACTH release as part of the stress response. However, CRF receptors and peptide are distributed much more widely in the brain. If CRF is injected into the lateral ventricles of rats it produces a complex behavioural state consisting of insomnia, impaired eating and impaired grooming. The pattern of this reaction is very similar to that seen following stress and is thought that CRF may actually be the peptide which mediates a full range of stress radiated behaviours (Fisher, 1989). A few CRF antagonists are becoming available and in rodents have been shown to reduce stress-related behaviours as well as being anxiolytic in other models. For this reason, some are currently under exploration as anxiolytics in humans.

The brain opiate receptor system is also sensitive to stress. It is thought acute stress causes the release of endorphins which suppress anxiety and produce behavioural changes that help the body resist stress. These peptides work predominantly through the mu class of opioid receptors. Blockade or down-regulation of this receptor can lead to a state similar to anxiety. This is best seen in opioid withdrawal where a down-regulation of opiate receptors and second messengers leads to anxiety, agitation and peripheral autonomic activation.

NEUROCHEMICAL APPROACHES TO ANXIETY

Exploring the brain substrates and the pharmacology of anxiety in humans is not easy. It is not generally possible to conduct the sort of invasive procedures that have given us such a clear view of the animal circuit in receptors involved in anxiety-like behaviours in animals. Figure 16.2 shows some of the approaches which have been used up till now to address this issue.

In general, the obvious place to begin a biological investigation of any psychiatric disorder is with peripheral measures either in plasma or urine. Plasma levels of amines such as noradrenaline, adrenaline and the main neuronal noradrenaline metabolite MHPG have been used. Although there was generally agreement that anxiety would be associated with a rise in these neurochemicals, it is proved harder to demonstrate a primacy of this effect. Some recent work examining the spillover of noradrenaline from sympathetic nerves suggested that patients with severe anxiety disorders e.g., panic disorder, probably do have some disregulation of this system which may predispose the paroxysmal changes in some of this activity such as are occurring in panic attacks (Roy-Byrne et al., 1989). By and large, urinary measures have proved relatively unfruitful.

Because noradrenaline and other amines are polar they do not cross the

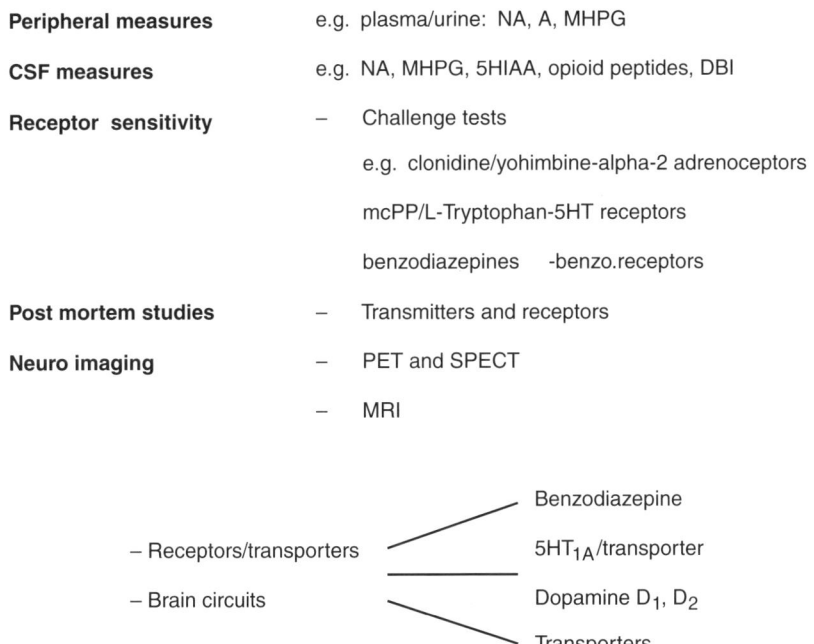

Peripheral measures	e.g. plasma/urine: NA, A, MHPG
CSF measures	e.g. NA, MHPG, 5HIAA, opioid peptides, DBI
Receptor sensitivity	– Challenge tests
	e.g. clonidine/yohimbine-alpha-2 adrenoceptors
	mcPP/L-Tryptophan-5HT receptors
	benzodiazepines -benzo.receptors
Post mortem studies	– Transmitters and receptors
Neuro imaging	– PET and SPECT
	– MRI

– Receptors/transporters — Benzodiazepine / 5HT$_{1A}$/transporter

– Brain circuits — Dopamine D$_1$, D$_2$ / Transporters

FIGURE 16.2   Neurochemical approaches

blood–brain barrier which means that studies of their concentration in cerebrospinal fluid are more direct measures of what may be happening in the brain. There have been relatively few such studies, however, in anxious patients. This is predominantly due to the fact that such patients are relatively phobic of the procedure and therefore do not readily give informed consent to undertake it. Nevertheless, some studies have been done with variable results, but at least one has shown an increased level of CSF noradrenaline in anxiety disorder patients (George et al., 1990). Additionally, during alcohol withdrawal (another state of high anxiety) CSF Na levels are elevated and correlate to symptoms (Hawley et al., 1985). Attempts have been made to look at other potentially important chemical messengers in CSF of anxious patients such as CSF levels of opioid peptides and diazepam binding inhibitor (BDI). Neither have shown particular abnormalities in anxiety.

A more direct measure of the possibility of receptor disfunction underlying anxiety disorders can be obtained by using challenge tests (see Figure 16.3). The principle is that the population of patients of interest are administered an agent which acts on a specific receptor and the consequences of this are studied. These consequences can be psychological changes or other dynamic measures such as body temperature and endocrine response. The challenge paradigm concept previously has been very well worked out in the study of depression and a number of these paradigms have been applied to anxiety disorders. For instance, tests of alpha-adrenergic dysfunction, to examine the involvement of the brain noradrenergic system, have been performed either using the agonist clonidine (which switches it off) or antagonists such as idazoxan and yohimbine (which switch it on). Both approaches have shown abnormalities in severe anxiety disorder such as panic. For instance, there is evidence of presynaptic noradrenergic hyperreactivity. Clonidine-induced presynaptic responses such as lowering of blood pressure and reductions in plasma MHPG are exaggerated in these patients whereas the effects of the antagonists to produce the opposite actions, e.g. an increase in the blood pressure, are also exaggerated (Nutt, 1989; Charney et al., 1990). Treatment with drugs to prevent panic such as tricyclic

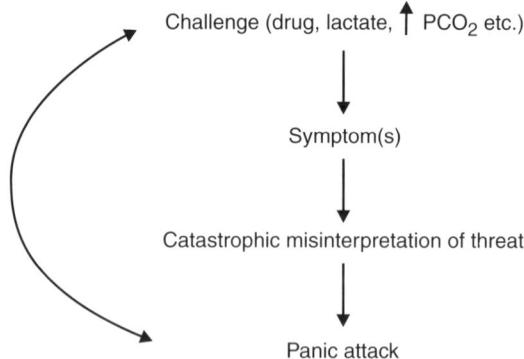

FIGURE 16.3 Cognitive gain

antidepressants or the SSRIs normalise the hyperreactivity of noradrenergic neurons.

A number of probes are now available to study the brain serotonin system and several have been used in anxiety disorders. MCPP is a 5-HT2 agonist drug which as well as causing endocrine stimulation will also induce restless and anxiety. Responses in both of these dimensions are exaggerated in patients with panic disorder (Charney et al., 1987; Kahn et al., 1988). Fenfluramine is a releasing agent for 5-HT which, when used in patients with panic disorders, tends to increase anxiety although it may reduce the likelihood of panic. This paradox is still a subject of much debate. It most probably reflects the fact that there are different brain 5-HT systems which serve to mediate the different forms of anxiety. For instance, the fronto cortex and amygdala projections may increase anxiety whereas the projection to the brain stem, particularly the periaqueductal grey matter, may inhibit panic (details in Bell and Nutt, 1998).

There is considerable evidence that the brain natural inhibitory system in the brain (the GABA-A receptor) may be involved in anxiety (see Kalueff and Nutt, 1997). Although it is not easy to directly stimulate these receptors, the GABA-A system is modulated by the benzodiazepine receptors and various benzodiazepine agonists have been given to humans in order to get a response from this receptor system. Benzodiazepine agonists will increase the effects of GABA and thus cause sedation and reduce anxiety. Such challenge tests have revealed sub-sensitivity of panic disorder patients to benzodiazepine agonists (Cowley et al., 1991). Thus these patients present less sedation, less slowing of saccadic eye movements and less of an inhibition of noradrenaline turnover (Roy-Byrne et al., 1989).

Alternatively, it has proved possible to challenge patients with an antagonistic benzodiazepine at this receptor, e.g. flumazenil. These studies have shown that patients with panic disorder tend to become more anxious and sometimes panic and the antagonist flumazenil is given (Nutt et al., 1990). The reasons for this are discussed in more detail later.

One of the more traditional ways of exploring neurochemistry of disease has been post-mortem studies. Such studies have been very fruitful in developing hypotheses about conditions such as schizophrenia, depression and dementia, however, there appear to have been no studies of the anxiety disorders. The reasons for this probably are that anxiety disorders occur predominantly in young people who are unlikely to die of natural causes or even of suicide. For this reason much interest has been directed towards developing new neuro-imaging techniques in order to study the living human brain.

Neuro-imaging techniques fall into two main groups. The first of these are radioactive procedures such as PET and SPECT, and the second are the MRI/CT techniques, particularly functional MRI. Both techniques allow the study of brain circuits and receptors. In general, brain circuits are studied using a technique called activation. This relies on the fact that when a part of the brain is engaged in a process such as anxiety there will be a change in metabolism. This in turn will lead to a change in blood flow. Changes in metabolism can be directly measured using the metabolic tracer ^{18}F-deoxyglucose (FDG). This is an analogue of glucose which is not metabolised. As cells are active, their metabolism rises so they increase their glucose uptake. Therefore, FDG levels rise in the cell and, as it is not metabolised, it remains, thus allowing quantification of uptake. This is the only direct measure of metabolic activity. However, a number of measures of blood flow have now been developed. In most normal situations when the brain tissue is functioning normally there is a strong linear relationship between local metabolic activity and blood flow. Hence traces of blood flow such as oxygen[15] PET and technetium[99] in HMPAO SPECT give very good, though indirect, measures of regional brain activation.

Very recently an MRI technique called functional MRI (fMRI) has been developed to allow blood flow to be determined without the use of radioisotopes. The technique relies on the fact that as haemoglobin is desaturated its magnetic signal changes. Thus areas of increased metabolic activity will initially show a change of magnetic signal due to loss of oxygen. However, quite rapidly the change in metabolic activity leads to a local increase in blood flow which then produces contrasting and opposite changing magnetic signal. When measuring these changes it is possible to get almost real-time measurements of local blood flow. The time resolution of MRI is impressive and has been used to prove circuits involved in many cognitive processes. However, the claustrophobic nature of the fMRI machine and the intense noise generated means it is extremely difficult to study anxious patients, thus in the foreseeable future it is likely that PET/SPECT techniques will be the mainstay of these studies. SPECT has the real advantage that the HMPAO tracer can be administered outside the scanner, for instance, during an exposure paradigm. It enters the brain and gives a snap-shot of the regions of the brain activated at the time of the injection and patients can then be taken to the scanner at some suitable time in the next few hours in order to be scanned.

A number of neuroimaging studies have examined the brain circuits of anxiety. By and large they have supported the earlier animal work which used both lesion and recording techniques. It is clear there is an anxiety circuit which involves the limbic system (particularly amygdala, hypothalamus, hippocampus) as well as cingulate and prefrontal cortex and probably some brain stem structures such as the PAG. A detailed review of this area is available (Malizia and Nutt, 1998).

Although there are fewer studies of receptors in anxiety disorders than of circuits, this area is also growing. Most workers focused on the benzodiazepine receptor as there is excellent PET (^{11}C flumazenil) and SPECT (^{123}I iomazenil) tracers. To date, there is a growing consensus of a down-regulation of this receptor system in panic disorder (see later). Effective tracers also exist to study some elements of the 5-HT system, particularly the 5-HT1A receptor (WAY100635) and the 5-HT transporter (Beta CIT). In the dopamine system PET tracers for the D1 and D2 receptor have been made as well as several tracers for the transporter. It is also possible to measure both serotonin and dopamine turnover using a precursor. There have been virtually no studies of these systems in anxiety disorders. The only exception is that of the dopamine transporter. A SPECT study from Finland has recently reported a reduced number of these uptake sites in patients with social phobia (Tiihoner et al., 1997). This is a rather unexpected finding but one which does, however, accord with some of the animal literature showing that mice with low levels of the dopamine are anxious.

It also may help explain why social anxiety can commonly occur with or precede Parkinson's disease (reviewed in Nutt, 1998).

WHAT INFORMATION CAN WE GET FROM THE STUDY OF EFFECTIVE TREATMENTS?

Until recently direct study of neurochemistry in patients with anxiety disorders has been very difficult. For this reason many therapists have had recourse to more inferential techniques. One of the most fruitful ways of thinking about possible pathophysiology disorder is to attempt to understand the mode of action of effective treatments and then extrapolate this knowledge to theories of brain dysfunction in the disorder. Such approaches have developed some interesting hypotheses in anxiety, some of which have already been touched on. Table 16.1 shows the two main classes of anxiety treatments whose actions have to be incorporated into such a schema. In essence, anxiolytic drugs can be classified into those which work immediately or at least very fast (in the order of less than one hour) and those which have a delayed action (generally two to six weeks).

The immediate or fast-acting drugs, with the exception of the Beta Blocker drugs, all act on the GABA-A receptor. These include the benzodiazepines, the barbiturates and a variety of alcohols including ethanol and chlormethiazole. In fact, the only other drugs that work quickly are the betablockers which have a limited role in the treatment of anxiety, only being effective in some forms of specific performance anxiety such as playing music in public. Their means of action is well known— preventing the peripheral activation caused by excessive sympathetic activity and noradrenaline release. There is little evidence of a major central component in the anxiolytic actions of betablockers and indeed their central actions to impair sleep may exacerbate symptoms.

The slow inset anxiolytics include a variety of different classes of drugs and psychotherapies. The tricyclic antidepressants are effective anti-panic agents that do have some role in GAD has well. They work by increasing the synaptic availability of both serotonin and noradrenaline by blocking re-uptake. The MAOIs similarly increase noradrenaline and serotonin by blocking metabolism. These are the first drugs to be successfully shown to work in anxiety disorders and they may be more

TABLE 16.1 Immediate and delayed anxiolytics

Immediate	Delayed
GABA-A receptor drugs:	
benzodiazepines	tricyclic antidepressants
barbiturates	MAOIs
alcohols (chlormethiazole)	buspirone
beta-blockers	SSRIs/SNRIs
	all psychotherapies

efficacious in these patients than in depression. Taken together with the tricyclic data, they point to either noradrenaline or serotonin being important in anxiety. More recently new treatments have been discovered. Buspirone is a 5-HT$_{1A}$ agonist which inhibits the firing of 5-HT cells but also stimulates postsynaptic 5-HT$_{1A}$ receptors. Buspirone is effective in the treatment of GAD (but not panic or social phobia) and it is not yet fully clear whether its mode of action is pre- or post-synaptic. The SSRIs and more recently the SNRIs (serotonin and noradrenaline re-uptake inhibitors) have recently been shown to be very effective in a variety of anxiety disorders. A number are now licensed for the treatment of panic disorder and more recent studies have showed efficacy in conditions such as OCD and social phobia. We presume that the effect of the SSRIs is predominantly through increasing serotonin levels in some parts of the brain. However, it may be that post-synaptic receptor desensitisation is a major factor in some of their anxiolytic actions. This is an area of considerable research interest and controversy at present which is reviewed in Bell and Nutt (1998).

EXPERIMENTAL ANXIETY PRODUCTION

Anxiety is unique among psychiatric disorders as it is easily amenable to laboratory study. Anxiety can be produced in controlled conditions by a variety of different processes, each of which have helped develop our understanding of the basic mechanisms of anxiety. Table 16.2 shows the three main approaches: pharmacological, physiological and psychological.

Pharmacological approaches predominantly refer to challenge tests with anxiogenic agents such as have already been mentioned. For instance, mCPP can reduce anxiety as can fenfluramine both through 5-HT stimulation. CCK4 analogues are also anxiogenic. As discussed later, it is also possible to provoke anxiety by withdrawing from pharmacological agents such as precipitating withdrawal from benzodiazepines with the antagonist flumazenil. Another classic example of pharmacologically mediated anxiety through withdrawal is opiate and alcohol dependence.

Physiologically challenged paradigms essentially centre on the respiratory system. Suffocation is highly anxiogenic in both animals and human and increasing levels of carbon dioxide in brain stems centres is very aversive. Experimental paradigms using either a rebreathing technique, or continued breathing of 5% CO_2 will cause a progressive rise in anxiety. Panic disorder patients find this particularly unsettling and will abort the experiment sooner than other patients with other anxiety disorders or normal volunteers. The alternative approach is to give one or two deep breaths of high concentration (35%) carbon dioxide. This will cause marked anxiety in normal volunteers as well as patients.

Paradoxically hyperventilation, which lowers blood CO_2, can also cause anxiety, particularly in patients with panic disorder. It is now thought that these patients have a hyperreactive respiratory centre just as their noradrenergic system is hyperreactive. Thus either increases in or decreases of CO_2 trigger off physiological changes in the brain stem, possibly locally which then leads to activation of higher limbic and cortical structures and panic attacks (Klein, 1993).

Psychological approaches to induction of anxiety are very well documented. One kind of psychological approach is the behavioural approach which includes the application or threat of pain or exposure to phobic situations. A classic way of inducing anxiety in neuro-imaging studies is to use the fear of an electric shock. Volunteers are told that when a signal occurs (e.g., change of colour on a VDU screen) they will get a painful electric shock to a limb. Scanning is performed before they get a shock so the effects of pain do not confound the effects of anxiety (Malizia and Nutt, 1998).

Another psychological approach is to use cognitive induction. This has been particularly prominent in the field of depression but more recently has been adapted to the generation of anxiety. For example, patients with panic disorder can be made very anxious by making them read scripts which tap into their fear cognitions, such as having a heart attack, fainting, dying, etc. Similarly, patients with social anxiety can be made anxious by reading to them recordings of their own scripts describing their own socially embarrassing episodes.

There is considerable controversy over the role of cognitive factors in other forms of anxiety provocation. Many challenge tests done on panic disorder patients will lead to anxious cognitions (so-called catastrophic cognitions such as "I'm going to die") as well as physiological and other psychological changes. For this reason, some cognitive psychologists believe that there is no such thing as a direct anxiogenic panic provocation and believe that they all work through a cognitive loop which involves generation of symptoms with secondary catastrophic misinterpretation of these (see Figure 16.3). The pure pharmacological view would be that there are challenge paradigms which directly induce the panic attack, and that the cognitions and peripheral symptoms are a secondary consequence of the initial central action.

This debate has also extended into the issue of clinical treatment. Cognitive therapy is a very effective treatment for uncomplicated patients with panic disorder (i.e., those who are not depressed) and this has strengthened the view of some clinical psychologists that catastrophic cognitions are a central feature of the disorder. However, there are a number of independent pieces of evidence which suggest that this theory is overstated, for example, some panic attacks occur in sleep, often waking people in a state of terror. Obviously these must occur without any conscious cognition and claims by cognitive therapists that there must be sub-conscious

TABLE 16.2 Experimental anxiety provocation

Method	Treatment
Pharmacological	
Physicological	5% and 35% CO_2
	hyperventilation
Psychological	behavioural—pain, phobic situations
	cognitive—induced mood

cognitive processes are very hard to substantiate. A list of problems with a solely cognitive explanation of panic attacks is as follows:

1. Panic attacks in sleep.
2. Peripherally-acting agents, e.g. betablockers inactive.
3. Drugs, e.g. FG 7142, cause anxiety beyond conscious control.
4. Spontaneous unprovoked panics can occur.
5. Anxiety precedes peripheral symptoms in challenge paradigms.
6. Biological abnormalities in panic patients to non-threatening challenges, e.g. clonidine.
7. Cognitions must have a biological basis.

A major peripheral component to panic attacks can be excluded by the fact that peripheral acting agents such as betablockers are relatively ineffective in this disorder. Moreover, some drugs, particularly FG 7142 (see later), which are centrally acting can cause anxiety which is beyond any kind of cognitive control. Other, slightly less well-founded arguments are that many patients have spontaneous and provoked panics without any negative cognitions other than feelings such as "Oh no, here it comes again". Also, in some challenge paradigms its been possible to show that the central anxiety preceded the peripheral symptoms (for a more detailed discussion, see Nutt and Lawson, 1992).

Perhaps the most important argument is that even if cognitions are the major cause of panic disorder, they must still have a biological basis. The fact that there is clear evidence of pharmacological abnormalities in patients with panic disorder supports the idea of an underlying neurobiological abnormality.

PHARMACOLOGICAL ANXIOGENIC CHALLENGES

It is important to try to make sense of the variety of mechanisms and the variety of different agents which have been reported to provoke anxiety in normal volunteers and in patients. One way of doing this is suggested in Figure 16.4. It involves dividing anxiogenic drug challenges into two groups, universal and selective. Universal challenges can be defined as those which cause anxiety in normal controls as well as in patients with one or more anxiety disorders. Selective challenges are those which work only in patients, most generally those with panic disorder. These are all-or-none challenges: either patients respond or they do not. In contrast, universal challenges often show a dose response effect which is different between patients and controls, in that a lower dose of drug is required to provoke anxiety in patients.

Universal challenges work by a range of mechanisms. Drugs which block GABA function such as pentylenetetrazol and benzodiazepine receptor inverse agonists (e.g. FG 7142) are highly anxiogenic. More details of this are given in the next section. Caffeine and very high doses (e.g. over 300 mg per person) can cause anxiety and occasionally panic although the mechanism is not clear (Bruce et al., 1991). It may

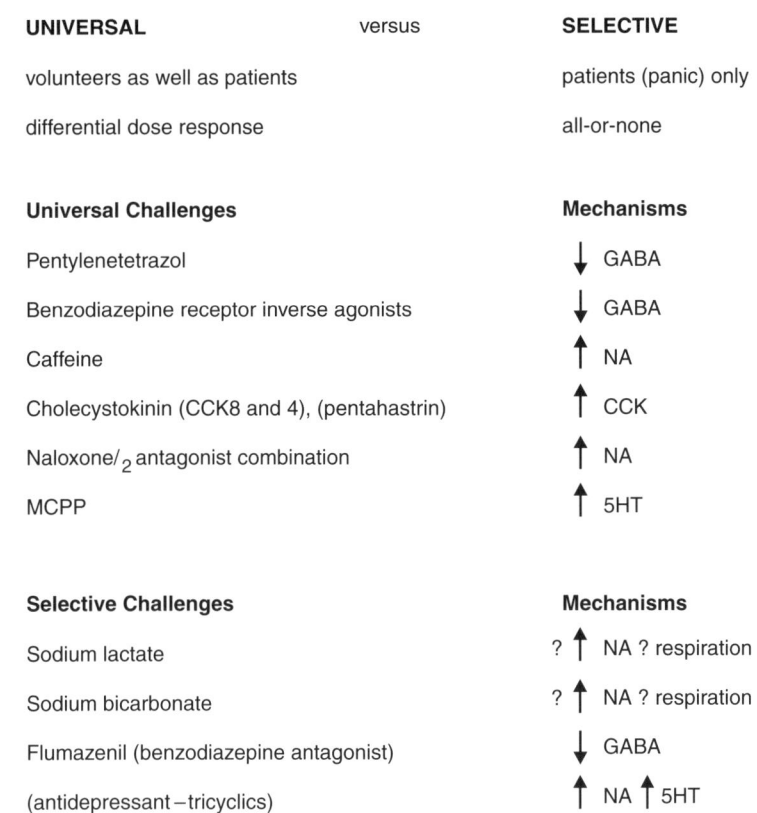

UNIVERSAL	versus	SELECTIVE
volunteers as well as patients		patients (panic) only
differential dose response		all-or-none

Universal Challenges	Mechanisms
Pentylenetetrazol	↓ GABA
Benzodiazepine receptor inverse agonists	↓ GABA
Caffeine	↑ NA
Cholecystokinin (CCK8 and 4), (pentahastrin)	↑ CCK
Naloxone/$_2$ antagonist combination	↑ NA
MCPP	↑ 5HT

Selective Challenges	Mechanisms
Sodium lactate	? ↑ NA ? respiration
Sodium bicarbonate	? ↑ NA ? respiration
Flumazenil (benzodiazepine antagonist)	↓ GABA
(antidepressant – tricyclics)	↑ NA ↑ 5HT

FIGURE 16.4 Pharmacological anxiogenic challenges

involve increasing brain or peripheral noradrenaline release. The anxiogenic effects of CCK4 and pentagastrin have already been mentioned—panic patients are most sensitive to these agents, with social phobics being somewhat less so and normal volunteers even more resistant. Nevertheless, high doses can cause severe anxiety even in volunteers. Increasing brain noradrenaline function with alpha$_2$-antagonists that disinhibit presynaptic auto-receptor control can raise arousal and cause anxiety. It is likely that both central and peripheral components contribute to this (Southwick et al., 1993). Moreover, there has been one report that combining an alpha$_2$ antagonist (yohimbine) with an opiate antagonist (naloxone) produces more profound anxiety (Charney and Heninger, 1986). Presumably this reflects the fact that both mu opioid and a$_2$-inhibitory receptors are found on locus coeruleus neurons, and removing the inhibitory effects of both causes marked noradrenergic activation. Finally, mCPP the 5-HT$_{2C}$ agonist will raise anxiety in all people and its not clear whether the increased sensitivity in panic patients is due to their having super-sensitive receptors or merely being more sensitive to the rather aversive experiences that this drug can cause (see earlier).

Selective challenges also have rather a varied pharmacology. In the classic panic provocation paradigm, sodium lactate probably works through affecting the respiratory centre with a secondary activation of brain noradrenergic systems. IV infusions of sodium bicarbonate are also anxiogenic probably through a similar mechanism (see Nutt and Lawson, 1992).

Flumazenil, the benzodiazepine antagonist, is anxiogenic in patients with panic disorder and to a considerably lesser extent in those with social phobia. It does not cause anxiety in normal volunteers. This is discussed in more detail in the next section. Finally, it is important to realise that other agents that are not generally used as challenge tests can significantly cause anxiety in patients with a predisposition. In particular, the antidepressant drugs when used early in the treatment of anxiety conditions, especially panic disorder, may cause an exacerbation of symptoms. This is true both of drugs which work on the 5-HT systems, such as the SSRIs, as well as the older tricyclic antidepressants which increase both serotonin and noradrenaline levels as well as blocking post-synaptic histamine H_1 receptors. On occasions intravenous infusions of these drugs have been used as challenge tests for endocrine studies and have provoked anxiety in patients directly (George et al., 1995). More usually in clinical practice we see an exacerbation of anxiety early in treatment. This has important clinical consequences, necessitating the use of low dose, usually half the standard dose of SSRI or as low as 10 mg of tricyclic for the first week of treatment. By about three to four weeks the anxiogenic affect is fully remitted and clear antipanic anxiolytic effects are seen (Nutt and Glue, 1991).

THE ROLE OF GABA IN ANXIETY

GABA is the main inhibitory neurotransmitter in the brain. Up to 40% of all brain synapses and the majority of interneurons use it as their transmitter. The function of GABA is to inhibit the activity of surrounding cells thus preventing excessive excitation which would lead to seizures and subsequent death. All sensory inputs to the brain activate in a feedforward manner GABA interneurons which modulate the degree of excitation. Similarly, most output neurons have collateral feedback GABA inhibition to limit the duration of their firing.

A huge body of experimental animal data links the GABA system with anxiety (reviewed in Kaluef and Nutt, 1997). Although there are much less direct human experimental tests of the GABA theory, there is strong indirect evidence that this neurotransmitter is involved in human anxiety. The first such evidence came through the use of pentylenetetrazol—PTZ (also called leptazol, metrazol or cardiazol) in the production of therapeutic seizures before the development of ECT. Judging the appropriate dose of PTZ for a particular individual was not easy: too much and the person could go into status epilepticus, too little and they would not convulse. When too little was given, so seizure was not induced, patients experienced severe anxiety described as feeling as if they were going to die. This led them to try to escape from the clinic and there are descriptions of patients having to be dragged down from the

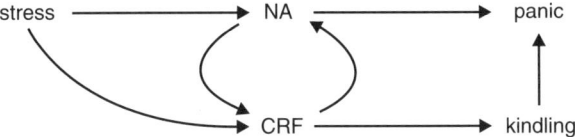

FIGURE 16.5   Stress and panic attacks

roofs of buildings by fire crew or hospital police. In addition, the memory of the anxiety and its association with the clinic led to huge resistance to returning to therapy. Thus pentylenetetrazol produces the three main components we see in anxiety disorders—anxiety, escape behaviour and subsequent conditioned avoidance (Nutt, 1990). Much later it was discovered that PTZ acts to block the chloride channel in the centre of the GABA-A receptor (see Figure 16.5).

Decades later other drugs which reduce GABA function were shown to be anxiogenic in humans. One of the classic papers is the one in which the benzo-diazepine inverse agonist FG 7142 was given to experienced human volunteers on the supposition that because it bound to the benzodiazepine receptor it would be anxiolytic. In fact, the opposite happened; at high doses it produced severe panic-like anxiety in two of the volunteers. This was not amenable to psychological override and one of the volunteers requested intravenous benzodiazepine to abort it, which it did successfully (Dorow et al., 1983). Subsequently, it became apparent that FG 7142 was an inverse agonist at the receptor and acted to switch off GABA. Another similar compound, Ro 15-3505, was also used in humans on the mistaken belief it was antagonist like flumazenil. However, it also caused marked anxiety due to its weak partial inverse agonist properties (Gentil et al., 1990).

The largest body of clinical evidence relating to reduced GABA-A function and anxiety comes from withdrawal states, from alcohol and benzodiazepines particular-ly, but also other similar compounds. One of the characteristic features of these states is severe anxiety which often leads to re-use of the drug. It now appears that much of the tolerance seemed to a down-regulation of GABA function, which when the drugs are removed as in withdrawal, leads to a relative deficiency of brain inhibition. The resultant excess exitation leads to anxiety, as well as seizures in severe cases (Cowen and Nutt, 1982). Finally, it should be remembered that in panic disorder flumazenil can be anxiogenic either because in these individuals it behaves as a weak universal agonist or because it blocks an endogenous anxiolytic benzodiazepine-like substance (Nutt et al., 1990). Recent PET and SPECT scanning studies in panic disorder have shown that this action of flumazenil may be associated with an apparent down-regulation of the benzodiazepine receptor in these patients, thus providing hard evidence of a biological abnormality in at least this one anxiety syndrome (Malizia et al., 1998).

If alterations in brain GABA-A function are of major aetiological importance in anxiety, how could they occur? In order to understand the possible mechanisms, it is important to realise that the GABA-A receptor system can show considerable variability. One reason for this is that each receptor is made up of five protein

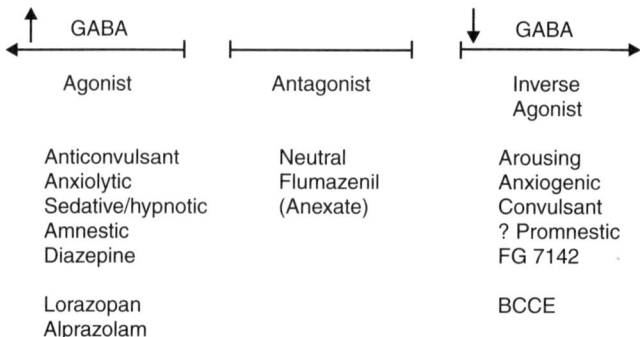

FIGURE 16.6 Benzodiazepine receptor ligands

sub-units which each come from a superfamily of at least 16 different proteins so that many different combinations can exist. In practice, only about 10 are thought to be found in mammalian brains, but these have quite marked differences in sensitivity to GABA and modulators such as the benzodiazepines. Another important factor is that each sub-unit can be phosphorylated and this will change the function of the complex. There is considerable evidence that short-term changes in GABA receptor function (as can be induced by stress, for example) are due to this type of mechanism whereas the adaptive changes which underlie tolerance to benzodiazepines and alcohol probably reflect changes in gene expression that alter the sub-unit composition of GABA receptors. If either change leads to receptors which are relatively less sensitive to GABA then anxiety would result. Recent data with mice in which the gene for the gamma 2 sub-unit was knocked out confirm that genetic alterations can cause anxiety. Although the homozygous KO: KO mice are not viable, the hetero-zygous KO: gamma 2 mice do live but are much more anxious than the wild type. It is not yet possible to measure gene expression in humans but we would predict similar alterations in sub-unit composition may result in some forms of anxiety.

The theory that alterations in brain GABA-A function may be of pathophysiologi-cal importance in anxiety has considerable explanatory power as many of the aetiological processes in anxiety affect this receptor system. This is shown in Figure 16.6. What is not yet known is the central site at which reduced GABA function could produce anxiety. It could be at the level of detection of threatening stimuli or in the output-response pathways or in the core emotional circuit itself. Of course changes in several of these sites might also be feasible. The PET studies mentioned earlier suggest a relatively global change but with maximal reductions in limbic cortical regions such as orbitofrontal and temporal cortex as well as insula.

CONCLUSIONS

In the century since the first scientific discussions on the biological basis of anxiety began there has been much progress. We now have a great deal of pharmacological evidence that anxiety can be increased as well as reduced by drugs. These studies have shown that there must be a number of different transmitters and possibly brain circuits involved in anxiety. Significant progress has been made towards understanding the mode of action of fast-acting anxiolytics such as the benzodiazepines and this has led to good evidence that abnormalities in brain GABA systems may underlie panic anxiety. Further studies are needed to elucidate the mode of action of slow-acting drugs and when such insights are made they are likely to generate new ideas about the biology of anxiety, and hopefully lead to new treatments. (A more detailed appraisal of many of the issues described here is available in Nutt, 1990 and Nutt and Lawson, 1992.)

REFERENCES

Bell CJ, Nutt DJ (1998) Serotonin and panic. *Br J Psychiatry* **172**: 465–471.

Bruce M, Scott N, Shine P, Lader M (1991) Anxiogenic effects of caffeine in patients with anxiety disorders. *Arch Gen Psychiatry* **49**: 867–869.

Charney DS, Heninger GR (1986) Alpha 2-adrenergic and opiate receptor blockade: Synergistic effects on anxiety in healthy subjects. *Arch Gen Psychiatry* **43**: 1037–1041.

Charney DS, Woods SW, Goodman WK, Heninger GR (1987) Serotonin function in anxiety: II. Effects of the serotonin agonist MCPP in panic disorder patients and healthy subjects. *Psychopharmacol* **92**(1): 14–24.

Charney DS, Woods SW, Goodman WK, Heninger GR (1990) Neurobiological mechanisms of panic anxiety: biochemical and behavioral correlates of yohimbine induced panic attacks. *Am J Psychiatry* **15**: 217–224.

Cowen PJ, Nutt DJ (1982) Abstinence symptoms after withdrawal of tranquillizing drugs: Is there a common neurochemical mechanism? *Lancet* **ii**: 360–362.

Cowley DS, Roy-Byrne PP, Hommer D, Greenblatt DJ, Nemeroff C, Ritchie J (1991) Benzodiazepine sensitivity in anxiety disorders. *Biol Psychiatry* **29**, 57A.

Dorow R, Horowski R, Paschelke G, Amin M, Braestrup C (1983) Severe anxiety induced by FG 7142, a b-carboline ligand for benzodiazepine receptors. *Lancet* **ii**: 98–99.

Fisher LA (1989) Corticotrophin-releasing factor: Endocrine and autonomic integration of responses to stress. *Trends Pharmacol Sci* **10**: 189–193.

Gentil V, Tavares S, Gorenstein C, Bello C, Mathias L, Gronich G, Singer J (1990) Acute reversal of flunitrazepam effects by Ro 15-1788 and Ro 15-3505: Inverse agonism, tolerance and rebound. *Psychopharmacology* **100**: 54–59.

George DT, Adinoff B, Ravitz B, Nutt DJ, De Jong J, Berrettini W, Mefford IN, Costa E, Linnoila M (1990) A cerebrospinal fluid study of the pathophysiology of panic disorder associated with alcoholism. *Acta Psych Scand* **820**: 1–7.

George DT, Nutt DJ, Rawlings RR, Phillips MJM, Eckhardt MJ, Potter WZ, Linnoila M (1995) Behavioural and endocrine responses to clomipramine in panic disorder patients with or without alcoholism. *Biol Psychiatry* **37**: 112–119.

Hawley RJ, Major LF, Schulman E, Linnoila M (1985) Cerebrospinal fluid 3-methoxy-4-hydroxyphenylglycol and norepinephrine levels in alcohol withdrawal. *Arch Gen Psychiat* **42**: 1056–1062.

Kahn RS, Asnis GM, Wetzler S, van Praag H (1988) Neuroendocrine evidence for serotonin receptor hypersensitivity in panic disorder. *Psychopharmacol* **96**: 360–364.

Kalueff AV, Nutt DJ (1997) The role of GABA in memory and anxiety. *Anxiety* **4**(3): 100–110.

Klein DF (1993) False suffocation alarms, spontaneous panics, and related conditions: An integrative hypothesis. *Arch Gen Psychiatry* **50**: 306–317.

Malizia AL, Cunningham VJ, Bell CM, Liddle PF, Jones T, Nutt DJ (1998) Decreased brain GABA$_A$-benzodiazepine receptor binding in panic disorder: Preliminary results from a quantitative PET study. *Arch Gen Psychiatry* **55**: 715–720.

Malizia AL, Nutt DJ (1998) Brain mechanisms and circuits in panic disorder. In Nutt DJ, Ballenger JC, Lépine JP (eds) *Panic Disorder: Clinical Diagnosis, Management and Mechanisms.* London: Martin Dunitz Publishers, pp. 55–77.

Montigny CD (1989) Cholecystokinin tetrapeptide induces panic-like attacks in healthy volunteers. *Arch Gen Psychiatry* **46**: 511–517.

Nutt DJ (1989) Altered central alpha-2-adrenoceptor sensitivity in panic disorder. *Arch Gen Psychiatry* **46**: 165–169.

Nutt DJ (1990) The pharmacology of human anxiety. *Pharmacology and Therapeutics* **47**: 233–266.

Nutt, DJ (1998) Antidepressants in panic disorder: Clinical and preclinical mechanisms. *J Clin Psychiatry* **59**(8): 24–29.

Nutt DJ, Glue P (1991) Clinical pharmacology of anxiolytics and antidepressants: A psychopharmacological perspective. In File S (ed.) *Psychopharmacology of Anxiolytics and Antidepressants.* New York: Pergamon Press, pp. 1–28.

Nutt DJ, Glue P, Lawson CW, Wilson SJ (1990) Flumazenil provocation of panic attacks: Evidence for altered benzodiazepine receptor sensitivity in panic disorder. *Arch Gen Psychiatry* **47**: 917–925.

Nutt D, Lawson C (1992) Panic attacks: A neurochemical overview of models and mechanisms. *Br J Psychiatry* **160**: 165–178.

Roy-Byrne PP, Lewis N, Villacres E, Diem H, Greenblatt DJ, Shader RI, Veith RC (1989) Preliminary evidence of benzodiazepine subsensitivity in panic disorder. *Biol Psychiatry* **26**: 744–748.

Southwick SM, Krystal JH, Morgan A, Johnson D, Nagy LM, Nicolaou A, Heninger GR, Charney DS (1993) Abnormal noradrenergic function in posttraumatic stress disorder. *Arch Gen Psychiatry* **50**: 266–274.

Tiihonen J, Kuikka J, Bergstrom K, Lepola U, Koponen H, Leinonen E (1997) Dopamine reuptake site densities in patients with social phobia. *Am J Psychiatry* **154**(2): 239–242.

Clinical Testing of Anxiolytic Drugs

M. Bourin

University of Nantes, Nantes, France

INTRODUCTION

This chapter defines the methodological problems associated with testing anxiolytic drugs in humans. The original indication of anxiety in all its forms is no longer acceptable because anxiety disorders have been dissected into a number of distinct entities no matter which classification has been used (DSM-IV or ICD-10). Tricyclic antidepressants or inhibitors of the uptake of serotonin (SSRIs) are still largely used to treat panic attacks, social phobia, obsessive-compulsive disorder or even post-traumatic stress disorder (Bourin and Baker, 1996). Nevertheless, the development of anxiolytic drugs almost inevitably passes by the treatment of generalised anxiety disorder (GAD) or adjustment disorder with anxious mood (ADAM). The lifetime prevalence of GAD is between 4% and 6% (Blazer et al., 1991), slightly less prevalent than phobia. However, the lack of pathognomonic symptoms and the heterogeneity of the symptoms associated with a frequent comorbidity with the diseases of axis-1 of DSM-IV lead to major diagnostic problems which can compromise the clinical studies for new drugs (DiNardo and Barlow, 1990; Noyes et al., 1992). Thus, GAD can be diagnosed by exclusion after elimination of all the forms of anxiety. However, DSM-III-R and DSM-IV have improved diagnostic reliability by focusing on the presence of worry (or fear), but the duration of symptoms must be for at least six months.

Patients suffering from transient or subsyndromic levels of anxiety are classified as ADAM. According to the DSM-IV the essential feature of this disorder is a maladaptive reaction to an identifiable psychosocial stressor. It is one of the most frequent psychiatric diagnoses made in serious physically ill patients (Schatzberg, 1990) and in older patients (Tueth, 1993). A final classification issue concerns the value of entering only patients who meet the three-month duration criteria. In both cases of GAD and ADAM an illness duration of three months may represent a fair compromise for some drug trials.

The problem of comorbidity in anxiety represents a serious methodological difficulty. Patients presenting "pure" symptoms of anxiety without an associated

Anxiety Disorders: An Introduction to Clinical Management and Research. Edited by E. J. L. Griez, C. Faravelli, D. Nutt and J. Zohar. © 2001 John Wiley & Sons, Ltd.

pathology are rare and probably not very representative of the general population. Several authors have insisted on the frequency of associated depression and particularly of associated dysthymia (Breier et al., 1985; Perugi et al., 1988; Lépine et al., 1989).

The cumulation of these difficulties in defining recruitable patients leads to major problems in the development of new drugs for the treatment of anxiety. Furthermore, benzodiazepines (BZD) are the gold standard in the treatment and the clinical tools available such as the Hamilton anxiety scale (HAM-A) (Hamilton, 1959) were developed subsequent to (and dependent on) the demonstration of the use of BZD. Thus, use of these scales may not always be appropriate for new types of anxiolytic drugs.

Finally, the modification of the different classifications (DSM or ICD) over time has not helped the development of psychotropic agents, in particular anxiolytics, because the criteria of inclusion, and therefore the patient populations, have changed with time. The concept of "all forms of anxiety" is no longer acceptable either as an operational concept or a therapeutic entity. The clinical methodology proposed in this chapter takes into account the different clinical and pharmacological constraints without forgetting that since the discovery of the BZDs, no anxiolytic apart from buspirone, has reached the market. At the present moment, the clinical studies in this area have been forced to favour antidepressants expanding their therapeutic reach into GAD.

PHASE I STUDIES

The goal of phase I studies is to find in human volunteers the maximum tolerated dose and to study the pharmacokinetic profile of the drug in question. The Food and Drug Administration (FDA) guideline of 1977 proposes that the first dose administrable to man is 1/5 to 1/10 of the maximal non-toxic dose in the rat. The first dosing studies are carried out in an open, single dose fashion. The doses are then progressively increased while assuring that the previous dose was well tolerated until the first side-effects are observed.

For anxiolytics it is possible to define in healthy volunteers potential sedative effects allowing the choice of non-sedative doses for study in phase II. The different tests which may be used in phase I are listed below.

Test Procedures

The following psychomotor tests are used.

Pictures Test

This test is used to assess long-term memory. A set of 15 pictures is presented to each subject who is allowed 10 seconds to name and memorise them. Thirty minutes later, a free recall of the names of the pictures is performed, and the restitution score is reported at intervals of 30 seconds over a total time of 2 minutes. A new set of pictures is presented at each session.

Digit Symbol Substitution Test (DSST)

This test is adapted from the Wechsler Adult Intelligence Scale. On the top of the sheet is a list of symbols to be substituted for each digit. The subjects are required to complete as many digit-symbol substitutions as possible in 90 seconds by writing down the appropriate symbol. The number of correct substitutions is scored. Six parallel forms are used (Hindmarch, 1980).

Choice Reaction Time (CRT)

This test is used to assess sensorimotor performance (Hindmarch and Parrott, 1978) and performed with an electronic automatised apparatus, the Leeds Psychomotor Tester (LPT). Subjects are required to extinguish one of six red lights presented in a semicircle and randomly illuminated by touching the appropriate response plot. From a session of 50 stimuli, the mean score (in milliseconds) of three parameters is automatically tested by LPT: the latency of the perception to the visual stimuli (recognition reaction time, RRT); the time taken to extinguish the light (motor reaction time, MRT) and the sum of both measurements (total reaction time, TRT).

Critical Flicker Fusion (CFF)

This test assesses central integrative capacity (Hindmarch, 1982). The LPT, which is positioned one metre away from the subject, shows four red diodes flickering at an increasingly rapid frequency. When a certain frequency is reached, the signals appear as a continuous light, i.e. they are fused. The frequency (measured in Hertz) at which the lights seem continuous is recorded for each subject. Individual thresholds are determined by the psychologic method of limits on three ascending and three descending values.

Side-effects Questionnaire

This self-evaluation checklist of 26 items (e.g., nausea, blurred vision, modification of appetite, dizziness) is given to subjects to record the frequency and severity of side-effects from the treatment.

Subjective Rating Scales

At the end of the session, subjects self-rate their feelings by a mark across a series of three ungraded Visual Analog Scales of 100-mm lines with opposite statements at each end (e.g., calmness/agitation, tiredness/dynamism, improvement or deterioration of concentration capacity). Scores are measured in millimetres from the middle of the lines to the mark. These tests are administered in the same order throughout the experimental period. Each test session lasts 30 minutes.

Studies in healthy volunteers have reported that BZD can produce sedation, psychomotor impairment and anterograde amnesia (Curran, 1991). However, most of the studies have been carried out with single, immediate dosages (Shader et al., 1986; File et al., 1992; Ellinwood et al., 1993) using the therapeutic doses prescribed for anxious patients. Few ongoing studies investigating possible tolerance effect on cognitive performance have been reported (File and Lister, 1983; Jurado et al., 1989; Allen et al., 1991; Bourin et al., 1994).

It would appear that the doses of BZD normally used in clinical treatment prolong reaction time (Table 17.1) or reduces the threshold for critical flicker fusion (Table 17.2). The development of substances such as abecarnyl and alpidem, partial agonists at BZD receptors, did not take into account results obtained in healthy volunteers concerning sedative effects. It was hoped that tolerance would develop to the sedative effects to a greater extent than to the anxiolytic effects. However, this phenomenon remains to be demonstrated. It is quite possible that sedative and amnestic effects contribute to the anxiolytic effects of BZDs in man.

However, it has been shown in the test described above that lorazepam and alprazolam, when administered in low doses (0.25 mg and 0.125 mg, respectively, twice daily), can improve psychometric performance in healthy volunteers (Bourin et al., 1995; Bourin et al., 1998). These findings underline the problem of the clinical dose where either disinhibition (facilitating performance) or sedative effects may be seen. The pharmacokinetic assessment is not especially difficult for anxiolytics although it is interesting to determine if sedative effects are associated with peak plasma levels after dose administration.

TABLE 17.1 Benzodiazepines increasing CRT

Drug	Dosage
Fluazepam	15 and 30 mg
Flunitrazepam	1 and 2 mg
Lorazepam	1 and 2 mg
Diazepam	2.5 and 5 mg

Source: Reproduced by permission of Hindmarch, 1980.

PHASE II STUDIES

The main purpose of phase II studies is to solve an equation with two unknown parameters, i.e. to find the efficacious dose in a given pathology, in this case in GAD or ADAM. In fact, it is essential to identify an effective dosage range and obtain preliminary evidence of efficacy. Less and less often, initial phase II studies are open or single-blind because it leads to non-objective evaluation. In most cases, five-arm studies with three doses of the product to study, a placebo and a reference drug are proposed with 60 patients in each group.

Nowadays it can be a two-arm study which compares the drug under study (very often an antidepressant drug for which the dosage in the treatment of depression is known) and a placebo. In this case a single dose of the drug is used if we have an idea of its activity in another pathology. Then, 100 patients per group are recruited. This second option can lead to failures as the efficacious dose is not necessarily the same in different pathologies such as depression, obsessive-compulsive disorder, social phobia, etc.

Thus, the first of the major phase II designs is a parallel-group design, usually with three doses in non-overlapping dose ranges (e.g., low, medium and high) of the study drug compared with placebo and a reference drug. For the time being, in most cases, the reference substances are BZDs and especially, alprazolam, bromazepam, diazepam or lorazepam.

In the pattern described above, patients can be included with a final fixed dose, preceded by a progressive increase in dose, with one to two weeks at each dose level. However, it is important to point out that although the use of flexible doses at this early stage of development has proven to be problematic, it reveals serious problems of statistical analysis as it leads to too many sub-groups at different doses.

In contrast, the disadvantage of fixed doses is the inherent inflexibility and subsequent drop-outs for patients who do not support a dose which is too high and a lack of effectiveness if the dose is too low. Nevertheless, current practice favours fixed dose schedules.

Phase II has the aim of defining dose limits and the most difficult aspect is the definition of the lowest active dose. For anxiolytics, two methods have been used: either a neurophysiological effect on the electroencephalogram (EEG) or which is

TABLE 17.2 Benzodiazepines decreasing threshold of CFF

Drug	Dosage
Diazepam	5 mg
Nedazepam	15 mg
Oxazepam	20 and 40 mg
Lorazepam	0.5 and 1 mg
Temazepam	30 mg
Nitrazepam	5 mg

Source: Reproduced by permission of Hindmarch, 1980.

even more difficult, the lowest therapeutic effect possible. Under these conditions, the minimum effective dose is often defined as the dose below which one can show a significant difference against placebo. However, this difference between placebo is problematic because in GAD or in ADAM the placebo response after a month's treatment is close to 50% which practically means that it would be difficult to show a response of 60%, i.e., only 10% superior to placebo! The question, then, is to know how long a clinical trial must be programmed for (one month or more) to show a difference in defining the minimal effective dose.

PHASE III STUDIES

After the definition of the effective dose range in phase II, the goal of phase III studies is to confirm these results on a larger patient population in comparison to a variety of reference drugs. Actually for GAD or for ADAM, the currently accepted reference products are antidepressants SSRIs, SNRIs, etc., and it would be interesting to compare the efficacity of the different types of antidepressants available. The main problem is to find a positive control which is active against placebo, given the extensive nature of the placebo response. Phase III studies can also be of longer duration than phase II studies, with a long-term evaluation after eight weeks of treatment. GAD is a chronic illness with a high level of relapse and it is important that this factor be programmed into long-term treatment trials. Here, at the beginning of the programme, one can plan to divide the treated patients into two groups at the end of eight weeks of treatment, one of the groups then being treated with placebo and the other maintained on the active drug. Under these conditions it is necessary at the start of the study to have approximately 100 to 250 patients per group. The evaluation criteria for relapse or for withdrawal phenomenon are listed below.

INCLUSION CRITERIA FOR PHASE II OR PHASE III CLINICAL TRIALS

The subjects included in the studies are non-hospitalised patients of either sex (18 to 65 years). Hospitalisation is not needed for two reasons: GAD and ADAM rarely lead to hospital admittance and the phase I and early phase II studies are given sufficient safety information about the product. Nevertheless, the patient must present the diagnostic criteria for GAD and ADAM. One difficulty with GAD is the fact that the disease may evolve over the six months placebo period which leads to real practical difficulties where the subject may want treatment prior to the end of the six months period.

The score of the HAM-A scale must be greater than 20 and remain stable during the "run-in" period, which includes the wash-out period and the immediate entry period. Furthermore, this score should not differ by more than 10% (2 points) between two tests during the same run-in period.

The patients must additionally have a score on the Covi scale greater than that of the Raskin scale to ensure that the patients are anxious rather than depressed. The two scales are easy and quick to use being made up of three items scored between 0 and 4.

EXCLUSION CRITERIA FOR PHASE II AND PHASE III CLINICAL STUDIES

An exhaustive list of the exclusion criteria is difficult to define. It is important to eliminate any pathology which might interfere with GAD or ADAM. An episode of major depression with a score superior to 15 on the Montgomery-Asberg (MADRS) scale (Montgomery and Asberg, 1979) is an exclusion criteria as is a major weight problem (bulimia or anorexia), any developing major organic disease or alcoholism. In addition, administration of psychotropic drugs in the two weeks prior to the trial is an exclusion. Further causes of exclusion are the presence of other anxious states as defined in DSM-IV which are not GAD, or ADAM.

Any associated treatment must be clearly defined in the protocol. The usual pharmacokinetic interactions (absorption, distribution, metabolism, elimination) must be considered as well as pharmacokinetic interactions common to anxiolytics. It is essential to eliminate co-administration of drugs which may be sedative or have effects on vigilance, for example, nasal vasoconstrictors may be problematic.

EVALUATION CRITERIA FOR PHASE II AND PHASE III CLINICAL STUDIES

Among all the evaluation criteria, it is necessary clearly to define the primary criteria in the protocol. However, there is no single scale which is ideal for evaluating anxiolytic activity. Among the different evaluation scales, ranking scales, etc. the principal criterion remains the HAM-A. Among all the ranking scales, the problem of the threshold for the presence of anxiety and particularly the percentage of improvement of a given score for an anxiolytic effect remains controversial.

Evaluation Scales for Anxiety

The oldest scale, the HAM-A, remains the most used and useful. It has 14 items of which only three are related to GAD: anxious mood, attention and behaviour during the test. The other items, particularly somatic ones, are not specific to anxious states. However, we previously defined that a score 20 on HAM-A is usually taken as an inclusion criterion. The global score of HAM-A reflects the total severity of the clinical syndrome but it is not an appropriate measure of anxiety such as GAD in the presence of other problems such as phobia or depressions. Again, we are confronted with the problem of comorbidity.

As we have previously seen, other scales can be associated with HAM-A such as the Covi scale for which a score of nine is commonly used as a criterion of inclusion. The Covi scale is a global evaluation tool which makes use of the overall judgement of the doctor. It consists of three items intended to evaluate speech, behaviour and the somatic complaints of the anxious subject (Covi et al., 1979). Each item is graded from 0 (absent) to 4 (very considerable). The total score for the scale therefore varies from 0 to 12. A score of ≥ 6 indicates the presence of anxiety, a score of ≤ 3 corresponds to mild or absent symptoms: a score of 3 or less is regarded as a success, a score of more than 3 is regarded as a treatment failure. This test is essentially used in the inclusion criteria to ensure that the patient is more anxious than depressed (see above).

The Tyrer scale is made up of 10 items of the Comprehensive Psychiatric Rating Scale (CPRS) which are frequently present in anxious patients: interior tension, hypochondria, hostile feelings, worry associated with hostility, general worry, phobia, neuro-vegetative disorders (1 and 2), reduction of sleep, pain and muscle tension (Tyrer et al., 1984). This scale is often used for secondary evaluation criteria because it is not specific to GAD.

These different scales are normally filled in by an assessor and it is necessary to train the assessors to give uniform responses to ensure there are no investigator differences. The translation of the scales and the questionnaires may also be problematic and require specific validation studies.

Anxiety Self-rating Scales

Anxiety self-rating scales are advantageous in that they reduce the variability associated with an external assessor. This is particularly important because of the large degree of subjectivity associated with anxiety.

The Sheehan incapacitation scale is a visual analogue scale on which the patient grades the repercussions of his or her anxiety syndrome between "not at all" and "very severely"; the patient evaluates the three areas of his or her personal life: work, family life and social life. This provides a global reflection of the repercussions of the disorder on the patient's quality of life (Sheehan et al., 1996).

Global Rating Scales

CGI (Clinical Global Impression) is often used. A score of 4 on a scale of 7 is taken as inclusion criterion. A difference of 2 points is a criterion of therapeutic success (Rickels, 1990). The CGI is the scale most commonly used in association with HAM-A.

In conclusion, it is essential to ensure homogeneity between the ratings of the clinical investigators. Group sessions uniting the different investigators are required to ensure a standard score for a given degree of anxiety. During these sessions, videos are presented showing patients being assessed using the relevant scale. It is important that the assessment be stable with time and also that there are not large differences in the scores between investigators. Thus while the score allows quantification, it is also essential for inclusion in a clinical study for an anxiolytic because the global score on HAM-A must be superior to 20.

DISCONTINUATION, DEPENDENCE AND WITHDRAWAL

Rebound, recurrence, withdrawal and dependence are closely related phenomena but these terms are not synonymous. The definition of dependence includes the presence of withdrawal symptoms leading to an inability to discontinue the drug and by itself is enough to qualify patients for the new DSM- III-R (APA, 1987) diagnosis of "psychoactive substance dependence" (Roy-Byrne and Hommer, 1988). However, a distinction must be made between BZD addiction and anxious patients who use BZD (Dupont, 1990). Addiction is a complex concept which refers to a pattern of drug use that is out of control, with social, medical, legal or economic harm resulting from drug use (Roy-Byrne and Hommer, 1988; Dupont, 1990).

Anxious patients are by definition dependent on their drug because they experience withdrawal symptoms on discontinuation, and the term "physiological dependence" implies that biological adaptation to the effects of the drug occurs (Lader and File, 1987; Greenblatt et al., 1990; Teboul and Chouinard, 1991). In those patients, three basic kinds of discontinuation syndromes have been identified on clinical and theoretical grounds, based on the character, time course and intensity of the symptomatology following discontinuation of treatment (Burrows et al., 1990; Greenblatt et al., 1990; Roy-Byrne and Cowley, 1991b).

Recurrence refers to symptoms similar in character to premorbid symptomatology and should be no more severe in intensity than the original symptoms. It occurs slowly over a period of weeks or months after stopping treatment. Rebound refers to symptoms more intense than those observed before drug treatment; it usually develops within hours or days of drug discontinuation. Withdrawal refers to symptoms different from those originally treated by BZD which occur in a time-limited fashion corresponding to the expected decline in blood level of the drug.

Theoretically, these symptoms constitute a corrective physiological reaction to the absence of the drug. Factors that contribute to greater withdrawal severity include a higher daily dose of BZD, a duration exceeding six months, the use of short half-life BZD, and abrupt discontinuation of the treatment (Roy-Byrne and Hommer, 1988; Rickels et al., 1990; Schweizer et al., 1990; Roy-Byrne and Cowley, 1991b).

For the withdrawal phase of an anxiolytic, the same methodological design as previously described is used, stressing the EEG because tonic-clonic seizures during BZD discontinuation are a rare phenomenon but have been reported for several agents. EEG has to be performed because there is insufficient epidemiological information on the risk factors, although withdrawal seizures occur more often in subjects with predisposing factors such as a history of brain damage, alcohol addiction or abnormal electroencephalograms (Fialip et al., 1987; Teboul and Chouinard, 1991), or in patients who are receiving drugs which lower the seizure threshold (Marks, 1985). Mellman and Uhde (1988) have shown that a subject has a significant increase in anxiety during BZD withdrawal, together with increased plasma corticol level, a change indicating the presence of neuroendocrine disturbance and arousal during this process. Therefore, this is further evidence that endocrinological tests are relevant. The emphasis will be on the sleep scales, which are the first to be disturbed during the withdrawal phase.

In addition to weekly assessments of anxiety, it is necessary to measure the efficacy of treatment to detect a recurrence or a rebound effect (for example, a 50% increase on the Hamilton anxiety scale is in favour of a rebound effect). A weekly withdrawal assessment including both patient-rated and physician-rated measurements is added to this design.

Physician-rated Measurements

- The Tranquilizer Withdrawal Scale (Peturson and Lader, 1984), translated and validated in French (Bourin, 1988). There are 11 items rated 0–3.
- The Benzodiazepine Withdrawal Check-list (Pecknold et al., 1982), a binary 16-item check-list.

Patient-rated Measurements

- The Benzodiazepine Withdrawal symptom questionnaire (Tyrer et al., 1990): a 20-item self-rating scale rated 0-2 on a severity scale.
- The Withdrawal symptom score (Merz and Ballmer, 1983): a 14-item self-rating scale rated on a four-point severity scale. Example: Buspirone shows less withdrawal symptoms than BZD and seems to be free of addiction potential (Lader, 1987).

REFERENCES

Allen D, Curran HV, Lader M (1991) The effects of repeated doses of clomipramine and alprazolam on physiological, psychomotor and cognitive functions in normal subjects. *Eur J Clin Pharmacol* **40**: 355–362.

American Psychiatric Association (1987) *Diagnostic and Statistical Manual of Mental Disorders* 3rd edition, revised. Washington, DC: American Psychiatric Association.

Blazer DG, Hughes D, George LK, Swartz M, Boyer R (1991) Generalized anxiety disorder.

In Robins L, Regier DA (eds) *Psychiatric Disorder in America*. New York: Free Press, pp. 180–203.

Bourin M (1988) Une échelle pour évaluer le sevrage induit par les anxiolytiques. *Encéphale* **14**: 283–285.

Bourin M, Baker GB (1996) The future of antidepressants. *Biomed Pharmacother* **50**: 7–12.

Bourin M, Colombel MC, Guitton B (1998) Alprazolam 0.125 mg twice a day improves aspects of psychometric performance in healthy volunteers. *J Clin Psychopharmacol* **18**: 364–372.

Bourin M, Colombel MC, Malinge M (1995) Lorazepam 0.25 mg twice a day improves aspects of psychometric performance in healthy volunteers. *J Psychopharmacol* **9**: 251–257.

Bourin M, Couëtoux du Tertre A, Colombel MC, Auget JL (1994) Effects of low doses of lorazepam on psychometric tests in healthy volunteers. *Int Clin Psychopharmacol* **9**: 83–88.

Breier A, Charney DS, Heninger GR (1985) The diagnostic validity of anxiety disorders and their relationship to depressive illness. *Am J Psychiatry* **142**: 787–797.

Burrows G, Norman T, Judd F, Marriott P (1990) Short-acting versus long-acting benzo-diazepines: discontinuation effects in panic disorders. *J Psychiatr Res* **24** Suppl 2: 65–72.

Covi L, Lipman MC, Nair DM, Crezlinsky T (1979) Symptomatic volunteers in multicenter drug trials. *Progr Neuropsychopharmacol Biol Psychiatry* **3**: 521–528.

Curran HV (1991) Benzodiazepines, memory and mood: A review. *Psychopharmacology* **105**: 1–8.

DiNardo PA, Barlow DH (1990) Syndrome and symptom co-occurrence in the anxiety disorders. In Maser JD, Cloninger RC (eds) *Comorbidity of Mood and Anxiety Disorders*. Washington, DC: American Psychiatric Press, pp. 205–230.

Dupont R (1990) A practical approach to benzodiazepine discontinuation. *J Psychiatr Res* **24** Suppl 2: 81–90.

Ellinwood EH Jr, Nikaido AM, Guptas K, Heatherly DG, Hege S (1993) Comparison of the relationship between structure and CNS effects for alprazolam, clonazepam and al-prazolam. *J Psychopharmacol* **7**: 24–32.

Fialip J, Aumaitre O, Eschalier A, Maradeix B, Dordain G, Lavarenne J (1987) Benzo-diazepine withdrawal seizures: Analysis of 48 case reports. *Clin Neuropharmacol* **10**: 538–544.

File SE, Lister RG (1983) Does tolerance to alprazolam develop with once weekly dosing? *Br J Clin Pharmacol* **16**: 645–650.

File SE, Sharma R, Shaffer J (1992) Is alprazolam-induced amnesia specific to the type of memory or to the task used to assess it? *J Psychopharmacology* **6**: 76–80.

Greenblatt D, Miller L, Shader R (1990) Benzodiazepine discontinuation syndromes. *J Psychiat Res* **24** Suppl 1: 73–79.

Hamilton M (1959) The assessment of anxiety states by rating. *Br J Med Psychol* **32**: 50–55.

Hindmarch I (1980) Psychomotor function and psychoactive drugs. *Br J Clin Pharmacol* **10**: 189–209.

Hindmarch I (1982) Critical flicker fusion frequency (CFF): The effects of psychotropic compounds. *Pharmacopsychiatria* **15**: 44–48.

Hindmarch I, Parrott AC (1978) The effects of sub-chronic administration of three dose levels of 1,5 benzodiazepine, clobazam, on subjective aspects of sleep and psychomotor perform-ance the morning after night-time medication. *Arzneimittelforschung* **28**: 2169–2172.

Jurado JL, Fernandez-Mas R, Fernandez-Guardiola A (1989) Effects of 1 week administration of two benzodiazepines on the sleep and early daytime performance of normal subjects. *Psychopharmacology (Berl)* **99**: 91–93.

Lader M (1987) Long-term anxiolytic therapy: The issue of drug withdrawal. *J Clin Psychiatr* **48**: 12–16.

Lader M, File S (1987) The biological basis of benzodiazepine dependence. *Psychol Med* **17**: 539–547.

Lépine JP, Lellouch J, Lovell A et al. (1989) Anxiety and depressive disorders in a French population: Methodology and preliminary results. *Psychiatry Psychobiol* **4**: 367–374.

Marks J (1985) *The Benzodiazepines: Use, Overuse, Misuse, Abuse* (2nd edition). Lancaster: MTP Press.

Martinet JP, Trebon P, Meillard MN, Reymann JM, Moran P, Lieury A, Allain H (1989) Memory assessment in elderly healthy volunteers through a short-term double-blind clinical trial. *Fund Clin Pharmacol (Abstr)* **3**: 465–466.

Mellman A, Udhe W (1988) Withdrawal syndrome with gradual tapering of alprazolam. *Am J Psychiatr* **45**: 444–450.

Merz WA, Ballmer U (1983) Symptoms of the barbiturate withdrawal syndrome in healthy volunteers: Standardized assessment by a newly developed self-rating scale. *J Psychoact Drugs* **15**: 71–84.

Montgomery SA, Asberg M (1979) A new depression scale designed to be sensitive to change. *Br J Psychiatry* **134**: 382–389.

Noyes R Jr, Woodman C, Garvey MJ et al. (1992) Generalized anxiety disorder versus panic disorder: Distinguishing characteristics and patterns of comorbidity. *J Nerv Ment Dis* **180**: 369–379.

Pecknold J, McClure D, Fleuri D, Chang H (1982) Benzodiazepine withdrawal effects. *Prog Neuro Psychopharmacol Biol Psychiatr* **6**: 517–522.

Perugi G, Akiskal H, Deltito J et al. (1988) Beyond DSM-III: Re-evaluation of the concepts of panic, agoraphobic and generalized anxiety disorders. In *Handbook of Anxiety* vol. 1. Amsterdam: Elsevier Science Publishers, pp. 47–58.

Petursson H, Lader M (1984) Benzodiazepine withdrawal. In *Dependence on Tranquilizers*. Oxford: Oxford University Press.

Rickels K (1990) Evaluating antidepressants and anxiolytic. In Benker O, Maier W, Rickels K (eds) *Methodology of the Evaluation of Psychotropic Drugs. Psychopharmacology*, Series 8, Berlin and Heidelberg: Springer Verlag.

Rickels K, Schweizer E, Case G, Greenblatt D (1990) Long-term therapeutic use of benzodiazepines. I. Effects of abrupt discontinuation. *Arch Gen Psychiatr* **47**: 899–907.

Roy-Byrne P, Cowley D (eds) (1991a) Cognitive and psychomotor effects. In Roy-Byrne, P, Cowley D (eds) *Benzodiazepines in Clinical Practice: Risks and Benefits*. Washington, DC: APA Press, pp. 113–121.

Roy-Byrne P, Cowley D (eds) (1991b) Benzodiazepines: dependence and withdrawal. In *Benzodiazepine in Clinical Practice: Risks and Benefits*. Washington, DC: APA Press, pp. 133–153.

Roy-Byrne P, Cowley D (eds) (1991c) Use of benzodiazepines in the elderly. In Roy-Byrne P, Cowley D (eds) *Benzodiazepine in Clinical Practice: Risks and Benefits*. Washington, DC: APA Press, pp. 215–227.

Roy-Byrne PP, Hommer D (1988) Benzodiazepine withdrawal: Overview and implications for the treatment of anxiety. *Am J Med* **84**: 1041–1051.

Schatzberg AF (1990) Anxiety and adjustment disorder: A treatment approach. *J Clin Psychiat* **51**(11): 20–24.

Schweizer E, Rickels K, Case G, Greenblatt D (1990) Long-term therapeutic use of benzodiazepines. II. Effects of gradual taper. *Arch Gen Psychiatr* **47**: 908–915.

Shader RI, Dreyfuss D, Gerrein JR, Harmatz JS, Allison SJ, Greenblatt DJ (1986) Sedative effects and impaired learning and recall after single oral doses of alprazolam. *Clin Pharmacol Ther* **39**: 526–529.

Sheehan DV, Harnett-Sheehan K, Raj BA (1996) The measurement of disability. *Int Clin Psychopharmacol* **11**: 89–95.

Teboul E, Chouinard G (1991) A guide of benzodiazepine selection. Part II: Clinical aspects. *Can J Psychiatr* **36**: 62–73.

Tueth MJ (1993) Anxiety in the older patient: Differential diagnosis and treatment. *Geriatrics* **48**: 51–54.

Tyrer P, Murphy S, Riley P (1990) The benzodiazepine withdrawal symptom questionnaire. *J Affect Dis* **19**: 53–61.

Tyrer P, Owen RT, Cicetti DV (1984) The brief scale for anxiety: A subdivision of the Comprehensive Psychopathological Rating Scale. *J Neurol Neurosurg Psychiatry* **47**: 970–975.

Methods of Experimental Psychiatry

A Case Study of the 35% CO_2 Challenge

K. Verburg, G. Perna and E.J.L. Griez

MEDIANT, Locatie Helmerzijde, Enschede, The Netherlands;
Istituto Scientifico Ospedale San Raffaele, Vita-Salute University, Milan, Italy;
Maastricht University, Maastricht, The Netherlands

INTRODUCTION

In this chapter, we will discuss the methodology of the 35% CO_2 challenge, as an example of how research using these kinds of techniques can be done and has been done in the past. Some general introductory comments will help put the experimental approach in the broader perspective of psychiatric research. Then the story of the 35% CO_2 challenge will be told. It will illustrate how an experimental model eventually emerged from an unexpected observation. The assumption that CO_2 vulnerability is closely related to the underlying mechanisms of panic, rapidly raised a number of basic problems regarding the validity of the model under investigation. The methods section will detail these issues, and show to which extent challenge tests may be validly used in psychiatric research, again using our own research as an example. We will end with a discussion on the possible implications of our findings, with a few remarks on possible future research.

Thus this chapter deals with experimental research in psychiatry. To the extent that a method can be defined as a procedure useful for the solution of problems, the experimental method refers to the use of experiments to solve the problems we are faced with. In science these problems are specifically related to the knowledge of the observable world where we live and the rules this world is governed by. Thus an experimental method is a procedure developed to confirm or falsify predictions (hypotheses) about links and causal relationships between observable phenomena. Basically, an experiment is the observation of the change induced in variable B (the dependent variable) after the deliberate modification of variable A (the independent variable). It helps to improve our knowledge of the "real" world by manipulating models of this world inside the laboratory. In medicine, such experimental methods most often involve a laboratory model of the clinical disorder. Animal models are a well-known example. Although animal models are widely used, they obviously have their limitations, particularly when subjective experiences such as affects and

Anxiety Disorders: An Introduction to Clinical Management and Research. Edited by E. J. L. Griez, C. Faravelli, D. Nutt and J. Zohar. © 2001 John Wiley & Sons, Ltd.

cognitions are involved. Therefore, the reproduction of certain aspects of pathology necessarily involves humans in experimental situations. Using human subjects in such studies demands high ethical and safety standards, but it also offers the great advantage that it provides a model as close as possible to the real clinical situation in which subjects can be asked about their subjective experience during the experimental procedure.

Tremendous progress can be expected from this type of research in the specific case of psychiatry. Currently, our diagnoses are based on the identification of clinical syndromes. These syndromes are clusters of related symptoms with a characteristic time course. Further criteria are the presence of abnormal behavior and/or distressing experiences. However, even though this process has led to a high reliability of in the current diagnostic systems (e.g. the DSM-IV: APA, 1994), we should be aware of the limits of psychiatric diagnoses. Current diagnostic entities rely on the consensus of experts interpreting epidemiological data. We miss any information at all on the validity of most of our diagnostic concepts. For instance, diagnoses in different hospitals and different countries may be fairly consistent, and two patients may be diagnosed as having a panic disorder both in Paris and New York on the basis of DSM criteria. However, this says nothing about the underlying mechanisms at work in these patients. It is just a statement that both subjects have some signs and symptoms that fit our current consensual diagnostic classification. Contrary to other branches of medicine, our specific diagnoses do not at all refer to specific underlying mechanisms. Thus, the high reliability of or current worldwide diagnostic systems may be misleading: most psychiatric diagnoses are still in need of validation. That is the main reason for the low credibility of psychiatric illnesses in medicine, and there is still a long way to go to elucidate underlying etiopathogenetic mechanisms of disordered behaviors. Nevertheless solid diagnostic criteria, genuine "gold standards" in psychiatric diagnoses cannot exist without a clear scientific insight in causal processes that underlie the clinical picture. As early as 1970, Eli Robins and Samuel B. Guze proposed a five-phase approach to the problem of diagnostic validity in psychiatric illness (Robins and Guze, 1970). They proposed different types of external validators for psychiatric diagnoses: (a) clinical description; (b) laboratory studies; (c) delimitation from other disorders; (d) longitudinal follow-up studies; and (e) family studies. Although this approach stands as one of the most influential models in the development of the most used psychiatric diagnostic systems (i.e. DSM III, III-R and IV), psychiatric diagnoses are still mainly based on clinical descriptions and epidemiological criteria.

Among external validators, as included by Robins and Guze, laboratory measures and experimental models might play a central role in improving validity of psychiatric diagnoses by relating diagnoses to the "real entities", coupling diagnoses to known underlying mechanisms. Experimental models of a disease might go beyond clinical and epidemiological features and deepen our insight into the mechanisms underlying pathological diagnostic entities, with major implications for the treatment and prevention of psychiatric illnesses.

As stated above, in the present chapter we will try to disentangle the many different aspects and difficulties of the development of an experimental model in anxiety disorders, from the very beginning (the idea), across the involvement of many different researchers and research centers, to its theoretical and practical effects.

Among anxiety disorders, panic disorder, and in particular the psychobiology of panic, has been widely studied. One of the main reasons for the interest of investigators in this disorder is the possibility of reproducing panic attacks, the core phenomenon of the clinical picture, in a laboratory. Many different agents, most of them probably triggering a central nervous system dysfunction in the mid-brain, have been reported to induce acute anxiety (see Chapter 16 in this volume). Among these, carbon dioxide is to date one of the closest to satisfy criteria for an ideal panicogenic model (Verburg et al., 1998a). Within the different methods of using carbon dioxide to provoke panic attacks, the 35% CO$_2$ challenge test is probably one of the most widely used. We will discuss the story of this model as it has developed across the last 15–20 years.

This discussion is relevant to the education of doctors in the field of mental disorders for the following reasons: first, from a clinical point of view, the understanding of the process that underlies the development of a good experimental model might be an example of a scientific approach to the practice of psychiatry, an approach that, unfortunately, does not have a central place in the daily care. We will try to show how some hypotheses regarding a particular disorder can be elaborated on the basis of laboratory observations, and how these hypotheses can be challenged and modified using an systematic methodology. With reference to evidence-based medicine, such a way of thinking should become standard even for clinicians in their dealings with patients, particularly when facing complex clinical syndromes. To this extend clinical practice should endorse the experimental method.

Second, from a research point of view, disentangling the complexity of the model will serve the understanding of the real disease and bring us closer to diagnoses and treatments based on the best available evidence.

THE EARLY CASE STORY

Although inhalation of carbon dioxide has a long (and strange) history in psychiatry (Griez and Van den Hout, 1984), the use of carbon dioxide in recent research started with the discovery that inhalation of carbon dioxide may trigger anxiety. Early observations on the anxiogenic properties of carbon dioxide had been done in the past (Cohen and White, 1951) but they went largely unnoticed. The current interest in the use of carbon dioxide as a probe for experimental anxiety originates by coincidence, simultaneously in two different places.

Gorman et al. (1984) investigated the once popular theory that hyperventilation may cause acute anxiety attacks. They designed an experiment in which subjects with a panic disorder had to go into forced hyperventilation. To control for the hyperventilation condition, they conceived a procedure that mimics the rapid respiration seen in hyperventilation, but in which subjects inhale a mixture with 5% carbon dioxide,

TABLE 18.1 Protocol for 35% CO_2 inhalation used at the Maastricht Academic Anxiety Center. Challenges may be either air-placebo controlled or not

Subjects

Patients are selected from among those referred to the clinic for treatment. Controls are recruited either through word of mouth or by advertisements placed throughout the city

Inclusion criteria

Patients
• DSM IV criteria, with agreement of diagnosis by at least 2 experienced clinicians
• and/or according to a structured interview
Controls
• good physical health
• absence of any present or past psychiatric illness

Exclusion criteria

A full physical examination is carried out and clinical history ascertained in search of the following exclusion criteria:

Absolute exclusion criteria

• Important cardiovascular history, or suspicion of infarct, cardiomyopathy, cardiac failure, TIA, angina pectoris, cardiac arrhythmias, CVA
• Important respiratory history, including asthma and lung fibrosis
• Personal or familial history of cerebral aneurysm
• Hypertension systolic press. > 180, diastolic press > 100 mmHg
• Pregnancy

Relative contraindications

• < 15 or > 60 years of age
• Epilepsy
• Non invalidating COPD

Procedure

1. **Informed consent** obtained and cosigned by 2 staff members in the Case Record File
2. **Vital capacity** measured
3. **Restrictions**
   • 2 weeks medication free of any central acting drugs including Beta Blockers, with occasional exception made of incidental use of low doses of benzodiazepines (i.e. single doses equivalent to 5 mg of diazepam)

• 36 hours of no excessive alcoholic consumption prior to gas inhalation
• 8 hours of no significant consumption of xanthine containing beverages prior to gas inhalation
• 2 hours of no xanthine, food or smoking prior to gas inhalation, if at all possible

4. **The first gas turned on** (either air or 35% CO_2–65% O_2, according to a randomisation table), by an assistant who does not attend steps 4 to 7

5. **Questionnaires** filled out
   • VAAS, a Visual Anxiety Analogue Scale with values ranging from "0" (no anxiety at all) to "100" (the worst anxiety ever imaginable)
   • DSM IV symptom list, with a total of 13 symptoms, each with a possible value ranging from "0" (not at all) to "4" (very intensive) giving a total maximum possible score of 52.

6. **Explanation** given
   Experimenter places the subject in a comfortable arm-chair and gives the following explanation:
   "You will be inhaling 2 different mixtures of O_2 and CO_2. These are harmless, physiological compounds, but, depending on individual susceptibility and on concentration, you may notice short-lived effects which may range from hardly perceptible sensations to frank anxiety"
   Explain some terms if necessary.
   Panic attacks are never referred to as such.

7. **Inhalation**
   • Subject takes the mask for self-administration.
   • Exhales as deeply as possible.
   • Presses the mask against face.
   • Inhales deeply (Experimenter assures that a minimum of 80% of the total vital capacity is inhaled)
   • Experimenter counts aloud 4 seconds (watch).
   • Subject exhales.

8. **Questionnaires** filled out (see 5)

9. Participants leave the laboratory for 15 minutes

10. Steps 4–8 are carried out again for the second gas mixture

to prevent a decrease in the pCO_2 in the blood. In fact subjects became slightly hypercapnic. To the investigators' surprise, more panic attacks occurred in the 5% CO_2 condition than in the hyperventilation procedure. This finding has been replicated repeatedly.

At the same time, Griez and Van den Hout (1984) also worked with carbon dioxide inhalation, but from a totally different perspective. They used a single breath inhalation of 35% carbon dioxide, a technique that had been advocated years before by the behavior therapist Joseph Wolpe (1958) in the treatment of free floating anxiety. Wolpe believed hypercapnic inhalations to have anxiolytic properties. In fact, full breath inhalations of a 35% CO_2 mixture in oxygen proved to lack any anxiolytic effect. On the contrary, when tested on patients with anxiety disorders, CO_2 appeared to trigger rather than to block anxious feelings. For a time, Griez and Van den Hout explored whether CO_2 may be used to teach patients to cope more effectively with an impending anxiety attack, using the exposure paradigm of behavior therapists. Although this appeared to work in one study (Van den Hout et al., 1987), the finding has never been replicated. Clinically, the beneficial effects of this method appeared to be short-lived and of little use. However, it appeared that a single inhalation of 35% CO_2–65% O_2 not only causes strong autonomic sensations in all subjects, mimicking those of a panic attack, but specifically triggers an immediate feeling of anxiety in subjects with a DSM-III diagnosis of panic disorder (PD) (APA, 1980). All panic disorder patients showed a brief, though definite anxiety response to the challenge, a response that they felt was similar to their naturally occurring panic attacks (Griez et al., 1987). Thus, research that originally intended to find a method to reduce anxiety led to a laboratory method that induces anxiety symptoms.

Indeed, carbon dioxide eliciting anxiety immediately raised a number questions. Is there response specificity? Are panic patients the only group of people who show this particular response to inhalation of carbon dioxide, or are there others who are equally responsive? If so, does this response occur in every panic disorder patient? Is the observed response a *reliable* phenomenon? How do panic disorder patients respond to repeated challenges? Is the response *sensitive* to preventive interventions? For instance, is it possible to block the response with effective anti-panic medication? If so, can this model be used to test new drugs? What is the *face validity* of the observed CO_2-induced effect? Are CO_2-induced PAs true PAs? Do they phenomenologically resemble real-life PAs? Does the mechanism that leads to CO_2 induced panic bear a relationship to the mechanism that causes real-life panic attacks?

The early studies showed that inhalation of carbon dioxide did exactly induce the physical symptoms of what had just been described as panic attacks (PAs), but, in susceptible patients, led to the subjective sensation of anxiety as well, triggering a very short-lived PA in the laboratory. The findings suggested that it was worthwhile to continue research with carbon dioxide in order to get a better insight into the mechanisms that caused anxiety in vulnerable individuals.

The first step that was taken to answer these questions was to compare the response of panic disorder patients to the response of normal controls, free from any type of psychopathology. Griez et al. (1987) challenged 12 panic disorder patients and 11 healthy controls. They found that the panic disorder patients experienced high levels of subjective anxiety, and more panic symptoms than the normal controls.

Such a study, in which subjects with the highest possible vulnerability are compared with subjects, believed to have the lowest vulnerability, is a first logical step. In case of no clear-cut difference between these two groups, the model would have lost most of its heuristic value. Griez et al. did find PD patients responded differently from normals. The next step was to challenge groups of patients that also might have a positive response to this challenge, namely, other anxiety disorder patients. A simple hypothesis to explain the above contrast between PD subjects and normals was to point to the baseline condition. One could conceive the response as a matter of baseline arousal, any type of highly aroused individual (as are PD patients), subjected to a strong autonomic stimulus as CO_2 administration, being supposed to display a severe reaction, i.e. an increase in anxiety. Therefore, a mixed group of anxious patients, all of them selected on the basis of high baseline ratings on a standardised scale, regardless of their specific diagnoses, underwent a CO_2 challenge. The CO_2 procedure affected only those with a diagnosis of PD (Griez et al., 1990b). Then we started to examine the CO_2 vulnerability of each category of anxiety disorder. The first study in that line compared the responses of panic disorder patients, obsessive-compulsive disorder patients and normal controls. In this study, obsessive-compulsive disorder patients appeared to react more like normal controls, rather than like panic disorder patients (Griez et al., 1990a). Since PD, characterized by acute bursts of anxiety, was originally delineated against GAD, a condition devoid of PAs, it was of prime importance to know whether the CO_2 challenge would support the distinction between PD and GAD. That was tested in a small study comparing PD patients and subjects with a GAD, who had no lifetime history of PAs. Only the former group reported high post-CO_2 ratings on subjective anxiety (Verburg et al., 1995).

The investigation of the specificity across anxiety disorders continued with the administration of a 35% CO_2 challenge to a group of people with specific phobias. Interestingly, while animal phobics displayed a normal response, subjects with situational phobias, as claustrophobics, were vulnerable to CO_2, though less than PD patients (Verburg et al., 1994). In that respect, it was noted that situational phobias, both from an epidemiological and a psychopathological point of view, are believed to have links with PD, which is acknowledged in the current edition of the DSM. Finally, investigation turned towards social phobia. The results were not clear-cut: after a first study suggesting social phobics to be CO_2-sensitive (Caldirola et al., 1997), another work showed discrepant results (Verburg et al., 1998b). Investigation into the specificity of the 35% CO_2 challenge is therefore a matter of ongoing concern.

While it is still unknown how carbon dioxide inhalation induces panic, it has become clear that hyperventilation is not the causal mechanism. Obviously, a single inhalation of an hypercapnic mixture induces a strong hyperventilatory reaction. Therefore, the hypothesis that a 35% CO_2 challenge may act by inducing acute hyperventilation was tested in two studies from the same group (Griez et al., 1988; Zandbergen et al., 1990). Both experiments clearly showed that hypocapnia resulting from forced hyperventilation fails to induce any clinically significant anxiety in patients with PD. Another early hypothesis was that PD patients might be hypersensitive to inhaled CO_2 because they have hypersensitive chemoreceptors. The *ventilatory response* is a physiological parameter, describing the increase in ventilation (frequency × volume) in response to the inhalation of increasing concentrations of carbon dioxide. No study has so far been successful in proving disturbed chemosensitivity in PD, but this could be the consequence of methodological problems (for an overview, see Griez and Verburg, 1999).

Most of the above studies with 35% CO_2 mentioned so far were performed in the Maastricht laboratory. The model made a big step forward when it was also introduced in Milan. Perna et al. (1994a) started replicating the most important studies conducted in The Netherlands. In one experiment, comparing 71 panic disorder patients with 44 normal controls, the Italian investigators found results that compared well with the Dutch data. The fact that the effects of the challenge are now replicated in many countries on different continents (Europe, Asia, North and South America, Australia) underscores that the original data were quite robust and adds to the validity of the findings.

Besides, the introduction of the model in Italy had another important consequence. The Milan department had a strong tradition in genetic studies. Knowledge from this field gave a strong impetus in a new direction, combining the experimental, challenge-based approach with expertise in the field of genetics. This conjunction of methodologies proved particularly fruitful. Both family and twin studies were started, using the 35% CO_2 challenge as a probe to explore the constitutional predisposition to CO_2 vulnerability (Perna et al., 1995a; Perna et al., 1996; Bellodi et al., 1998). The results support that 35% CO_2 hypersensitivity could be a laboratory marker associated with familial loading in PD. These findings have been replicated by research teams in USA (Coryell, 1997) and Europe (van Beek and Griez, 2000). The Milan research team performed a segregation study of panic disorder using 35% CO_2 hyperreactivity as an objective diagnostic validator with the aim of reducing the influence of phenocopies (Cavallini et al., 1999). Finally, Schmidt et al. (in press) reported an association between a functional polymorphism in the serotonin transporter gene and 35% CO_2 subjective reactivity. The 35% CO_2 challenge has been also used as a laboratory model to study the role of cognitive factors in panic disorder with particular reference to anxiety sensitivity (Eke and McNally, 1996; McNally and Eke, 1996; Schmidt et al., 1999; Schmidt et al., in press; Shipherd et al., in press).

Other areas of research with the 35% carbon dioxide model have also proven to be successful. These include, beside finding out which groups of patients and healthy subjects are vulnerable to the challenge, conducting pharmacological studies on the influence of medication on CO_2 vulnerability, and using this approach to screen for potential new panicolytics. A more detailed mention of these recent developments will be made later.

SOME METHODOLOGICAL CONCERNS

The methods of the 35% carbon dioxide challenge are fairly simple, however, there are a number of important issues. The main issue is to make sure that the effects are indeed due to the inhalation of carbon dioxide. Alternative explanations are that the laboratory setting, the investigators themselves, the nurses and/or the machinery cause or influence the amount of anxiety. Also, in consideration of the bulk of work that has been done on cognitive factors and panic, the instruction, mentioning to a panic patient that he/she possibly may have a panic attack, needs to be controlled for: genuine PAs might be induced by cognitive manipulation (see, for instance, Clark, 1986).

To control for these factors, every patient or control subject who is about to undergo the panic provocation is given a standardised instruction. Subjects are informed about what is going to happen, that they may experience some level of anxiety, depending on their individual vulnerability, and that they also may experience some physical symptoms usually associated with anxiety. It is, however, stressed that any discomfort that may occur will be short-lived, not exceeding a matter of a minute. In the procedure of the 35% CO_2 challenge, the word panic is deliberately not mentioned. The procedure is explained in detail to every subject. All preparations are made in the same order, all laboratory procedures are under the control of experienced and well-trained persons. However, the most important method to ensure that the effects that are seen are really induced by carbon dioxide is the use of a placebo condition. In the 35% carbon dioxide challenge subjects are asked to take a breath of two different mixtures, the active condition (35% CO_2 and 65% O_2) and the placebo mixture (80% N_2 and 20% O_2, almost the composition of normal air). These two inhalations are given in a randomised order, according to a double blind procedure. A strongly related issue is that of assessing the dependent variables. If we do induce anxiety and panic attacks, we have to be able to make reliable measurements.

Let us try to understand the problems related to measurement by looking at the 35% CO_2 challenge. In most 35% CO_2 studies so far, the dependent variables are as follows. Immediately before and immediately after (a matter of 30 seconds) each inhalation (both the placebo and the active condition) assessments are made by means of (a) a Visual Analogue Scale for Anxiety (VAS-A) describing the degree of global subjective anxiety on a continuum from 0 ("no anxiety present at all") to 100 ("the worst anxiety you can imagine"), and (b) a so-called "Panic Symptom List" which is a self-rating questionnaire assessing, on a 5-point scale, the 13 panic symptoms described, in DSM III-R and DSM IV. The key issue is: "What do we want to measure for what aim?" Such a simple question brings out several problems. Not all of them have been solved in a totally satisfactory way.

Do the Scales Really Measure the "Disease-specific Reactivity" of Patients?

The fact that we can detect some response is not sufficient to infer that the performed measure is a valid measure. For example, if we would like to evaluate heart rate response to physical effort, measuring sweating might provide a response, but is not an appropriate way to measure heart rate. The scales that we described do measure a behavioural response to panicogenic challenges. However, are we really sure, for instance, that "panic" = "anxiety"? So far, we assume that it is, but there is evidence in favour of heterogeneity, and measuring anxiety while meaning panic may be not entirely valid.

We have to decide what dimension exactly among the scales used is to be considered as the best measure. This pertains to the aims of our studies. If we want to demonstrate a difference between PDs and healthy controls or, say, between PD and patients with other disorders, we are searching for the very best measure to differentiate our target group (patients with PD) from the others (healthy controls). This measure will be the variable that provides the highest sensitivity (ability to detect the target, i.e. the "true positives") together with the highest specificity (ability to avoid detecting noise, i.e. "false negatives"). For a diagnostic test, for instance, sensitivity is defined as having a positive measurement among those patients with a positive diagnosis, and specificity as the probability of having a negative measurement among those who have a negative diagnosis. In medicine and psychology, the ideal measurement always has both the maximum sensitivity and the maximum specificity. However, in fact, most tests lose specificity when gaining sensitivity and vice versa.

A rather sophisticated method of addressing this issue is to make use of the so-called Receiver Operating Characteristic Analysis (ROC). ROC allows us to choose among different measurements and to find out the variable that is best able to differentiate true positives and true negatives. In a ROC analysis, sensitivity and specificity of a test at different cut-off points (the point above which a response is considered to be positive) are plotted against each other. Two recent studies from our groups suggest that a VAS for anxiety is better at distinguishing patients with PD from healthy controls and patients with other anxiety disorders. The ROC analysis also tells us at which cut-off point the discriminatory ability of a test is at its highest (see Battaglia and Perna, 1995; Verburg et al., 1998c).

How Can We Measure the "Reactivity"?

Most of the researchers use delta scores (post-scores minus pre-scores). This method gives a simple measure of increase in anxiety due to the challenge test. However, this method does not take into account the "ceiling" effect. If the scale ranges between 0 and 100, and the subject starts at a baseline value of 90 there is little room to increase, and it is impossible to have a delta score higher than 10. Is going from 0 to 10 the same as going from 90 to 100? This problem is not yet solved even if some solutions have been proposed. For example, we have tried (Perna et al., 1994b) to overcome the use of simple delta scores, calculating a "% score" on the VAS scale. This percentage score represents the percentage of maximum increment or decrement possible for a particular subject, taking into account the maximum increase or decrease that was possible seeing the baseline value. It is simply calculated as follows:

1. If VAS-A (post-CO_2 VAS-A values minus pre-CO_2 VAS-A values) was positive, then % VAS-A = VAS-A × 100/(100- VAS-A before CO_2).
2. If VAS-A was negative, then % VAS-A = VAS-A × 100/VAS-A before CO_2.

However, even if this measure overcomes the "ceiling" effect by taking into account baseline anxiety, it is possible to find some paradoxical score (i.e. VAS score before $CO_2 = 0$, VAS score after $CO_2 = 99$; %VAS = 99 while if VAS score before $CO_2 = 99$ and VAS score after $CO_2 = 100$; %VAS = 100).

We have also considered simply using the VAS after CO_2 as the measure of CO_2 reactivity. But in this way we do not take in account baseline anxiety and in some studies (pharmacological studies) this might be a problem (Pols et al., 1996a) since by applying this measure differences related to baseline anxiety are masked. Once again, ROC analysis can help to choose between these measures and we have suggested that VAS scores after CO_2 might be more valid than VAS and %VAS in distinguishing patients with PD from patients with other anxiety disorders (see Verburg et al., 1998c). However, the limitations of this measure do not allow us to consider this problem as solved.

A major issue in every challenge procedure, or better, in every study involving human subjects, is safety. Safety pertains to ethics, although the last dimension is not reduced to safety. Safety in panic provocation procedures has several aspects.

Just as any medical intervention, the challenge should not induce any physical or psychological damage both in the short and the long term. Needless to say, it should not worsen the clinical condition of the subject participating to the procedure. It is a *conditio sine qua non* that all experimentally induced effects are completely reversible and stay under full control of the physician at any point of the procedure. Any induced discomfort should be as least disturbing as possible, both in intensity and duration. Investigators in experimental psychiatry will make sure that the applied procedure does not increase any risk of developing any type of psychiatric symptoms with particular reference to those with a possible underlying susceptibility (e.g. relatives of patients with panic disorder). For the 35% CO_2 challenge, both absolute and relative exclusion criteria have been developed throughout the years. A full list of current criteria is available from the authors upon request. These criteria are not based on observed accidents but on the evaluation of the well-known physiological effects of CO_2. So, even in the absence of evidences of adverse effects, all subjects with significant cardiovascular and respiratory disorders, personal or family history of cerebral aneurysm, significant hypertension (systolic > 180 mmHg, diastolic > 100 mmHg) or epilepsy are on the exclusion list. Also, women who are (possibly) pregnant are excluded from the challenge studies. Although, there have been no reports in the scientific literature of significant adverse effects following a 35% CO$_2$ challenge. Finally, three recent studies (Harrington et al., 1996; Perna et al., 1997b; Perna et al., 1999) have shown that the challenge was not able to prime or potentiate any anxiety disorder in both healthy controls and in healthy first-degree relatives of patients with panic disorder.

The issues mentioned so far, (1) being sure that the reaction is indeed induced by carbon dioxide; (2) being able to measure the response correctly; and (3) being sure the procedure is safe, are the basic conditions to conduct panic provocation studies.

From a heuristic point of view, other important issues come into play for those investigators trying to elaborate experimental models of psychiatric disorders. The validity of a laboratory model cannot simply rely on the ability of triggering some idiosyncratic reaction in a specific group of patients. Constructing a valid laboratory model requires a more complex and integrated approach. Several authors (Guttmacher et al., 1983; Gorman et al., 1987; Uhde and Tancer, 1990) have proposed specific criteria for an ideal model. In general, four main criteria have been identified by most of the authors. They are: symptom convergence, specificity, reliability and clinical validation.

Symptom Convergence

This refers to the requirement that the sensations that are experimentally induced must be similar in quality, duration and severity to those experienced by patients during natural, spontaneous panic attacks covering both cognitive and somatic symptoms. Having in mind an experimental model of panic we should be able to reproduce the genuine symptoms of a naturally occurring panic attack. The 35% CO$_2$ challenge seems to fulfil this criterion as most patients with PD (Perna et al., 1994a) reported that the reaction induced by the challenge was qualitatively very similar, or even the same of what they experienced during their naturally occurring attacks. This is particularly important since it allows the researchers to study in the laboratory the core phenomenon of panic disorder and thus to accelerate the knowledge of both the biological and psychological mechanisms underlying this disease. Some studies underway in our laboratories do prove that the symptoms' profile of induced panic attacks are very similar to those of naturally occurring panic attacks. A beneficial side-effect is that symptom convergence helps participant patients to gain a better insight in the symptoms of his/her disease; also the ability to reproduce the patients' symptomatology in the laboratory might help psychiatrists/psychologists to gain a stronger alliance with patients from a therapeutic perspective.

Specificity

A challenge may show either "complete" or "threshold" specificity. Complete specificity implies that only patients with a PD do panic in reaction to the challenge.

Healthy controls and patients with other psychiatric disorders are not affected at all by the procedure. Threshold specificity implies that although healthy controls and patients with psychiatric disorders other than panic may be affected by the challenge, there is a difference in the amount of the stimulus necessary to affect PDs, on one hand, and others, on the other hand. The issue of specificity is of particular import-ance since, as we already suggested, the value of experimental models and laboratory markers may be related to their ability to trigger specific pathophysiological mechan-isms underlying specific nosological entities. In the near future, some laboratory markers might even outshine some of our current diagnostic "gold standards" based on consensus rather than on true objective validators. For instance, when looking at studies using the 35% CO_2 challenge, we can subdivide subjects tested in two different groups, those with a strong reactivity and those without a significant reactivity. Somewhat surprisingly, among those with a strong reactivity there were patients with disorders other than panic disorder, Especially social and specific phobia, pre-menstrual dysphoria and healthy subjects with sporadic panic attacks or with a familial vulnerability to PD. Patients with obsessive-compulsive disorder, generalised anxiety disorder or mood disorders are not (for an overview, see Verburg et al., 1998a). These findings suggest that there might exist a spectrum of disorders, all characterised by an abnormal sensitivity to CO_2, whatever the underlying mechan-isms may be, but sharing possibly a common pathogenic background. Should this be confirmed by further evidence, it would be a convincing illustration of an experimen-tal approach contributing to better validity of psychiatric nosology.

Reliability

The susceptibility to the challenge should be preserved even after repeated challenges as far as the clinical condition remains unchanged. This is another important criterion, too often insufficiently investigated. To date some studies suggest that the reliability of the 35% CO_2 challenge is good, but it must be recognised that results reported in literature are not completely in agreement.

Studies from the Milan's group (Perna et al., 1994b; Bertani et al., 1997) suggest that there is a good reliability for three challenges across a week using the %VAS as measure of the response. Verburg et al. (1998a) showed that the VAS scores and the PSL list are reliable measures when the challenge is repeated after one week. Coryell (1999) reported a reduction of provoked panic symptoms during a second challenge performed after a variable interval (1–52 days). Finally, Schmidt and co-workers (1997) suggest that the panic/anxiety reactivity to 35% CO_2 inhalations is reproduc-ible after 12 weeks. One of the main difficulties in evaluating these studies on reliability is the difference in the measures used as indicators of CO_2 reactivity. The absence of homogeneity makes it very problematic to draw definitive conclusions on this topic. Furthermore, it should be borne in mind that some early studies (Griez and van den Hout, 1986; van den Hout et al., 1987) have reported some desensitisation of the CO_2 response occurring after a prolonged series of intense exposure to the challenge.

Clinical Validation

Drugs or interventions that are effective in the treatment of the clinical condition are expected to reduce the reactivity to the provoking procedure. Conversely, drugs or procedures that are ineffective should not alter this reactivity. Several studies investigated the effects of psychotropic drugs on the response to CO$_2$ stimulation. There is clear evidence that treatment with clinically effective anti-panic agents (tricyclic antidepressants, selective serotonin re-uptake inhibitors, reversible monoamine oxidase inhibitors and high potency benzodiazepines) significantly reduces 35% CO$_2$ reactivity both measured from a behavioural and physiological point of view (Pols et al., 1991, 1993, 1996a, 1996b; Perna et al., 1994a; Bertani et al., 1997; Gorman et al., 1997; Nardi et al., 1997; Bocola et al., 1998). So it has been shown that effective anti-panic medication also blocks the response to CO$_2$. However, only few studies investigated the effects of compounds ineffective in the treatment of panic disorder, and these were only done on healthy subjects. Yohimbine, buspirone and propranolol, were not able to induce relevant modification of CO$_2$ induced symptomatology in healthy subjects (van den Hout and Griez, 1984; Pols et al., 1989, 1996). To draw definitive conclusions on this topic, studies on the effects of ineffective anti-panic compounds on 35% CO$_2$ reactivity in patients with panic disorder are needed.

As noticed, the value of experimental models and laboratory markers cannot be evaluated in another way than by reference to the "gold standard" for clinical diagnosis, currently DSM-IV, that provides the worldwide accepted diagnostic category of panic disorder. Given this, the paradox is that the model cannot perform better than clinical diagnosis. If this clinical diagnosis is imperfect, both in reliability and in validity (and we have many reasons to believe that it is), the interpretation of experimental/laboratory measures is compromised. Therefore, in the future, laboratory markers must prove themselves to be better diagnostic validators than the mere clinical criteria reached upon by consensual procedures. As a first step in this direction, an feedback process integrating both the clinical features and the laboratory probes might give a clue to the identification of valid clinical diagnostic entities.

CONCLUSION

This chapter describes the development and the use of a panic provocation model. We described how the initial discovery that carbon dioxide inhalation causes panic was made. There is an element of chance involved probably related to what is called "serendipity" (= "the faculty of making happy and unexpected discoveries by accident"). Gorman et al. (1984) found that their control condition was actually the most active condition, Griez and Van den Hout (1984) expected to reduce anxiety with carbon dioxide inhalations, but found a panic provocation model.

The chapter describes how initial hypotheses on alleged mechanisms were not confirmed, and how the research became gradually more systematic, including a more representative population in the studies and more carefully designed protocols.

As more data were gathered and results were becoming more robust, the emerging line of research was introduced in more laboratories. In turn, more convincing replication studies were performed adding to the gathered scientific evidence. The story also illustrates the validity of the results across ethnic and cultural dimensions. A most important advantage of collaborative studies between different centres of excellence is also illustrated when a cross-fertilisation occurred initially between the Dutch experimental expertise and the Italian experience in genetic research.

Briefly stated, what is the outlook in the case of the 35% CO_2 challenge? First of all, we now have a great deal of knowledge on the specificity of the challenge. Panic disorder patients are highly vulnerable. It has even been demonstrated that this vulnerability is still higher in panic disorder patients with a comorbid depression, (Verburg et al., 1997) although mood disorder patients are not sensitive (Perna et al., 1995a). There may be some increased vulnerability in some individuals with specific and/or social phobia. People with sporadic panic attacks, who do not fulfil the diagnostic criteria for panic disorder are also vulnerable (Perna et al., 1995c), as are first-degree relatives of panic disorder patients (Perna et al., 1995b; van Beek and Griez, 2000). We reported above that patients with GAD, OCD and animal phobia are not susceptible to CO_2.

It has also become clear that the essence of a "real" carbon dioxide-induced panic attack is not circumscribed to the mere physical symptoms of anxiety, but that the genuine experience of subjective fear belongs to the response, as far as susceptible individuals are concerned. Experiencing a transient brief sensation of subjective anxiety is pathognomonic for panic disorder (Verburg et al., 1998c).

Many studies have shown that the experimentally triggered response is affected by effective anti-panic medication. This opened the perspective to the use of the CO_2 model in the search for new anti-panic treatments.

In Milan, a number of interesting studies explored the genetic vulnerability to PD by using the 35% CO_2 inhalation model. Family studies on panic disorder have shown that first-degree relatives of panic disorder patients have an increased risk on panic disorder themselves. Estimates are that 7.8% to 20.5% of first-degree relatives of panic disorder patients suffer from panic disorder themselves. Monozygotic twin brothers or sisters of panic disorder patients have a higher chance of panic disorder than dizygotic twin brother or sisters. Although these results speak for themselves, until now, it has not been possible to establish the mode of transmission (autosomal dominant or recessive, single locus or multifactorial), perhaps because of a problem of invalid diagnostic categories. The same clinical picture currently covered by the diagnosis of panic disorder may be related to different diatheses. Carbon dioxide vulnerability may be the phenotypical manifestation of a genetic constitution predisposing to one type of PD, the so-called "respiratory" type. The 35% carbon dioxide challenge can be used to narrow the clinical picture down. For instance, genetic research can be done specifically in panic disorder patients who are CO_2 responsive. Consistent findings are underway to support the idea that CO_2 vulnerability may be linked to a family history of panic disorder. Conversely, it was shown that PD patients with a positive response to the 35% CO_2 challenge more often have family members who also suffer from panic disorder. Such studies open interesting perspectives for experimental work at the frontiers of nosology, genetics and pathophysiology.

REFERENCES

American Psychiatric Association (1980) DSM-III. *Diagnostic and Statistical Manual of Mental Disorders* 3rd edition. Washington, DC: APA.

American Psychiatric Association (1987) DSM-III-R. *Diagnostic and Statistical Manual of Mental Disorders* 3rd edition revised. Washington, DC: APA.

American Psychiatric Association (1994) DSM-IV. *Diagnostic and Statistical Manual of Mental Disorders* 4th edition. Washington, DC: APA.

Battaglia M, Perna G. (1995) The 35% CO$_2$ challenge in panic disorder: Optimization by Receiver Operating Characteristic (ROC) analysis. *J Psychiat Res* **29**: 111–119.

Bellodi L, Perna G, Caldirola D, Arancio C, Bertani A, Di Bella D (1998) Carbon dioxide-induced panic attacks: A twin study. *Am J Psychiatry* **155**: 1184–1188.

Bertani A, Perna G, Arancio C, Caldirola D, Bellodi L. (1997) Pharmacologic effects of imipramine, paroxetine and sertraline on 35% Carbon dioxide hypersensitivity in panic patients: a double-blind, random, placebo-controlled study. *J Clin Psychopharmacol* **17**: 97–101.

Bocola V, Trecco MD, Fabbrini G, Paladini C, Sollecito A, Martucci N. (1998) Anti-panic effect of fluoxetine measured by CO$_2$ challenge test. *Biol Psychiatry* **43**: 612–615.

Caldirola D, Perna G, Arancio C, Bertani A, Bellodi L. (1997) The 35% CO$_2$ challenge test in patients with social phobia. *Psychiatry Res* **71**: 41–48.

Cavallini MC, Perna G, Caldirola D, DiBella D, Bellodi L (1999) A segregation study for panic disorder families in which probands are responsive to 35% CO$_2$ challenge test. *Biol Psychiatry* **46**: 815–820.

Clark DM (1986) A cognitive approach to panic. *Behav Res Ther* **24**: 461–470.

Cohen ME, White PD (1951) Life situations, emotions and neurocirculatory asthenia. *Psychosom Med* **13**: 335–357.

Coryell WH (1997) Hypersensitivity to carbon dioxide as a disease specific trait marker. *Biol Psychiatry* **41**: 259–263.

Coryell W, Arndt S (1999) The 35% CO$_2$ inhalation procedure: test–retest reliability. *Biol Psychiatry* **45**: 923–927.

Eke M, McNally, RJ (1996) Anxiety sensitivity, suffocation fear, trait anxiety, and breath holding duration as predictors of response to carbon dioxide challenge. *Behav Res Ther* **34**: 603–607.

Gorman JM, Askanazi J, Liebowitz MR, Fyer AJ, Stein J, Kinney JR, Klein DF (1984) Response to hyperventilation in a group of patients with panic disorder. *Am J Psychiatry* **141**: 857–861.

Gorman JM, Browne ST, Papp LA, Martinez J, Welkowitz L, Coplan JD, Goetz RR, Kent J, Klein DF (1997) Effect of anti-panic treatment on response to carbon dioxide. *Biol Psychiatry* **42**: 982–991.

Gorman JM, Fyer MR, Liebowitz MR, Klein DF (1987) Pharmacologic provocation of panic. In Meltzer HY (ed.) *Psychopharmacology: The Third Generation of Progress.* New York: Raven Press.

Griez E, De Loof C, Pols H, Zandbergen J, Lousberg H (1990a) Specific sensitivity of patients with panic attacks to carbon dioxide inhalation. *Psychiatry Res* **31**: 193–199.

Griez E, Lousberg H, Van den Hout MA, Van der Molen GM (1987) CO$_2$ vulnerability in panic disorder. *Psychiatry Res* **20**: 87–95.

Griez E, Van den Hout MA (1984) Carbon dioxide and anxiety: an experimental approach to a clinical claim. Thesis.

Griez E, Van den Hout MA (1986) CO_2 inhalation in the treatment of panic attacks. *Behav Res Ther* **24**: 145–150.

Griez E, Verburg K (1999) The current status of respiration in panic disorder. In Nutt DJ, Ballenger JC, Lépine JP (eds) *Panic Disorder, Clinical Diagnosis, Management and Mechanisms*. London: Martin Dunitz Ltd.

Griez E, Zandbergen J, Lousberg H, Van den Hout MA (1988) Effects of low pulmonary CO_2 on panic anxiety. *Comp Psychiat* **29**: 490–497.

Griez E, Zandbergen J, Pols H, De Loof C (1990b) Response to 35% CO_2 as a marker of panic in severe anxiety. *Am J Psychiatry* **145**: 796–797.

Guttmacher LB, Murphy DL, Insel TR (1983) Pharmacological models of anxiety. *Compr Psychiat* **24**: 312–326.

Harrington PJ, Schmidt NB, Telch MJ (1996) Prospective evaluation of panic potentiation following 35% CO_2 challenge in non-clinical subjects. *Am J Psychiatry* **153**: 823–825.

Nardi AE, Valenca AM, Zin WA, Figuiera I, Marques C, Versiani M. (1997) Short-term clonazepam treatment in carbon dioxide induced panic attacks. *J Bras Psiq* **46**: 611–614.

Perna G, Barbini B, Cocchi S, Bertani A, Gasperini M (1995b) 35% CO_2 challenge in panic and mood disorders. *J Affect Disord* **33**: 189–194.

Perna G, Battaglia M, Garberi A, Arancio C, Bertani A, Bellodi L. (1994a) 35% CO_2/65% O_2 inhalation test in panic patients. *Psychiatry Res* **52**: 159–171.

Perna G, Bertani A, Caldirola D, Bellodi L (1996) Family history of panic disorder and hypersensitivity to CO_2 in panic disorder. *Am J Psychiatry* **153**: 1060–1064.

Perna G, Caldirola D, Arancio C, Bellodi L (1997a) Panic attacks: A twin study. *Psychiatry Res* **66**: 69–71.

Perna G, Cocchi S, Allevi L, Bussi R, Bellodi L (1999) . A long-term prospective evaluation of first-degree relatives of panic patients who underwent the 35% CO_2 challenge. *Biol Psychiatry* **45**: 365–367.

Perna G, Cocchi S, Bertani A, Arancio C, Bellodi L (1994b) Pharmacological effect of toloxatone on reactivity to 35% CO_2 challenge: A single blind, random, placebo controlled study. *J Clin Psychopharmacol* **14**: 414–418.

Perna G, Cocchi S, Bertani A, Arancio C, Bellodi L (1995b) 35% CO_2 challenge in healthy first-degree relatives of patients with panic disorder. *Am J Psychiatry* **152**: 623–625.

Perna G, Cocchi S, Politi E, Bellodi L (1997b) CO_2 challenge in non clinical subjects. *Am J Psychiatry* **154**: 886–887.

Perna G, Gabriele A, Caldirola D, Bellodi L (1995c) Hypersensitivity to inhalation of carbon dioxide and panic attacks. *Psychiatry Res* **57**: 267–273.

Pols H, Hauzer RC, Meijer JA, Verburg K, Griez E (1996b) Fluvoxamine attenuates panic induced by 35% CO_2 challenge. *J Clin Psychiatry* **57**: 539–542.

Pols H, Lousberg H, Zandbergen J, Griez E (1993) Panic disorder patients show decrease in ventilatory response to CO_2 after clomipramine treatment. *Psychiatry Res* **47**: 295–296.

Pols H, Verburg K, Meijer J, Hauzer R, Griez E (1996a) Alprazolam premedication and 35% carbon dioxide vulnerability in panic patients. *Biol Psychiatry* **40**: 913–917.

Pols H, Zandbergen J, De Loof C, Griez E (1991) Attenuation of carbon dioxide-induced panic after clonazepam treatment. *Acta Psychiatr Scand* **84**: 585–586.

Robins E, Guze SB (1970) Establishment of diagnostic validity in psychiatric illness: Its application to schizophrenia. *Am J Psychiatry* **126**: 983–987.

Schmidt NB, Trakowski JH, Staab JP (1997) Extinction of panicogenic effects of a 35% CO_2 challenge in patients with panic disorder. *J Abnorm Psychol* **106**: 630–638.

Schmidt NB, Storey J, Greenburg BD, Santiago HAT, Li Q, Murphy DL (in press) Evaluation gene × psychological risk factor in the pathogenesis of anxiety: a new model approach. *J Abnormal Psychology*.

Shipherd JC, Beck JG, Ohtake PJ (in press) Relationship between the anxiety sensitivity index, the suffocation fear scale and responses to CO_2 inhalation. *J Anxiety Disorders*.

Uhde TW, Tancer ME (1990) Chemical models of panic: A review and critique. In Tyrer P (ed.) *Psychopharmacology of Anxiety*. Oxford: Oxford University Press.

Van den Hout MA, Van der Molen M, Griez E, Lousberg H, Nansen A (1987) Reduction of CO_2-induced anxiety in patients with panic attacks after repeated CO_2 exposure. *Am J Psychiatry* **144**: 788–791.

Verburg K, Griez E, Meijer J, Pols H (1995) Discrimination between panic disorder and generalized anxiety disorder by 35% carbon dioxide challenge. *Am J Psychiatry* **152**: 1081–1083.

Verburg K, Klaassen T, Pols H, Griez E (1997) Comorbid depressive disorder increases vulnerability to the 35% carbon dioxide (CO_2) challenge in panic disorder patients. *J Affect Disord* **49**: 195–201.

Verburg K, Perna G, Bellodi L, Griez E (1998c). The 35% CO_2 panic provocation challenge as a diagnostic test for panic disorder. In Bellodi L, Perna G (eds) *The Panic Respiration Connection*. Milan: MDM Medical Media Srl.

Verburg K, Pols H, De Leeuw M, Griez E (1998a) Reliability of the 35% carbon dioxide panic provocation challenge. *Psychiatry Res* **78**: 207–214.

Verburg K, Pols H, Hauzer R, Meijer J, Griez E (1998b) The 35% carbon dioxide challenge in social phobia, in Who Panics? K. Verburg, thesis.

Wolpe J (1958) *Psychotherapy by Reciprocal Inhibition*. Stanford, CA: Stanford University Press.

Zandbergen J, Lousberg H, Pols H, De Loof C, Griez E (1990) Hypercarbia versus hypocarbia in panic disorder. *J Affect Disord* **18**: 75–81.

The Tryptophan Depletion Technique in Psychiatric Research

S.V. Argyropoulos, J.K. Abrams and D.J. Nutt

University of Bristol, School of Medical Sciences, Bristol, UK

INTRODUCTION

Serotonin (5-HT) neurotransmission in the brain is thought to play a central role in panic, and anxiety in general. Perhaps the strongest evidence for 5-HT involvement in anxiety disorders is that they are amenable to treatment with pharmacological agents acting upon the 5-HT system, such as the selective serotonin re-uptake inhibitors (SSRIs). A number of double-blind, placebo-controlled trials have demonstrated the efficacy of SSRIs in panic disorder (Hoehn-Saric et al., 1993; Oehrberg et al., 1995; Londborg et al., 1998; Michelson et al., 1999), social phobia (Van Vliet et al., 1994; Katzelnick et al., 1995; Stein et al., 1998; Allgulander, 1999), obsessive-compulsive disorder (OCD) (McDougle et al., 1993; Montgomery et al., 1993; Jenike et al., 1997), and post-traumatic stress disorder (PTSD) (van der Kolk et al., 1994). Comparative studies in generalised anxiety disorder (GAD) also look promising (Rocca et al., 1997). However, the exact mechanism by which changes in central 5-HT function affect anxiety levels is still unclear.

Competing theories exist, attempting to account for the available data. The "classic" or "excess" theory proposes that 5-HT excess in some parts of the brain causes anxiety, and that patients with anxiety or panic disorder have either increased 5-HT release or supersensitive postsynaptic receptors. Antidepressant treatment with selective serotonin reuptake inhibitors (SSRIs), therefore, temporarily exacerbates anxiety by acutely increasing the available 5-HT in the synaptic cleft, but gradually reduces it by down-regulating the supersensitive postsynaptic receptors. A second theory, or the "deficit" hypothesis, suggests that the presence of 5-HT restrains anxiety, and especially panic, in particular brain regions, the periaqueductal grey matter (PAG) (Deakin and Graeff, 1991), the amygdala (Stutzmann et al., 1998), and the medial hypothalamus (Graeff, 1994), and when this restraint is removed, panic results. In this model, antidepressant exacerbation of anxiety results from an initial decrease in synaptic 5-HT, through its action on the inhibitory 5-HT_{1A} autoreceptor,

Anxiety Disorders: An Introduction to Clinical Management and Research. Edited by E. J. L. Griez, C. Faravelli, D. Nutt and J. Zohar. © 2001 John Wiley & Sons, Ltd.

temporarily causing more panic. In time, this inhibitory receptor is desensitised and 5-HT release at the synapse increases. Evidence for and against these theories has been discussed elsewhere (Bell and Nutt, 1998; Kent et al., 1998). In short, the exact relationship between 5-HT function and anxiety remains to be unravelled.

It is generally believed that the SSRIs exert their anxiolytic properties through their modulation of 5-HT function. However, direct modulation of the serotonin systems is not a sufficient condition to induce anxiolysis, as evidenced by the effectiveness of other classes of drugs in treating anxiety disorders. For example, the benzodiazepines (BDZs) exert their effect through modulation of the γ-aminobutyric acid (GABA)/BDZ receptor complex (Argyropoulos and Nutt, 1999). Similar to depression, noradrenergic pathways are also thought to be playing a part in creating or maintaining anxiety. The presence of noradrenergic heteroreceptors on serotonergic neurones (Frazer, 1997) suggests that the picture is much more complicated than the simple presence or absence of 5-HT in various areas, although the possibility of a common final pathway for the different pharmacological agents cannot be excluded either.

The question also arises, whether the presence of 5-HT is a necessary condition for the SSRIs to bring around improvement of the disorders they are used in. Researchers can now call on a variety of tools to try and solve this conundrum. Tryptophan depletion is one such relevant technique, which has been applied in clinical settings easily and at a relatively low cost. Studies in depression (Delgado et al., 1990; KA Smith et al., 1997b) have shown that the maintenance of the antidepressant-induced remission depends on the presence of serotonin. Researchers were intrigued whether this holds true for other SSRI responsive conditions, especially the anxiety disorders.

5-HT SYNTHESIS AND THE TECHNIQUE OF TRYPTOPHAN DEPLETION

At present, the most direct way of studying the anatomical distribution and function of neurotransmitters and their receptors, in health and disease states, involves highly sophisticated and expensive neuroimaging techniques, such as positron emission tomography (PET) and functional magnetic resonance imaging (fMRI). The availability of these research methods is still rather restricted to few large centres. The study of the neurotransmitter metabolites in the cerebrospinal fluid (CSF), an indirect measure of central neurochemical activity, involves a lumbar puncture, a technique that has many problems. An alternative to these inconveniences is tryptophan depletion. While it cannot substitute for the precision of a PET scan, it does allow temporary and reversible manipulation of 5-HT levels in a minimally invasive manner; and as such, it opens up the possibility of answering a wide range of questions.

Tryptophan depletion (TD) aims at acutely reducing the available serotonin in the brain. It achieves that by restricting temporarily the synthesis of 5-HT. Tryptophan (TRP), an essential amino acid, is the precursor of 5-HT. Serotonin synthesis is a two-step process: TRP is first converted into 5-hydroxytryptophan (5-HTP) by the enzyme tryptophan hydroxylase, after which the 5-HTP is decarboxylated by aromatic acid decarboxylase to 5-HT (Green and Grahame-Smith, 1975). The step catalysed by tryptophan hydroxylase determines the rate of 5-HT synthesis. This enzyme is only about 50% saturated in the CNS (Wurtman et al., 1981), so the 5-HT synthesis rate depends on the availability of its substrate, free plasma TRP.

Most plasma TRP is bound to protein, leaving only about 5% available for transport into the central nervous system (CNS). The rest is diverted to the liver for protein synthesis along various pathways. The free TRP level depends on the balance between dietary TRP intake and its depletion by protein synthesis. An active protein shuttle, for which five other large neutral amino acids (LNAA) i.e. valine, leucine, isoleucine, phenylalanine and tyrosine compete, transports tryptophan across the blood-brain barrier (BBB) (Olendorf and Szabo, 1976; Purdridge, 1986). It is thought that the free plasma TRP/LNAA ratio is the most important factor in determining central TRP availability (Menkes et al., 1994; Weltzin et al., 1994).

In summary, three factors determine total 5-HT synthesis (Figure 19.1): (a) the total amount of free plasma TRP; (b) how much of that free TRP crosses the BBB; and (c) the activity of tryptophan hydroxylase. Tryptophan hydroxylase can be inhibited with parachlorophenylalanine (PCPA), which has been shown to antagonise the therapeutic effects of antidepressants (Shopsin et al., 1975). PCPA is, however, too toxic for ethical use in human subjects. Therefore, interest is focused on techniques affecting the first two factors. Free plasma TRP levels vary with the amount of dietary TRP, but merely stopping TRP intake reduces plasma TRP by only 15–20% (Delgado et al., 1989), making any effects on central TRP levels questionable. Central TRP can be reduced by loading subjects with the LNAAs that compete with TRP for transport into the brain, although this alone does not produce

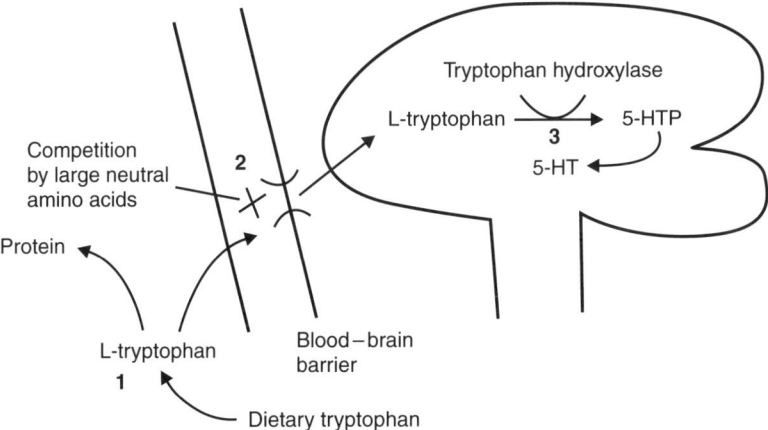

FIGURE 19.1   Depletion of brain 5-HT
Notes: Points at which 5HT synthesis may be controlled: 1. TRP availability: dietary restriction; 2. shuttle; 3. Synthesis: inhibition of tryptophan hydrolyase. Best TD results are achieved using a combination of control at points 1 and 2

dramatic effects on TRP levels or behaviour (Williamson et al., 1995). Maximal brain TD is achieved with a combined technique: a low-protein diet plus a TRP-deficient protein load containing large amounts of LNAAs that compete with TRP for transport across the BBB. In addition, the LNAA load stimulates protein synthesis in the liver, using up plasma TRP to further reduce its availability in the brain.

While details vary, a common TD procedure includes a low-TRP (160 mg/day) diet for 24 hours followed by an overnight fast extending through the test day and a 100 g load of 15 amino acids, plus or minus TRP. The best experimental design is one in which subjects undergo the same procedure on two different days one week apart, in a double blind fashion. On the experimental day the TRP-free depletion drink is given, and on the control day an otherwise identical TRP-containing drink is consumed, while on both days the subject undergoes the special diet. With the combined low-protein diet plus a TRP-deficient protein load, total plasma TRP levels may be reduced up to 80% (Delgado et al., 1990).

Evidence for the effectiveness of tryptophan depletion in reducing central TRP and 5-HT levels is accumulating. A robust though non-linear correlation has been found between lowered plasma TRP level during TRP depletion and lowered levels of the 5-HT metabolite 5-hydroxyindolacetic acid (5HIAA) in CSF (Carpenter et al., 1998; Williams et al., 1999). Lowered nocturnal melatonin secretion has also been observed during TD in healthy volunteers. Since 5-HT is the precursor of melatonin, this is good indirect evidence for lowered central 5-HT (Zimmermann et al., 1993a; Zimmermann et al., 1993b). Attenuated prolactin responses to challenge with fen-fluramine (a 5-HT releasing agent) have also been noted (Coccaro et al., 1998), and preclinical studies show that lowered L-tryptophan levels lead to lowered 5-HT release (Sharp et al., 1992).

How plasma and central TRP levels correspond to each other remains unclear though. Plasma TRP reaches its minimum approximately five hours after TD. However, in studies where monitoring was continued past that point, the lowest mood ratings occurred 7–9 hours after ingestion of the depletion drink, suggesting that central TRP levels continue to drop (Carpenter et al., 1998; Dierks et al., 1999; Williams et al., 1999).

TRYPTOPHAN DEPLETION STUDIES IN HEALTHY VOLUNTEERS

Low 5-HT has been associated with depression, therefore the prediction of early studies was that TD would cause depressive symptoms in healthy volunteers. These studies used men with depression scores at the high end of the normal range and did not include a low-TRP diet in their experiments. The subjects in these early studies did report mild mood lowering during TD, though none approached clinically significant depression (Young et al., 1985; SE Smith et al., 1987). Most of the later studies, conducted in the 1990s, used truly euthymic subjects with no personal or family history of depression. They found no or little mood lowering in healthy men

(Abbott et al., 1992; Benkelfat et al., 1994; Salomon et al., 1997; Carpenter et al., 1998; Knott et al., 1999) but a tendency to non-clinical mood lowering in healthy women (Ellenbogen et al., 1996; KA Smith et al., 1997a). This may reflect different serotonin processing between the sexes (Nishizawa et al., 1997; Arató and Bagdy, 1998).

Just as TD cannot elicit clinical depression in healthy volunteers, it cannot elicit anxiety either, at least when used on its own. No effects whatsoever were seen on resting anxiety following TD (Carpenter et al., 1998; Kent et al., 1996). Various neurochemical challenges have been used to complement tryptophan depletion. Healthy volunteers did not panic when given the α-adrenergic antagonist yohimbine at the time of minimum plasma TRP, although 5 out of 11 subjects rated themselves as "more nervous" after the infusion (Goddard et al., 1995). Inhalation of 5% CO_2 did not increase anxiety or panic (Miller et al., 2000), but in another study, there was a small but significant increase in anxiety on the Spielberger State Anxiety Inventory (STAI), and an increase in reporting neurovegetative symptoms of panic, when the subjects were depleted and made to breathe 35% CO_2 (Klaassen et al., 1998). This result was interpreted as evidence of increased "nervousness". However, true panic was not seen. The neuropeptide cholecystokinin (CCK-4) causes panic in normal volunteers whether tryptophan-depleted or not (55% in the TD group and 65% in controls) (Koszycki et al., 1996). The qualitative effect of CCK-4 was virtually identical in both groups. Clearly, it takes more than simple lack of 5-HT or even a combination of low 5-HT with challenges that cause anxiety or panic in anxious patients, in order to cause panic in normal volunteers.

TRYPTOPHAN DEPLETION IN ANXIETY DISORDERS

Most TD studies in the anxiety disorders have been performed in panic disorder and OCD. There are ongoing studies in social phobia (including one in our lab) and there is at least one planned in GAD. To our knowledge, this technique has not been applied in PTSD so far.

Panic Disorder

Untreated patients with this disorder experience panic when given panicogens such as flumazenil or CO_2 inhalation (Nutt et al., 1990; Kent et al., 1996; Miller et al., 1995), but patients recovered with SSRI antidepressants do not. When treated patients stop their medication, however, their vulnerability returns (Miller et al., 2000). Unmedicated panic patients showed increased ventilatory response (Kent et al., 1996) when subjected to TD, but in another study there was no significant change in anxiety (Goddard et al., 1994). Further, when drug-free patients where depleted and subjected to 5% CO_2 inhalation, they reported increased rate of panic attacks (Miller et al., 2000).

To test whether increased 5-HT availability is responsible for the antipanic effect of serotonergic antidepressants, eight panic disorder patients, treated with the SSRI paroxetine and remitted for at least three months, were put through TD, and then given flumazenil and normal saline challenge, in a double-blind fashion. During the non-TD day, none of the patients experienced change in their anxiety scores when challenged with flumazenil or normal saline. In contrast, during the TD day, five out of eight patients experienced an anxiety increase and/or panic with flumazenil, but none showed anxiety increase with normal saline (Table 19.1) (Nutt et al., 1999). This implies that chronic SSRI treatment ameliorates panic by increasing 5-HT transmission through the synapse. If 5-HT availability is reduced, as during TD, this effect is negated, a finding supporting the PAG model of panic restraint (see the Introduction). Further studies are needed to replicate this finding.

Obsessive-compulsive Disorder (OCD)

PET scans have implicated a specific orbitofrontal cortex—head of caudate nucleus—thalamus pathway in OCD, in contrast to the brainstem—amygdala—hypothalamic circuits thought to be involved in anxiety and panic (Insel, 1992). Treatment with clomipramine (a serotonergic tricyclic antidepressant) or SSRIs is effective in OCD (Uhlenhuth et al., 1999), but larger doses and a longer period of treatment than in panic/anxiety or depression are needed. This may be because presynaptic $5-HT_{1A}$ autoreceptor desensitisation (the proposed therapeutic mechanism) occurs later in the orbitofrontal cortex and/or head of caudate nucleus (Blier and de Montigny, 1998). It is reasonable, therefore, to assume that TD would worsen OCD symptoms.

There have been four studies on TD in OCD, on patients either taking medication (Barr et al., 1994) or remitted and drug-free (Smeraldi et al., 1996; Rasmusson et al., 1997; Hohagen et al., 1998). There was no effect noted on OCD or Tourette symptoms in any of them, although some mood lowering and sleep changes were seen. As yet, no challenge studies have been performed in OCD during TD, and it may be that provocation of symptoms would reveal an effect, as in panic disorder.

TABLE 19.1 Response of eight panic patients, remitted with paroxetine, on flumazenil challenge during tryptophan depletion

	Control day	Tryptophan depletion
Depression	1/8	3/8
Panic/anxiety with flumazenil challenge	0/8	5/8
Panic/anxiety with normal saline	0/8	0/8

Source: Modified from Nutt et al., 1999.

TABLE 19.2   Tryptophan depletion (TD) studies in healthy volunteers, mood and anxiety disorders

Condition	TD applied	Medication status	Challenge test	Effect
Healthy volunteers	Yes	Drug-free (Carpenter et al., 1998; Kent et al., 1996)	No	No effect on mood or anxiety
		Drug-free (Salomon et al., 1997)	TD combined with AMPT (NA depletion)	No effect on mood
		Drug-free (Knott et al., 1999)	Fenfluramine	No effect on mood
		Drug-free males vs. females (KA Smith et al., 1997b)	Mood induction procedure	No clinical mood lowering in males vs. slight but non-clinical mood lowering in females
		Drug-free (Goddard et al., 1995)	Yohimbine	Increased nervousness/ anxiety, no panic
		Drug-free (Klaassen et al., 1998)	35% CO_2	Increased nervousness, no panic
		Drug-free (Miller et al., 2000)	5% CO_2	No effect on anxiety
Depression	Yes	Untreated depressed patients (Delgado et al., 1994)	No	Worsening of mood
		Patients remitted, on SSRIs (Delgado et al., 1990)	No	Transient relapse of depression
		Patients remitted, drug-free (KA Smith et al., 1997a)	No	Transient relapse of depression
OCD	Yes	Drug-free patients (Smeraldi et al., 1996)	No	No effect on mood or OCD symptoms
		Patients remitted, on SSRIs (Barr et al., 1994)	No	Increase in depressive symptoms, no change in OCD
		Drug-free Tourette patients, with OCD or OCD symptoms (Rasmusson et al., 1997)	No	No worsening of tics, mood or OCD symptoms

TABLE 19.2 (*cont.*)

Condition	TD applied	Medication status	Challenge test	Effect
Panic disorder	Yes	Unmedicated patients (Goddard et al., 1994)	No	Not anxiogenic
		Unmedicated patients (Kent et al., 1996)	No	Increased ventilatory response, but no panic
		Unmedicated patients (Miller et al., 2000)	5% CO_2	Anxiogenic response, increased rate of panic attacks
		Patients remitted, on paroxetine (Nutt et al., 1999)	Flumazenil	Increased anxiety/panic
Social phobia	Under way	Patients remitted, on paroxetine	Autobiographical script/verbal task	?
PTSD	No	—	—	?
GAD	No	—	—	?

SSRI: selective serotonin reuptake inhibitor, AMPT: a-methyl-para-tyrosine, NA: noradrenaline, OCD: obsessive-compulsive disorder, PTSD: post-traumatic stress disorder, GAD: generalised anxiety disorder.

CONCLUSION

Although TD is at this point familiar, if not exactly established in the study of depression, these are still early days for anxiety disorders. This may, in part, reflect the fact that research in the area of anxiety disorders lags behind that of depression, not least because of the changes in diagnostic criteria and differentiation of syndromes in the past 20 years. Now that conditions such as social anxiety disorder and generalised anxiety disorder have "matured" into an independent status, they have attracted more attention from researchers and the balance is in the process of being redressed. Panic and OCD, as the most easily identified of the anxiety disorders, have been the first to undergo TD investigations.

In summary (see Table 19.2), tryptophan depletion has established that the availability of serotonin is necessary for the action of SSRIs in depression. The evidence in bulimia also points to the same direction, although it is not as strong. The picture in panic disorder appears to be similar, but the initial findings need replication, perhaps with the use of different chemical challenges. On the contrary, TD studies have been negative in OCD, perhaps because challenge tests have not been performed in this condition during TD. Studies are currently carried out in other anxiety disorders. The work done so far in anxiety disorders, although exciting, can only be seen as preliminary.

REFERENCES

Abbott FV, Etienne P, Franklin KBJ et al. (1992) Acute tryptophan depletion blocks morphine analgesia in the cold-pressor test in humans. *Psychopharmacology* **108**: 60–66.

Allgulander C (1999) Paroxetine in social anxiety disorder: A randomized placebo-controlled study. *Acta Psychiat Scand* **100**: 193–198.

Arató M, Bagdy G (1998) Gender difference in m-CPP challenge test in healthy volunteers. *Int J Neuropsychopharmacology* **1**: 121–124.

Argyropoulos SV, Nutt DJ (1999) The use of benzodiazepines in anxiety and other disorders. *Eur Neuropsychopharmacology* **9** Suppl 6: S407–S412.

Barr LC, Goodman WK, McDougle CJ et al. (1994) Tryptophan depletion in patients with obsessive-compulsive disorder who respond to serotonin reuptake inhibitors. *Arch Gen Psychiatry* **51**: 309–317.

Bell CJ, Nutt DJ (1998) Serotonin and panic. *Br J Psychiatry* **172**: 465–471.

Benkelfat C, Ellenbogen MA, Dean P et al. (1994) Mood lowering effect of tryptophan depletion: Enhanced susceptibility in young men at risk for major affective disorders. *Arch Gen Psychiatry* **51**: 687–697.

Blier P, de Montigny C (1998) Possible serotonergic mechanisms underlying the antidepressant and anti-obsessive-compulsive disorder responses. *Biol Psychiatry* **44**: 313–323.

Carpenter LL, Anderson GM, Pelton GH et al. (1998) Tryptophan depletion during continuous CSF sampling in healthy human subjects. *Neuropsychopharmacology* **19**: 26–35.

Coccaro EF, Kavoussi RJ, Cooper TB et al. (1998) Acute tryptophan depletion attenuates the prolactin response to d-fenfluramine challenge in healthy human subjects. *Psychopharmacology* **138**: 9–15.

Deakin JFW, Graeff F (1991) 5-HT and mechanisms of defence. *J Psychopharmacology* **5**: 305–315.

Delgado PL, Charney DS, Price LH et al. (1989) Neuroendocrine and behavioral effects of dietary tryptophan restriction in healthy subjects. *Life Science* **45**: 2323–2332.

Delgado PL, Charney DS, Price LH et al. (1990) Serotonin function and the mechanism of antidepressant action: Reversal of antidepressant-induced remission by rapid depletion of plasma tryptophan. *Arch Gen Psychiatry* **47**: 411–419.

Delgado PL, Price LH, Miller HL et al. (1994) Serotonin and the neurobiology of depression: Effects of tryptophan depletion in drug-free depressed patients. *Arch Gen Psychiatry* **51**: 865–874.

Dierks T, Barta S, Demisch L et al. (1999) Intensity dependence of auditory evoked potentials (AEPs) as biological marker for cerebral serotonin levels: Effects of tryptophan depletion in healthy subjects. *Psychopharmacology* **146**: 101–107.

Ellenbogen MA, Young SN, Dean P et al. (1996) Mood response to acute tryptophan depletion: Sex differences and temporal stability. *Neuropsychopharmacology* **15**: 465–474.

Frazer A (1997) Pharmacology of antidepressants. *J Clin Psychopharmacology* **17** Suppl 1: 2S–18S.

Goddard AW, Charney DS, Germine M et al. (1995) Effects of tryptophan depletion on responses to yohimbine in healthy human subjects. *Biol Psychiatry* **38**: 74–86.

Goddard AW, Shlomskas DE, Walton KE et al. (1994) Effects of tryptophan depletion in panic disorder. *Biol Psychiatry* **36**: 775–777.

Graeff FG (1994) Neuroanatomy and neurotransmitter regulation of defensive behaviors and related emotions in mammals. *Braz J Med Biol Research* **27**: 811–829.

Green AR, Grahame-Smith DG (1975) 5-Hydroxytryptamine and other indoles in the central nervous system. In Iverson LL, Iverson SD, Snyder SH (eds) *Handbook of Psychopharmacology* vol. 3, *Biochemistry of Biogenic Amines*. New York: Plenum Press, pp. 169–245.

Hoehn-Saric R, McLeod DR, Hipsley PA (1993) Effect of fluvoxamine on panic disorder. *J Clin Psychopharmacology* **13**: 321–326.

Hohagen F, Huwig-Poppe C, Voderholzer U et al. (1998) Effects of acute tryptophan depletion on sleep in patients with obsessive-compulsive disorder. *J Sleep Research* **7** Suppl. 2: 119.

Insel TR (1992) Toward a neuroanatomy of obsessive-compulsive disorder. *Arch Gen Psychiatry* **49**: 739–744.

Jenike MA, Baer L, Minichiello WE et al. (1997) Placebo-controlled trial of fluoxetine and phenelzine for obsessive-compulsive disorder. *Am J Psychiatry* **154**: 1261–1264.

Katzelnick DJ, Kobak KA, Greist JH et al. (1995) Sertraline for social phobia: A double-blind, placebo-controlled crossover study. *Am J Psychiatry* **152**: 1368–1371.

Kent JM, Coplan JD, Gorman JM (1998) Clinical utility of the selective serotonin reuptake inhibitors in the spectrum of anxiety. *Biol Psychiatry* **44**: 812–824.

Kent JM, Coplan JD, Martinez J et al. (1996) Ventilatory effects of tryptophan depletion in panic disorder: A preliminary report. *Psychiat Research* **64**: 83–90.

Klaassen T, Klumperbeek J, Deutz NEP et al. (1998) Effects of tryptophan depletion on anxiety and on panic provoked by carbon dioxide challenge. *Psychiat Research* **77**: 167–174.

Knott VJ, Howson AL, Perugini M et al. (1999) The effect of acute tryptophan depletion and fenfluramine on quantitative EEG and mood in healthy male subjects. *Biol Psychiatry* **46**: 229–238.

Koszycki D, Zacharko RM, Le Melledo J-M et al. (1996) Effects of acute tryptophan depletion on behavioral, cardiovascular, and hormonal sensitivity to cholecystokinin-tetrapeptide challenge in healthy volunteers. *Biol Psychiatry* **40**: 648–655.

Londborg PD, Wolkow R, Smith WT et al. (1998) Sertraline in the treatment of panic disorder: A multi-site, double-blind, placebo-controlled, fixed-dose investigation. *Br J Psychiatry* **173**: 54–60.

McDougle CJ, Goodman WK, Price LH (1993) The pharmacotherapy of obsessive-compulsive disorder. *Pharmacopsychiatry* **26** Suppl 1: 24–29.

Menkes DB, Coates DC, Fawcett JP et al. (1994) Acute tryptophan depletion aggravates premenstrual syndrome. *J Affect Dis* **32**: 37–44.

Michelson D, Pollack M, Lydiard RB et al. (1999) Continuing treatment of panic disorder after acute response: randomised, placebo-controlled trial with fluoxetine. The Fluoxetine Panic Disorder Study Group. *Br J Psychiatry* **174**: 213–218.

Miller H, Anderson IM, Deakin JFW (1995) Acute tryptophan depletion increases panic anxiety in panic disorder patients. *J Psychopharmacology* **9** Suppl 3: A18.

Miller HEJ, Deakin JFW, Anderson IM (2000) Effect of acute tryptophan depletion on CO_2-induced anxiety in patients with panic disorder and normal volunteers. *Br J Psychiatry* **176**: 182–188.

Montgomery SA, McIntyre A, Osterheider M et al. (1993) A double-blind, placebo-controlled study of fluoxetine in patients with DSM-III-R obsessive-compulsive disorder. The Lilly European OCD Study Group. *Eur Neuropsychopharmacology* **3**: 143–152.

Nishizawa S, Benkelfat C, Young SN et al. (1997) Differences between males and females in rates of serotonin synthesis in human brain. *Proc Nat Ac Sci USA* **94**: 5308–5315.

Nutt DJ, Forshall S, Bell C et al. (1999) Mechanisms of action of selective serotonin reuptake inhibitors in the treatment of psychiatric disorders. *Eur Neuropsychopharmacology* **9** Suppl 3: S81–S86.

Nutt DJ, Glue P, Lawson C et al. (1990) Flumazenil provocation of panic attacks. *Arch Gen Psychiatry* **47**: 917–925.

Oehrberg S, Christiansen PE, Behnke K et al. (1995) Paroxetine in the treatment of panic disorder: A randomised, double-blind, placebo-controlled study. *Br J Psychiatry* **167**: 374–379.

Olendorf WH, Szabo J (1976) Amino acid assignment to one of three blood–brain barrier amino acid carriers. *Am J Physiology* **230**: 94–98.

Purdridge WM (1986) Blood–brain barrier transport of nutrients. *Nutr Review* **15** Suppl: 214.

Rasmusson AM, Anderson GM, Lynch KA et al. (1997) A preliminary study of tryptophan depletion on tics, obsessive-compulsive symptoms, and mood in Tourette's syndrome. *Biol*

Psychiatry **41**: 117–121.

Rocca P, Fonzo V, Scotta M et al. (1997) Paroxetine efficacy in the treatment of generalized anxiety disorder. *Acta Psychiat Scand* **95**: 444–450.

Salomon RM, Miller HL, Krystal JH et al. (1997) Lack of behavioral effects of monoamine depletion in healthy subjects. *Biol Psychiatry* **41**: 58–64.

Sharp T, Bramwell SR, Grahame-Smith, DG (1992) Effect of acute administration of L-tryptophan on the release of 5-HT in rat hippocampus in relation to serotoninergic neuronal activity: An in-vivo microdialysis study. *Life Science* **50**: 1215–1223.

Shopsin B, Gershon S, Goldstein M et al. (1975) Use of synthesis inhibitors in defining a role for biogenic amines during imipramine treatment in depressed patients. *Psychopharm Communications* **1**: 239–249.

Smeraldi E, Diaferia G, Erzegovesi S et al. (1996) Tryptophan depletion in obsessive-compulsive patients. *Biol Psychiatry* **40**: 398–402.

Smith KA, Clifford EM, Hockney RA et al. (1997a) Effect of tryptophan depletion on mood in male and female volunteers: a pilot study. *Hum Psychopharmacology* **12**: 111–117.

Smith KA, Fairburn CG, Cowen PJ (1997b) Relapse of depression after rapid depletion of tryptophan. *Lancet* **349**: 915–919.

Smith SE, Pihl RO, Young SN et al. (1987) A test of possible cognitive and environmental influences on the mood lowering effect of tryptophan depletion in normal males. *Psychopharmacology* **91**: 451–457.

Stein MB, Liebowitt MR, Lydiard RB et al. (1998) Paroxetine treatment of generalised social phobia (social anxiety disorder): A randomised controlled trial. *JAMA* **280**: 708–713.

Stutzmann GE, McEwen BS, LeDoux JE (1998) Serotonin modulation of sensory inputs to the lateral amygdala: dependency on corticosterone. *J Neuroscience* **18**: 9529–9538.

Uhlenhuth EH, Balter MB, Ban TA, Yang K (1999) International study of expert judgement on therapeutic use of benzodiazepines and other psychotherapeutic medications: VI. Trends in recommendations for the pharmacotherapy of anxiety disorders, 1992–1997. *Depr anxiety* **9**: 107–116.

van der Kolk BA, Dreyfuss D, Michaels M et al. (1994) Fluoxetine in post-traumatic stress disorder. *J Clin Psychiatry* **55**: 517–522.

van Vliet IM, den Boer JA, Westenberg HGM (1994) Psychopharmacological treatment of social phobia: A double-blind, placebo-controlled study with fluvoxamine. *Psychopharmacology* **115**: 128–134.

Weltzin TE, Fernstrom JD, McConaha C et al. (1994) Acute tryptophan depletion in bulimia: Effects on large neutral amino acids. *Biol Psychiatry* **35**: 388–397.

Williams WA, Shoaf SE, Hommer D et al. (1999) Effects of acute tryptophan depletion on plasma and cerebrospinal fluid tryptophan and 5-hydroxyindoleacid in normal volunteers. *J Neurochemistry* **72**: 1641–1647.

Williamson DJ, McTavish SFB, Park SBG et al. (1995) Effects of valine on 5-HT-mediated prolactin release in healthy volunteers and on mood in recovered depressed patients. *Br J Psychiatry* **167**: 238–242.

Wurtman RJ, Hefti H, Melamed E (1981) Precursor control of neurotransmitter synthesis. *Pharmacol Review* **32**: 315–335.

Young SN, Smith SE, Pihl RO et al. (1985) Tryptophan depletion causes a rapid lowering of mood in normal males. *Psychopharmacology* **87**: 173–177.

Zimmermann RC, McDougle CJ, Schumacher M et al. (1993a) Effects of acute tryptophan depletion on nocturnal melatonin secretion in humans. *J Clin Endocrin Metabolism* **76**: 1161–1164.

Zimmermann, RC, McDougle CJ, Schumacher M et al. (1993b) Urinary 6-hydroxymelatonin sulfate as a measure of melatonin secretion during acute tryptophan depletion. *Psychoneuroendocrinology* **18**: 567–578.

Index

Index compiled by Penelope Allport